SOCIAL WELFARE POLICY AND ADVOCACY

Advancing Social Justice through 8 Policy Sectors

Bruce S. Jansson

University of Southern California

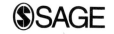

Los Angeles | London | New Delhi
Singapore | Washington DC | Boston

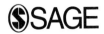

Los Angeles | London | New Delhi
Singapore | Washington DC | Boston

FOR INFORMATION:

SAGE Publications, Inc.
2455 Teller Road
Thousand Oaks, California 91320
E-mail: order@sagepub.com

SAGE Publications Ltd.
1 Oliver's Yard
55 City Road
London EC1Y 1SP
United Kingdom

SAGE Publications India Pvt. Ltd.
B 1/I 1 Mohan Cooperative Industrial Area
Mathura Road, New Delhi 110 044
India

SAGE Publications Asia-Pacific Pte. Ltd.
3 Church Street
#10-04 Samsung Hub
Singapore 049483

Copyright © 2016 by SAGE Publications, Inc.

Printed in the United States of America

Library of Congress Cataloging-in-Publication Data

A catalog record of this book is available from the Library of Congress.

ISBN: 978-1-4833-7788-9

This book is printed on acid-free paper.

Acquisitions Editor: Kassie Graves
Associate eLearning Editor: Lucy Berbeo
Editorial Assistant: Carrie Montoya
Production Editor: Libby Larson
Copy Editor: Rachel Keith
Typesetter: C&M Digitals (P) Ltd.
Proofreader: Sally Jaskold
Indexer: Sheila Bodell
Cover Designer: Leonardo March
Marketing Manager: Shari Countryman

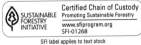

17 18 19 20 10 9 8 7 6 5 4 3

SOCIAL WELFARE
POLICY AND ADVOCACY

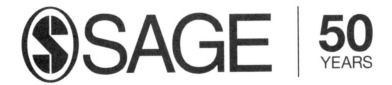

SAGE was founded in 1965 by Sara Miller McCune to support the dissemination of usable knowledge by publishing innovative and high-quality research and teaching content. Today, we publish more than 750 journals, including those of more than 300 learned societies, more than 800 new books per year, and a growing range of library products including archives, data, case studies, reports, conference highlights, and video. SAGE remains majority-owned by our founder, and after Sara's lifetime will become owned by a charitable trust that secures our continued independence.

Los Angeles | London | Washington DC | New Delhi | Singapore | Boston

CONTENTS

Chapter 10: Becoming Policy Advocates in the Mental Health Sector

Bruce S. Jansson, Judith A. DeBonis, and Eri Nakagami

Chapter 11: Becoming Policy Advocates in the Child and Family Sector

Bruce S. Jansson, James David Simon, and Anamika Barman-Adhikari

Chapter 12: Becoming Policy Advocates in the Education Sector

Bruce S. Jansson, Elaine Sanchez Wilson, and Vivien Villaverde

Chapter 13: Becoming Policy Advocates in the Immigration Sector

This book is dedicated to those social workers who embed policy advocacy in their work

PREFACE

S ocial workers work primarily in eight policy sectors, but no existing text gives them skills to engage in policy advocacy in each of those sectors despite the extensive analysis of problems that consumers experience in each of them.

Shortcomings in the *safety-net sector* are partly responsible for economic inequality approaching levels last seen in the Gilded Age of the 1890s. In the *child and family sector*, millions of children lack sufficient or adequate childcare and thousands of children graduate from foster care only to become homeless. In the *mental health sector*, individuals with chronic mental conditions still lack sufficient community-based services to help them. In many high schools within the *education sector*, roughly half of minority students fail to graduate. The nation has not prepared sufficient numbers of social workers, nurses, and gerontologists to help roughly 30 million baby boomers in the gerontology sector as they become older. The warehousing of inmates and a lack of preventive programs have contributed to high rates of recidivism in the *criminal justice sector.* In the *immigration and global sector*, the United States has readily used immigrants for labor in the agricultural, tourism, construction, and other economic sectors but has often failed to provide them with adequate human services and has often violated their human rights. In the *healthcare sector*, many Americans fail to receive preventive care, such as programs to reduce obesity, or receive inadequate assistance.

This text provides the first framework that links micro policy advocacy, mezzo policy advocacy, and macro policy advocacy—and demonstrates how these three kinds of advocacy can be used by social workers in the healthcare, gerontology, safety-net, child and family, education, immigration/global, mental health, and criminal justice sectors to promote social justice.

This text begins by making the case that advocacy is required by the National Association of Social Workers' Code of Ethics. It identifies 16 vulnerable populations that particularly need advocacy. It identifies seven core problems that advocates must confront to address the needs of their consumers and clients in each of the eight policy sectors. They should work to augment (a) ethical rights, human rights, and economic justice; (b) the quality of services and programs; (c) the cultural responsiveness of services and programs; (d) preventive strategies and programs; (e) the affordability and accessibility of social programs; (f) the scope and effectiveness of programs that address consumers' and clients' mental distress; and (g) linkages between social programs and services with consumers' and clients' households and communities.

Chapter 3 provides a multilevel advocacy intervention framework. It identifies and defines micro, mezzo, and macro advocacy interventions. If micro policy advocacy interventions aim to help specific clients and families obtain rights, opportunities, and benefits that will improve their well-being, mezzo and macro policy advocacy seek to reform dysfunctional policies in organizations, communities, and governments. The chapter describes eight challenges that advocates must address at each of these levels of policy advocacy; identifies specific advocacy skills needed by micro, mezzo, and macro policy advocates; and provides specific examples of micro, mezzo, and macro advocacy interventions. Chapters 4, 5, and 6, respectively, are devoted to analyzing the challenges that micro policy advocates, mezzo policy advocates, and macro policy advocates address—and the skills that they need to do so.

This text uniquely discusses how micro, mezzo, and macro policy advocates use their skills to improve policies in each of the eight policy sectors addressed in Chapters 7 through 14. Each of these chapters provides learning objectives, analyzes the historical evolution of the sector under discussion, identifies client problems within the sector that are caused by economic inequality, analyzes the political economy of the sector, and identifies key advocacy groups within the sector.

Each of these eight sector chapters is divided into seven sections that correspond to the seven core problems—that is, to the ethical, quality, cultural, prevention, and affordability issues consumers often confront as well as the difficulties they have in receiving assistance for their mental problems and the lack of linkage of services to their communities and households. Each of the chapters includes **Red Flag Alerts** that identify specific manifestations of the core problem. Resources such as statutes, court rulings, regulations, and programs that help advocates engage in advocacy at the three levels are discussed. At the beginning of each of the eight policy sector chapters, advocacy groups are identified that provide useful information on their websites about how to address Red Flag Alerts.

This text emphasizes a "hands-on" approach by providing many vignettes that describe micro, mezzo, and macro interventions undertaken by social workers and others as they help consumers deal with specific problems identified in the Red Flag Alerts.

Each chapter in this book begins with **Learning Objectives** and ends with **Learning Outcomes** that are linked to the Learning Objectives.

Each chapter includes links to **Video Interviews**, available on the book's companion website at http://study.sagepub.com/jansson, that offer first-person insights into key concepts from experts in the field. Look for the "play button" icon accompanied by labels in the margins of the book that signal when you can visit the companion website to watch the accompanying video.

Acknowledgments

Many people helped me develop innovations in this book that include identification of seven core problems that exist in each policy sector, "Red Flag Alerts," and the division of policy advocacy into three elements: micro policy advocacy, mezzo policy advocacy, and macro policy advocacy. They also helped me embed these innovations in specific policy sectors.

This text evolved from the bottom-up in my policy classes. I developed the seven core problems in MSW classes in health policy. I identified specific examples of the seven core problems in these classes. I linked case advocacy (or patient advocacy) with macro policy advocacy in these classes and in a book that emerged from them, *Improving Healthcare Through Advocacy* (John Wiley & Sons, 2011). I gathered empirical data from roughly 300 frontline health professionals in a research project funded by the Patient-Centered Outcomes Research Institute (PCORI) titled "Improving Healthcare Outcomes Through Advocacy"—and was delighted to find that these innovations were corroborated by empirical data.

I trial tested the concept of "Red Flag Alerts" with doctoral students, as well as the division of policy advocacy into micro policy, mezzo policy advocacy, and macro policy advocacy.

I would like to thank the following persons for demonstrating that policy advocacy can be embedded in specific policy sectors:

Dawn Joosten, Ph.D.; Eri Nakagami, Ph.D.; James David Simon, doctoral candidate; and Vivian Villaverde, MSW—all from the *School of Social Work, University of Southern California*

Judy DeBonis, Ph.D., *Department of Social Work, California State University at Northridge*

Gretchen Heidemann, Ph.D., Assistant Professor, *Department of Social Work, Whittier College*

Anamika Barman-Adhikari. Ph.D., *School of Social Work, University of Denver*

Elaine Sanchez, MPP, independent researcher and journalist

Thanks to Melissa Bird, doctoral candidate in the *School of Social Work, University of Southern California,* for her outstanding discussion of her macro policy advocacy as chief lobbyist for Planned Parenthood of Utah.

Elaine Sanchez facilitated this book in many ways.

Rafael Angulo, MSW of the School of Social Work, University of Southern California, developed many video clips for this book.

SAGE Publications and I thank the following reviewers:

Jitendra M. Kapoor, *Alabama A&M University*

Karen Morgain, *California State University Northridge*

Joyce Lee Taylor *Springfield College*

Joseph Wronka, *Springfield College*

Kassie Graves, the Editor of Social Work at SAGE Publications, facilitated this book's production in many ways.

Thanks to my wife, Betty Ann, for her constant support.

Chapter 1

ADVANCING SOCIAL JUSTICE IN EIGHT POLICY SECTORS

LEARNING OBJECTIVES

In this chapter, you will learn to:

1. Identify eight policy sectors that deliver services, resources, benefits, and opportunities to millions of residents of the United States

2. Define micro policy interventions, mezzo policy interventions, and macro policy interventions

3. Identify seven core problems that exist in each of the eight policy sectors

4. Recognize how advocacy allows social workers to follow the Code of Ethics of the National Association of Social Workers (NASW)

5. Define social policy and enumerate different kinds of social policies

6. Identify challenges and rewards encountered by policy advocates

7. Understand the reform traditions of the social work profession

Social workers, unlike many high-level officials and policy experts in government positions and think tanks, engage social policy in their daily work. They understand that policy impacts individuals and families because they see how it influences their lives. They see clients and families who do not receive benefits, services, resources, and rights to which they are entitled, such as clients who are wrongly declared ineligible for specific programs. They understand, too, that some policies are dysfunctional, such as those that disqualify women from using public welfare and food programs when they leave prison, even when they have children who depend on these resources. They understand that they are required by their code of ethics to be advocates of policies that advance ethical principles such as self-determination and social justice.

Social workers, then, interact with policies on three levels. They:

- Help specific clients, families, and communities obtain rights, benefits, opportunities, and services that they need and to which they are entitled (*micro policy interventions*)
- Reform dysfunctional policies at the organizational and community levels that may create the need for micro policy interventions (*mezzo policy interventions*)
- Reform dysfunctional policies at the legal and government levels that may create the need for micro policy interventions (*macro policy interventions*)

This book offers a unique empowerment framework to provide social workers with tools to develop micro policy, mezzo policy, and macro policy interventions in eight policy sectors. It also provides many vignettes that illustrate how social workers have empowered themselves and their clients to work for greater social justice.

VIDEO LINK 1.1
Ethics of Policy
Framing

REFORMING POLICIES IN EIGHT SECTORS

Most social workers work in eight policy sectors. They work in the *child and family sector* in child welfare agencies, childcare agencies, child guidance clinics, preschool programs, and other programs; the *health sector* in hospitals, community clinics, physician practices, public health programs, and other settings; the *gerontology sector* in hospitals, long-term care agencies, convalescent homes, hospice programs, palliative care programs, retirement homes, day treatment programs, and other settings; the *mental health sector* in counseling agencies, suicide prevention programs, mental hospitals, places of work, and other settings; the *education and job development sector* in public and private schools at the preschool, primary, and secondary levels as well as in community colleges, colleges, universities, and vocational education and other job training settings; the *corrections sector* in prisons, probation and parole agencies, community transition programs, gang-related programs, police departments, juvenile courts, and other settings, and the *safety-net sector* in local and federal offices of the U.S. Social Security Administration, local and state welfare offices, not-for-profit and faith-based programs that provide food banks and other services to low-income individuals, and other settings. Social workers also work with immigrants in the *global sector* as well as with international organizations such as agencies of the United Nations, not-for-profit agencies like Oxfam and the Gates Foundation, and faith-based organizations.

These eight sectors lie at the heart of the American network of social programs and policies. Most social workers work in them, and most programs "belong" to one of these sectors. Each sector has:

- Its own distinctive policies, sources of funds, agencies, programs, and literature
- Its own administrative arrangements
- Its own ways of selecting and deploying its staff
- Its distinctive mission, such as providing services (mental health, education, and health sectors), hard benefits (the safety-net sector), or law enforcement and rehabilitation (the corrections sector) or assisting immigrants and people of other nations (the global sector)
- Subdivisions within it (e.g., some mental health sector agencies address substance abuse while others help people with their overall mental health)

An extensive policy literature exists regarding policies in these sectors. It describes myriad policies within each of the sectors. It evaluates and discusses the historical evolution of a number of these policies. It identifies policy controversies in each of the eight sectors.

A notable omission exists, however, in current policy literature. It fails to sufficiently embed micro, mezzo, and macro policy interventions *within* each of these policy sectors by discussing how social workers can and should provide these policy interventions within them. It fails to discuss specific tasks and skills that empower social workers to become advocates in each sector. It fails to provide examples of social workers' policy interventions in these sectors. These omissions risk *disempowering* social workers who work in these various sectors. They may be able to describe and analyze specific policies in these sectors, but they may not be equipped to develop micro, mezzo, and macro policy interventions within them.

This book addresses these omissions in several ways. Chapter 2 discusses why social workers need to reform policies in the eight sectors. Chapter 3 draws upon an emerging literature on policy practice and policy advocacy to provide a policy advocacy framework describing specific tasks and skills that will allow social workers to develop advocacy interventions at the micro, mezzo, and macro policy levels in *any* sector, agency, or government. Chapter 4 defines *micro policy advocacy* as interventions to help clients, families, and communities obtain services, benefits, resources, rights, and opportunities that they need and to which they are entitled, but that they might not otherwise obtain. Chapter 5 defines *mezzo policy advocacy* as interventions to change dysfunctional policies in organizations and communities. Chapter 6 defines *macro policy advocacy* as interventions to change dysfunctional policies in court and government settings. And Chapters 7 through 14 discuss how social workers work to advance social justice in each of eight sectors.

This book discusses how micro policy advocacy can lead to mezzo and macro policy advocacy in these eight sectors. If Tip O'Neill, former Speaker of the House of Representatives, argued, "All politics is local," we can say that "all policies begin with specific individuals, families, and communities." As social workers provide micro policy interventions to help their clients gain access to Medicaid or the Supplemental Nutrition Assistance Program (SNAP, formerly known as food stamps), they may *also* decide that dysfunctional policies contribute to this adverse outcome and engage in, for example, mezzo policy advocacy to change the unnecessary complexity of application forms, the requirement that clients frequently recertify their eligibility, the lack of sufficient public service advertisements, and the inaccessibility of eligibility offices. Or they may battle to prevent cuts in SNAP in their states and in the U.S. Congress with macro policy advocacy.

REALIZING THAT MICRO, MEZZO, AND MACRO POLICY ADVOCACY ARE *REALLY* NEEDED

Social workers engage in policy advocacy as they realize that the well-being of individuals and families is threatened by dysfunctional policies in organizational, community, and government settings. Of course, many programs and policies *are* meritorious. Health systems save many lives and prevent the emergence or progression of many chronic conditions. Many individuals surmount serious mental problems such as depression and anxiety. The lives of many children who have been subjected to extreme neglect or abuse are saved due to the interventions of child welfare workers. Many elderly individuals are helped to contend with end-of-life issues by hospice and palliative care programs. Some criminal offenders are rehabilitated by community-based programs after they have been released from prisons. Some low-achieving students become high achievers due to help they receive from teachers and counselors.

Remarkable improvements have occurred in each of the policy sectors when they are viewed from a historical perspective. Life expectancy has increased from roughly 68 years for women and 65 years for men in 1960 to roughly 83 and 78 years, respectively, in 2014. Medications such as psychotropic drugs now ease the symptoms of people with severe mental illnesses like schizophrenia. Elderly individuals and people with mental conditions no longer languish for decades in the back wards of state hospitals. Violations of the civil rights of people of color have been reduced by enactment of civil rights legislation at federal and state levels.

Considerable research suggests, however, that seven challenges are often encountered by consumers in the eight policy sectors: (1) violation of their ethical rights, (2) failure to receive quality services, (3) lack of culturally responsive services, (4) insufficient preventive services, (5) lack of access to services and programs, (6) lack of attention to mental problems, and (7) receipt of services not sufficiently linked to consumers' households and communities.

IDENTIFYING SEVEN CORE PROBLEMS THAT CUT ACROSS EIGHT POLICY SECTORS

We now turn to the seven core problems that consumers of services encounter in each of the eight policy sectors.

Core Problem 1: Advancing Ethical Rights, Human Rights, and Economic Justice

Ethicists mostly agree that service providers, as well as nations, should meet individuals' basic survival needs, honor their self-determination, provide them with accurate and honest information, preserve the confidentiality of personal information, treat people equitably, honor individuals' human rights, and advance social justice (Holland, 2012).

Meeting Basic Survival Needs

The United States has made important strides in protecting basic survival needs during the past 60 years. It protected millions of Americans from starvation with cash relief and work relief in the Great Depression as well as formed federal welfare programs and unemployment insurance to supplement welfare programs. It established the Food Stamps Program in 1964 and expanded it in subsequent decades, recently changing its name to the Supplemental Nutrition Assistance Program (SNAP). It established the Medicaid and Medicare programs in 1965 to expand health coverage for low-income individuals and elderly people—and added the Children's Health Insurance Program (CHIP) for low-income children in 1997. It developed federal housing programs in the 1930s and added other rent subsidy programs in the 1970s. Many private organizations give cash, food, and shelter relief to Americans. The United States also established a federal minimum wage in 1938 that had risen to $7.25 by 2014, and many states have mandated higher wages, such as California with a minimum wage of $9 per hour. It will provide about 32 million additional Americans with health insurance when the Affordable Care Act (ACA) is fully implemented. The United States has developed federal emergency programs to help residents in the wake of natural disasters.

Much remains to be done to meet Americans' survival needs. Considerable numbers of people earn income just above, at, or below federal poverty levels (FPL), which are set very low, such as $19,790 for families of three and $23,850 for families of four in 2014. Disparities in income between the bottom fifth of the population and the top fifth have widened since 1978—and the gap between the income of the bottom fifth and that of the top 2% has widened even more since that date. Thomas Piketty, a French economist, published a book in 2014 that revealed that Americans with the top 1% of the nation's wealth, including their investments and capital, possess 20% of the nation's wealth—and the top 10% of them possess 50% of the nation's wealth. These wealth disparities are the most extreme America has seen since the Gilded Age, from roughly 1880 to 1900 (Piketty, 2014). Piketty's discovery led to widespread debates about the negative implications of extreme economic disparities and how to decrease them, such as by greatly increasing tax rates on the very rich and redistributing resources to people with less wealth. Many Americans are malnourished. Large numbers of Americans do not receive sufficient medical services. The mental health problems of many individuals are not addressed. Many Americans do not use social programs that could markedly improve their well-being. Only about half of eligible individuals use, for example, SNAP, the Medicaid Program, and the Earned Income Tax Credit, as well as the CHIP program—depriving low-income individuals of billions of dollars of income, food, and health resources.

Providing Individuals With Opportunities

If people do not receive education, job training, and employment, they can meet their survival needs only through assistance from government or from private charities. Many people rely on welfare and assistance from the private and public sectors during economic downturns, in the wake of disabling health and physical problems, and during bouts of unemployment, but most people should have education and skills to support themselves and their dependents through gainful employment. Their employment should provide sufficient wages to meet their survival needs and to provide them with other amenities, such as savings, recreation, and decent housing. Their employment, too, should give them the ability to steadily improve their wages through time—and should meet other personal needs such as creative expression and fulfillment.

Millions of Americans lack skills to find employment in the global economy. Individuals who possess only a high school education or less are seriously compromised in finding work or in finding employment that meets their basic needs.

The wages of many workers have been relatively stagnant during the past three decades. The quality of education varies widely in the United States. Inner-city schools often have more crowded classrooms and poorer teachers than suburban schools. Many students, particularly low-income, African American, Latino, and Native American students, do not achieve national norms in math and reading. In many inner-city high schools, more than 50% of students drop out; nationally, roughly 25% drop out. About 50% of students who enter community colleges drop out before the second year. Less than 60% of students who enter colleges graduate in six years. People of color disproportionately do not enter educational programs after high school and fail to graduate from them. The learning of many students is compromised by their lack of nutrition, homelessness, and mental conditions.

Many laws protect vulnerable populations from discrimination. The Americans with Disabilities Act (ADA) prohibits discrimination by employers against people with disabilities. The Civil Rights Acts of 1964 and 1965 prohibit discrimination by schools and employers against people of color and women. Some states prohibit discrimination against members of the lesbian, gay, bisexual, transgender, queer, and questioning (LGBTQQ) population in places of employment.

Honoring Self-Determination

Many court rulings, as well as writings of ethical philosophers and religious leaders, support the right of individuals to decide whether, when, and how to seek services or use social programs in the United States. The Supreme Court has ruled, for example, that individuals who are cognitively competent can decline medical treatments even when their physicians believe that this decision could cause them physical harm or even death. Specific laws, court rulings, and accreditation standards require agencies and programs to honor self-determination through "*informed* consent" that informs clients about:

- Likely outcomes of specific treatments
- Likely monetary costs of specific treatments
- Likely side effects or threats to their well-being from specific treatments or courses of action, including death and injury
- Alternative treatments or services
- Evidence-based findings relevant to their treatment

Providers who do not give individuals full and accurate information about treatment options so that they can make informed decisions are liable to incur penalties that can include loss of their licenses. Providers do not have to obtain informed consent in cases where a court has ruled that a specific client is mentally incompetent and where the court itself, or a guardian appointed by it, acts in the best interests of that person.

States usually allow parents or guardians to make decisions for minors as long as those decisions advance the children's well-being. Under the doctrine of *parens patriae*, however, public authorities can investigate whether parents or guardians are neglecting or abusing children and can take custody of them or order specific ameliorating actions or treatment when they discover that children have been harmed or might suffer harm.

Most states allow public authorities to commit individuals involuntarily to hospitals, correctional facilities, or other settings when they are suicidal or have already attempted to harm themselves. They also allow public authorities to restrain or incarcerate individuals who have threatened or harmed others. These actions of public authorities are circumscribed, however, by mandated legal representation for people who are involuntarily admitted to institutions, required reviews of their cases by courts, and other procedural safeguards.

Many obstacles exist to self-determination. Some providers fail to involve their clients sufficiently in the helping process. Providers may be less likely to provide informed consent to individuals from vulnerable populations, such as women and people of color. People with mental conditions, such as schizophrenia, may be viewed as unable to make specific choices even when they are capable of making them. Relatively submissive individuals may not assert their rights.

Honoring Consumers' Right to Accurate and Honest Information

People have an ethical right to know the nature of their mental, health, and other problems in clear and understandable terms. They need to know their prognosis. They need accurate and honest information throughout their treatments or services, such as knowledge of how their condition has changed, outcomes of their current treatments, and whether different treatments should be selected as they progress forward. People also need accurate and honest information from personnel in financial institutions, car dealers, landlords, and employers.

Many obstacles prevent the provision of accurate and honest information. Providers sometimes want to steer people to treatments and facilities that will financially benefit them by giving them higher reimbursements. They may give their patients or consumers false statistics about the success of their services or treatments in hopes that those individuals will be more likely to use them. They may overstate the seriousness of specific conditions or prognoses in order to frighten people into using their services or treatments. They may deceive individuals with low levels of education, such as when car dealers, landlords, and employers victimize their consumers. Providers sometimes do not divulge conflicts of interest. Many policies, court rulings, regulations, and laws protect people's right to accurate and honest information by, for example, prohibiting false advertising, requiring disclosure of conflicts of interest, and requiring disclosure of treatment options. Professionals may sometimes give inaccurate information because *they* are misinformed. Perhaps they are not aware of new research that identifies specific evidence-based treatments.

Protecting the Ethical Right to Confidentiality

Consumers of services are entitled to confidentiality—and would likely not seek assistance for many of their problems if they did not trust their providers to maintain it. The federal Health Insurance Portability and Accountability Act of 1996 (HIPAA) protects the confidentiality of clients' information in health systems. It requires health organizations and health personnel to adhere to numerous procedures to protect patients' confidentiality. Its standards extend to other service delivery systems, such as mental health. Other protections for confidentiality include state laws, accreditation standards, court rulings, and professional licensing standards as well as the Code of Ethics of the National Association of Social Workers (NASW). Other standards protect the confidentiality of students.

Exceptions to confidentiality exist. If someone threatens to injure or kill another person, for example, health and mental health providers are *required* to disclose this information to the specific external authorities, such as the police. Some health information, such as cases of HIV/AIDS infection and tuberculosis, must be disclosed to public health authorities. Social workers must sometimes verify to courts that specific individuals have actually received specific health and mental health services that the courts mandated them to use.

Many factors jeopardize the confidentiality of clients' information. Some providers are insufficiently aware of the hazards that specific consumers may experience if their private information is divulged to certain individuals or organizations—such as possible loss of employment or disruption of relationships or marriages. Providers are sometimes careless in the ways they transmit information about specific clients to others, such as by telephone in ways that allow third parties to listen in. Hackers can sometimes gain illicit access to clients' information that is stored electronically.

Providing Equitable Treatment

All people have a right to receive the same quality, kind, and duration of services, benefits, and treatments as those that other people with the same problems or conditions receive, regardless of their race, gender, sexual orientation, place of national origin, age, social class, level of intelligence, religion, disability status, literacy level, ability or inability to speak English, genetic characteristics, mental health, socioeconomic status, or other personal characteristics. Many state and federal civil rights policies prohibit inequitable treatment, including:

- The federal Civil Rights Acts of 1964 and 1965 that prohibit discrimination against people of color, women, and people born in other nations
- The Americans with Disabilities Act of 1990 (ADA) that bans discrimination against people with physical and mental disabilities
- State laws banning discrimination in housing and employment against individuals on the basis of sexual orientation
- State and federal laws banning discrimination in housing for many vulnerable populations
- State and federal laws banning discrimination against individuals with HIV/AIDS
- Policies that require affirmative action and quotas for women, people of color, and veterans
- State and federal laws that protect members of vulnerable populations from discrimination at their places of work

Professionals sometimes discriminate on the basis of prejudice against specific kinds of people. Individuals with schizophrenia often receive inferior healthcare, even when they possess heart disease. African Americans and women are less likely than Caucasians and males to obtain some types of advanced health technology. Disabled individuals are often treated paternalistically, with an emphasis on their physical limitations rather than their strengths. People with a history of criminal offenses are often subjected to discrimination in their places of work. Homeless youth often find it difficult to enroll in secondary education. People of color are more likely to be sentenced to death than Caucasians—and are incarcerated at higher rates and for longer periods that whites for specific offenses. African Americans who use illicit drugs are more likely than Caucasians to receive prison sentences. People of color are subject to more police brutality than Caucasians. Students of color are more likely to be expelled from secondary schools than Caucasian students. Employers often use "race" as a shortcut measure to assess applicants' capabilities for employment rather than objectively viewing their qualifications. Educators often convey their lower expectations to people of color and low-income whites.

Honoring Human Rights

Human rights are broadly defined as basic rights and freedoms, including the right to free speech, the ability to travel without restriction, protection from human trafficking, freedom from violence, and the right to free association. They include the right to humane treatment by employers and fellow employees in places of work. They prohibit genocide. They include protection of children and others from bullying in schools and places of employment. They include protection against sexual harassment in the workplace, verbal and physical abuse within families, and sex trafficking.

It is difficult to curtail violations of human rights for many reasons. Some behaviors are difficult to change, such as the bullying of children in schools, the sexual harassment of women in places of work, and gang violence. Many people profit monetarily from violating the rights of others, such as pimps and international traffickers of girls and women for prostitution. Violations of human rights often occur in developing nations, such as genocide in Rwanda, the Sudan, and Syria. They often occur in nations with dictatorships where freedom of speech, freedom of movement, and freedom of assembly are often curbed or prohibited.

The fundamental rights of human beings are embodied in international law; constitutions, statutes, and regulations; and court rulings (Barria & Roper, 2010; Gelb & Palley, 2009; Tomuschat, 2008). They include:

- Civil rights laws in local, state, and federal jurisdictions
- Article 1 of the United Nations Universal Declaration of Rights that defines "basic rights and freedoms" in response to atrocities during World War II
- The four treaties and three protocols of the Geneva Convention (1949), which defined rights of combatants and civilians during wars
- The UN Convention on the Elimination of All Forms of Discrimination Against Women (1981)
- The UN Convention Against Torture (1984)
- The International Convention on Protection of the Rights of All Migrant Workers and Members of Their Families (1990)
- The Convention on the Elimination of All Forms of Discrimination Against Women (1975)
- The UN Protocol to Prevent, Suppress, and Punish Trafficking in Persons (2000)
- The UN Convention on the Rights of the Child
- The Victims of Trafficking and Violence Protection Act of the United States (2000)

Provisions of the American Constitution include such rights as "due process," "equal protection under the law," freedom of speech, freedom of the press, and freedom of association in the Bill of Rights. Many state and federal laws protect human rights, such as anti-trafficking laws, laws prohibiting discrimination against individuals in their places of work, and laws protecting children and students from bullying in schools.

Promoting Social Justice

Social injustice occurs when specific populations, such as women, members of racial minorities, and low-income individuals, are subject to violations of civil and human rights, violations of equitable life conditions, and violations of access to opportunities. We have already discussed disparities in *civil and human rights* between people of color, women, and the mainstream population.

Social injustice also occurs when specific populations suffer *poorer life conditions* than others, such as when low-income individuals suffer from greater physical and mental illness, shorter life expectancy, more disabling conditions, higher rates of unemployment, and lower levels of school achievement than relatively affluent individuals. Disabled people have considerably less income, higher rates of unemployment, higher rates of mental illness, and shorter life expectancies than people who are not disabled. Individuals with schizophrenia have an average life expectancy of 63 years, compared to 77.9 years for other Americans. People of color are more likely to reside in crime-infested areas than white individuals, making life hazardous for them on a daily basis. Single female heads of households are among the poorest members of our society—to the point that an academic has coined the term *feminization of poverty*. They often work multiple jobs in a desperate effort to meet their children's basic needs, which wreaks a toll on their mental and physical health, not to mention their ability to obtain further schooling that might allow them to obtain a higher-wage job.

Social injustice imposes unnecessary costs on society. When specific vulnerable populations are denied equal access to opportunities, they are more likely than other people to need financial and medical assistance from the broader society. They are likely to contribute lower taxes to the revenues of local, state, and federal governments. Extreme inequality breeds social problems because it marginalizes large numbers of people who are acutely aware that they are poorer and sicker than mainstream populations. It breeds desperation in the case of individuals who cannot meet the survival needs of themselves and their children. It decreases participation in elections among low-income individuals—making it harder for them to elect public officials who would work to secure enhancements of their rights, life conditions, and opportunities.

Extreme inequality violates ethical standards established by many religions, professions, and ethicists. It is even more ethically problematic in industrialized nations, such as the United States, that possess sufficient resources to create more egalitarian economic and social systems.

We should not imply that members of vulnerable populations are passive victims of circumstances. Members of these groups often contend with adversity in many ways, such as through churches, small businesses, neighborhood associations, and advocacy groups. Many people better their condition by perseverance and resilience. Members of vulnerable populations often join forces to achieve legislative reforms, such as when African Americans and Latinos oppose efforts to curtail their voting rights.

Core Problem 2: Improving the Quality of Social Programs

Consumers of services have an ethical right to services and programs that ameliorate or solve social problems that they possess, but they often do not receive effective services. Perhaps providers give them interventions that have not been empirically evaluated. Perhaps service providers are not sufficiently skilled in providing specific services. Perhaps providers give consumers services that yield substantial revenues but are not effective.

Consumers of services, like taxpayers, have a right to *cost-effective services*—effective services delivered at a reasonable cost. Some medications may prolong life, for example, but only for several months at a cost exceeding $100,000. Some interventions are far more expensive than others that are just as effective or more effective, as was recently discovered when researchers found that acupuncture was more effective and less costly than surgery for some kinds of lower-back pain.

We can sometimes determine whether specific programs, treatments, interventions, or policies are effective or cost-effective by using research methodology. In so-called gold standard research, for example, researchers use randomized controlled trials (RCT) in which they compare the outcomes of groups of patients who receive specific assistance to those of groups that receive different kinds of assistance or no assistance. They might, for example, give one group a specific intervention for depression (the experimental group) and compare its outcomes with a group *not* receiving this intervention (the control group). Researchers sometimes cannot perform RCTs and instead conduct so-called quasi-experimental research in which they compare two or more groups that do and do not receive a specific intervention. Researchers sometimes use natural experiments to gauge the effectiveness of specific policies, such as determining if motorcyclists' death rate from accidents declines after the enactment of a state law requiring motorcyclists to wear helmets.

Surveys of consumers' satisfaction with services provide another measure of their quality. Medicare officials routinely ask patients to evaluate the Medicare services they receive from physicians and hospitals, for example, and place the results on the Internet so that patients can use this information to decide where to seek services.

The quality of services is often impeded by their fragmentation when consumers receive care from specific providers that is not coordinated. Assume, for example, that a child receives help with convulsions that sometimes accompany autism, but not for her emotional outbursts. Or perhaps an elderly person receives medication to control his depression that adversely interacts with other medications prescribed by other physicians. Case-management and navigation models of service have evolved to circumvent fragmentation. Case managers try to orchestrate a package of services for specific consumers, and patient navigators help individuals keep appointments, adhere to medications, and follow treatments. Only a small fraction of consumers of services receive such assistance, however, due to a lack of staff and funding to provide them, even for people with serious problems. Some state and federal laws require providers to develop comprehensive plans for certain clients, such as when they mainstream disabled or developmentally challenged children into the educational system. Comprehensive plans are ineffective, however, if schools and other agencies lack sufficient staff to implement them. Interagency collaborations, such as those developed between schools and mental health agencies, also curtail fragmentation.

Core Problem 3: Making Social Programs and Policies More Culturally Responsive

The United States has been an immigrant nation since its inception, its citizenry having originated from a mixture of forced immigration of slaves, subjugation of native peoples, and voluntary immigration from Europe, Russia, Mexico and Central America, Asia, the Middle East, Africa, and elsewhere over several centuries. In 2007, the U.S. population included 199 million non-Hispanic whites, 45 million Latinos, 37 million African Americans, 13.1 million Asians, 2 million American Indian and Alaska Natives, and 402,000 Native Hawaiians and other Pacific Islanders. Many people have limited English proficiency (LEP).

It is challenging to define "culturally responsive care" partly because it is difficult to define "culture." Brislin (2000) defines culture as the "shared values and concepts among people who most often speak the same language in proximity to each other . . . [that] are transmitted for generations, and . . . provide guidance for everyday behaviors" (p. 4). Culturally responsive care contains a language dimension. It requires that providers respect the cultural views about health and other social issues held by specific individuals, such as how they view specific health conditions, how they wish to receive healthcare, which terminology they prefer, how they wish to communicate with healthcare providers, and what treatments they wish to have. Culturally competent care is needed in every policy sector.

Culturally competent services must be provided not only to LEPs, but also to people from many groups that differ from mainstream ones, including illiterate or semiliterate individuals, LGBTQQ individuals, elderly people, disabled people, people from different religions, and women. Many people want complementary and alternative medicine (CAM) in healthcare, such as the use of herbs, acupuncture, meditation and yoga, and other nontraditional methods of preventing or treating health problems. They sometimes want CAM instead of traditional medicine and often use CAM and traditional medicine in tandem.

People who do not receive culturally competent services may suffer adverse consequences. They may not seek or return for needed services. They may not adhere to treatments that can improve their condition. They may sue providers, such as when they are not given translation services as required by federal and state laws. They may believe that they have not given informed consent when they are unable to communicate with providers.

Culturally competent care is enhanced when providers are self-aware, respect other cultures, have cultural awareness, possess cultural knowledge, and develop cultural skills where they "negotiate or facilitate relationships between consumers and providers" (Kao & Jansson, 2011, p. 184). Providers need skills that are described by Galanti (2008) as the "4 Cs of culture":

- CALL: What do you *call* the problem? What do you think is wrong?
- CAUSE: What do you think *caused* your problem?
- COPE: How do you *cope* with your condition? What have you done to make it better? Who else have you been to for treatment?
- CONCERNS: What *concerns* do you have regarding the condition? How serious do you think it is? What potential complications do you fear? How does it interfere with your life or your ability to function? What are your *concerns* regarding the recommended treatment?

Title VI of the federal Civil Rights Act of 1964 declares that no one in the United States can be excluded from participating in, or denied benefits of, any program or activity receiving federal financial assistance on the grounds of race, color, or *national origin*, which has been interpreted by courts to include an individual's primary language (Perkins & Youdelman, 2008; Perkins, Youdelman, & Wong, 2003). Subsequent presidential executive orders have required federal agencies and federally funded programs to provide "meaningful access" to LEP individuals (Kao & Jansson, 2011). Many states have enacted statutes and regulations that also require provision of translation services to LEP people. Accreditation standards of hospitals and clinics require the use of translation services, and in 2010 the ACA mandated collection of more data on race, ethnicity, gender, primary language, disability status, and underserved rural populations in health settings.

Service organizations should use census materials as well as analyses of their clients to determine their ethnicity and other demographic characteristics. They should hire people from various backgrounds and provide in-service training in cultural competence.

Core Problem 4: Developing Preventive Strategies to Decrease Social Problems

Theorists have distinguished between primary, secondary, and tertiary prevention. Primary prevention seeks to prevent the emergence of specific social problems such as cancer, diabetes, truancy, and mental illness. Secondary prevention aims to identify and treat specific problems early in their development, such as by slowing their progress or by curing them—for example, by helping someone slow the progress of his early-stage diabetes. Tertiary prevention has the same goals as secondary prevention, but for more advanced problems, such as helping someone slow the progress of an advanced medical or mental health problem.

Primary and secondary prevention often receive insufficient priority in health and human services. Providers are often diverted to people with advanced and serious problems due to their sheer number and the cost and time required to help them. People often find it difficult to modify lifestyle preferences that cause them to develop social problems, such as poor diet, lack of exercise, substance abuse, and smoking. Health insurance companies often do not fund preventive services at all—or they do so at lower rates than the actual cost of surgery and medications. Tobacco, industrial, and food interests have slowed or blocked policies related to smoking, pollution reduction, and food labeling. Elected public officials often focus on short-term policies rather than long-term preventive ones. They often slash funding for prevention during budget crises and recessions.

Researchers have made considerable progress in identifying promising preventive strategies. They identify "at-risk indicators" that allow them to predict with considerable accuracy who will and will not develop specific problems in future years, that is, "true positives." (At-risk indicators may include poor habits like smoking, low income, poor diet, obesity, poor lifestyle decisions such as inadequate exercise, abusive treatment by parents, poor education, genetic factors, and many other variables.) Their predictions are limited, however, in that some people who are predicted to develop a specific problem do not (false positives) while others predicted *not* to develop a problem actually *do* (false negatives).

We can distinguish between passive prevention and active prevention. Passive prevention seeks to change the human environment so that people are less likely to develop diseases like lung cancer *without requiring individuals to modify their behaviors*. When pollution is reduced in the air and water, for example, people achieve health benefits without taking action themselves. By contrast, active prevention succeeds only when individuals take specific actions, such as changing their diets or engaging in more exercise. They often have to work with other people to prevent a problem, such as by participating in a 12-step program to prevent substance abuse.

Policy advocates work on many levels to advance prevention. They convince organizations to fund and implement prevention programs. They convince legislators and government officials to develop regulations and enact statutes that promote prevention. They work with the mass media to publicize effective preventive strategies. They work with researchers to obtain evidence that specific preventive strategies are effective and cost-effective. They convince administrators and public officials to prioritize prevention—and to fund it adequately.

Core Problem 5: Improving Affordability and Access to Social Programs

People often encounter specific or multiple barriers to accessing services. They often find they cannot afford them, endure excessive waits, encounter complex and time-consuming eligibility processes, find services to be geographically distant, or possess health or mental health problems that make travel difficult. Accessibility may be hindered, as well, by a lack of advertising or publicity for specific services so that many people do not know they exist.

People in the United States pay greater out-of-pocket costs for health and human services than people in Europe and Canada, where governments foot a greater share of their costs. Even the ACA will leave about 16 million Americans uninsured in 2020. Many other services and programs require substantial payments from consumers, including most childcare and preschool programs, many medical services, many mental health services, and most postsecondary education programs. The inequities are often glaring: Affluent Americans often gain greater access to services and opportunities because they can afford out-of-pocket costs, unlike many low- and moderate-income individuals, who often refrain from using services or discontinue them prematurely. Out-of-pocket payments take many forms, including deductibles, payment for services excluded from coverage by insurance companies, fees for excluded or noncovered services, and sliding fees that adjust fees upward as personal income increases. These fees can cause hardships for people with low and moderate income, not only impeding their access to services but also decreasing their ability to pay rent, purchase food, or purchase medical and other kinds of care.

Many services require excessive waits, such as emergency rooms in many hospitals, public health and mental health clinics, substance abuse treatment programs, and subsidized housing. People who decide to seek help for substance abuse problems often encounter waits of six months or more. Waits often lead consumers to exit services even when they need them, such as when people prematurely leave emergency rooms.

Health and human services are not distributed equitably across the American landscape but are disproportionately located in relatively affluent areas, because organizations and professionals often seek locations where people are more likely to pay their fees. Individuals who cannot afford cars, cannot afford gasoline, lack public transportation, or cannot easily seek services during working hours find it particularly difficult to access services and programs not located their communities.

Policy advocates can decrease the cost and increase the accessibility of services and programs. They can propose changes in the fee structures of public programs, such as upward changes in their eligibility levels, inclusion of excluded services, and reduction of deductibles and copayments. They can pressure public agencies to make services more accessible in underserved areas. They can persuade agencies to establish outreach programs or storefront programs for people in underserved areas. They can station services in other agencies, such as in libraries, hospitals, or schools. They can establish outreach programs to homebound individuals. They can downsize their central or largest programs as they move staff and resources to smaller programs. They can publicize their programs by targeting messages to media, churches, libraries, or social media used by specific segments of the population.

Core Problem 6: Increasing the Scope and Effectiveness of Mental Health Programs

Many Americans have serious undetected health and substance abuse problems. These problems may be "hidden" *because* they are not the presenting problems when people use medical and other agencies. Many people do not volunteer that they have these problems due to the stigma often attached to them. Mental health or substance abuse problems may be caused by *other* social problems, such as experiencing foreclosure, performing poorly in school, or losing work.

Mental health services are often inadequately provided in settings beyond clinics and institutions that focus on them. Roughly 44% of males and 61% of females in federal prisons possess serious mental problems, but they often receive no, little, or substandard care for them. Primary care physicians provide the largest quantity of mental health services in community settings, but they often have little mental health training and are not usually supervised by mental health specialists. Publicly subsidized mental health clinics exist, but they often have insufficient resources despite funding from local, state, and federal governments; reimbursements from private insurance; funding from Medicaid and Medicare; and client fees.

Unlike physicians, the dominant providers in the healthcare system, many professionals provide mental health services, including primary care physicians, psychiatrists, psychologists, social workers, marriage and family counselors, and psychiatric nurses. Social workers provide more mental health services than members of any other mental health profession.

Mental health staff are often not present, or only peripherally present, in many settings where people present their mental health problems. Employee Assistance Programs (EAPs) provide mental health services in some corporate settings but reach only a small fraction of American workers. School systems employ relatively few social workers and psychologists despite the sheer number of students with depression, anxiety, autism, attention deficit disorder, and behavioral problems. Many hospitals and clinics employ relatively few social workers and psychologists. Mental health services are chronically underfunded in the United States, both for outpatient care and institutional care that is still needed for suicidal individuals and people who may present a threat to others.

Access to mental health services greatly increased after the enactment of the Mental Health Parity and Addiction Equity Act of 2008, which requires employers offering group health insurance plans to their employees to include coverage for mental health services. The ACA also requires private insurance companies as well as Medicaid and Medicare not to discriminate against mental health services relative to services for physical problems. Many state and federal laws protect the rights of people with mental and substance abuse problems, such as by protecting the confidentiality of patients' records, requiring legal counsel to represent individuals who are subject to involuntary commitments, and requiring conservatorship for people with serious cognitive deficits.

Core Problem 7: Making Social Programs More Relevant to Households and Communities

Assume a person receives care for a mental or physical problem in a clinic or hospital, but her providers are unaware of her home and community environment. Unable to obtain medications and food in her neighborhood because she lacks transportation and is barely ambulatory, she dies from inadequate nutrition—a problem that might have been avoided had professionals enrolled her in services offered by visiting nurses as well as Meals on Wheels.

Several strategies can improve the linkage of services to consumers' households and communities. Agencies can establish contracts or agreements with community-based agencies that provide specific services, such as from visiting nurses, case managers, transportation services, and many other agencies. Agencies can establish formal collaborations with one another to provide needed services to clients. Innovative electronic systems can be used to monitor and educate home-based individuals with disabilities, chronic diseases, and other conditions.

The ACA is increasingly vesting specific hospitals and clinics with the total care of their clientele in so-called medical homes. These hospitals and clinics are penalized if their discharged patients return to inpatient care or emergency rooms within 30 days after receiving surgeries, providing them with incentives to give patients home-based services.

The ADA requires public housing and other housing agencies to provide accommodations to people with disabilities.

RECOGNIZING THE SEVEN CORE PROBLEMS IN EIGHT POLICY SECTORS

In Chapters 7 through 14, we discuss how these seven core problems manifest themselves in each of the eight policy sectors. In healthcare, for example, specific patients' ethical rights are sometimes violated when they do not give their "informed consent" to specific medical procedures at the level of an individual or family (Core Problem 1). In the child and family sector, children with specific mental conditions sometimes do not receive evidence-based care at a child or family level, such as when professional staff members do not diagnose clinical depression or anxiety (Core Problem 2). Mental health staff may fail to give specific clients culturally competent care, such as when they do not adapt their services to the cultural needs of Latinos, who often want family members to be present during counseling sessions (Core Problem 3). In the gerontology sector, some elderly people do not receive preventive care from health providers for early-stage chronic diseases such as congestive heart failure (Core Problem 4). Many individuals cannot afford healthcare in the United States due to lack of insurance coverage, a situation that was partially addressed when the Affordable Care Act of 2010 was enacted (Core Problem 5). The mental distress of many prisoners is inadequately addressed in many prisons and correctional facilities (Core Problem 6). People who receive services from agencies in the gerontology sector often receive insular care not connected to their households and communities (Core Problem 7).

UNDERSTANDING THAT SOCIAL WORK'S CODE OF ETHICS REQUIRES ADVOCACY

Micro policy advocacy, mezzo policy advocacy, and macro policy advocacy are interventions that allow social workers to adhere to the NASW's Code of Ethics, which requires social workers to engage in "social and political action" (NASW, n.d., Section 6.04):

(a) Social workers should engage in social and political action that seeks to ensure that all people have equal access to the resources, employment, services, and opportunities they require to meet their basic human needs and to develop fully. Social workers should be aware of the impact of the political arena on practice and should advocate for changes in policy and legislation to improve social conditions in order to meet basic human needs and promote social justice.

(b) Social workers should act to expand choice and opportunity for all people, with special regard for vulnerable, disadvantaged, oppressed, and exploited people and groups.

(c) Social workers should promote conditions that encourage respect for cultural and social diversity within the United States and globally. Social workers should promote policies and practices that demonstrate respect for difference, support the expansion of cultural knowledge and resources, advocate for programs and institutions that demonstrate cultural competence, and promote policies that safeguard the rights of and confirm equity and social justice for all people.

(d) Social workers should act to prevent and eliminate domination of, exploitation of, and discrimination against any person, group, or class on the basis of race, ethnicity, national origin, color, sex, sexual orientation, age, marital status, political belief, religion, or mental or physical disability.

Social workers implement this Code of Ethics *whenever they engage in micro, mezzo, and macro policy advocacy.* They help people obtain rights, services, benefits, and opportunities that they might not otherwise obtain through micro policy advocacy. They advance the well-being of individuals, families, and communities when they engage in mezzo or macro policy advocacy to reform dysfunctional policies through social and political action. Social workers often prioritize the needs of vulnerable populations when they engage in advocacy.

DEFINING "SOCIAL POLICIES"

We define social policies as "collective strategies to prevent and address social problems." They are "collective" because they are *binding* on those individuals, populations, communities, companies, and jurisdictions to which they apply. For example, when Congress enacts and the president signs a statute such as the ACA, individuals, health providers, states, and others must adhere to its provisions under penalty of law because statutes *are* binding laws. They can challenge provisions of a federal law, such as the ACA, through the courts, but must adhere to relevant court rulings. When a state declares the growing and distribution of marijuana to be legal under certain circumstances, it allows growers and distributors to engage in this practice "under certain circumstances," such as for medical purposes—provided that officials in the federal government, which has its own laws that pertain to marijuana, allow people in a state to grow and distribute this drug.

Many kinds of social policies exist:

- *Constitutions* define the social policy powers of government at the federal and state levels. The failure of the federal Constitution to enumerate social welfare functions for the federal government was originally interpreted to mean that such functions should be left to state and local governments and to the private sector. As a result, the development of social welfare policies in this country was seriously delayed. States, too, possess constitutions that establish important duties of state governments, as well as how they govern themselves.
- Some social welfare strategies involve *public policies*, laws enacted in local, state, or federal legislatures. The Chinese Exclusion Act of 1882, the Social Security Act of 1935, the Adoption Assistance and Child Welfare Act of 1980, the Americans with Disabilities Act of 1991, and the Affordable Care Act of 2010 are examples of public laws, as are the state and local laws that established poorhouses and mental institutions in the 19th century.
- *Court decisions* play an important role in American social policy. By over-ruling, upholding, and interpreting the federal and state constitutions, statutes of legislatures, ordinances of local government, and practices of public agencies such as mental health, police, and welfare departments, courts establish policies that significantly influence the American response to social needs. For example, in the 1980s, the courts required the Reagan administration to award disability benefits to many disabled individuals even though many administration officials opposed this policy.
- *Budget and spending programs* are also an expression of policy, as are the budget priorities established by the nature of budget allocations and tax policies. For example, Americans chose not to expend a major share of the gross

national product on social programs prior to the 1930s but greatly increased levels of spending in the Great Depression and succeeding decades. Despite the large increases in spending on social programs in the 1960s and the 1970s, for example, the nation chose to devote a significant portion of its federal budget to military spending during the Cold War and also to make successive tax cuts—policies that much reduced the resources available for social programs.

- *International treaties, as well as policies of the United Nations,* govern an array of economic, social, migration, environmental, and national security issues in an era of globalization.
- *Stated or implied objectives* also constitute a form of policy. For example, the preambles and titles of social legislation suggest broad purposes or goals. Thus, as its title suggests, the Personal Responsibility and Work Opportunity and Reconciliation Act that Bill Clinton signed in August 1996 emphasized rules and procedures for getting welfare recipients off welfare rolls rather than providing training, education, or services.
- *Rules, procedures, and regulations* define the ways in which policies are to be implemented. Legislation often prescribes, for example, the rules or procedures to be used by agency staff in determining applicants' eligibility for specific programs. Courts often prescribe procedures that the staff of social agencies must employ to safeguard the rights of clients, patients, and consumers; the protections afforded to people who are involuntarily committed to mental institutions provide an example here. Government agencies issue administrative regulations to guide the implementation of policies—regulations that have the force of law.
- *Informal policies* as compared to *written or official policies* are subjective views of individuals and groups that influence whether and how they implement specific policies. If we want to know how the poorhouses of the 19th century worked—or how social agencies have implemented the ACA—we have to examine how their staff implemented formal policies that were given to them by legislatures and public officials. Informal and formal policies sometimes work in tandem, such as when the line staff of agencies fully understand and agree with official policies. They sometimes clash, however, when staff do not fully implement official policies because they disagree with them.

Social policy surrounds and envelops social workers, as well as the people and communities that they help, at virtually every point in their professional work. It describes the benefits their clients can receive from many social programs—whether material benefits from programs like SNAP or services from mental health, vocational, or education programs. It describes their clients' rights through regulations, legislation, and court rulings. It gives opportunities to their clients, such as educational, preschool, and vocational programs. It provides Americans with tax benefits that help them purchase homes and accumulate savings. It gives civil rights to people of color, women, and disabled individuals. It provides preventive services, such as primary care medical services and nutritional benefits to pregnant women. It helps people survive disasters like floods, hurricanes, and tornadoes. It funds social programs. It determines the purpose or mission of specific social programs and agencies.

Social policy shapes the nature of society itself. It helps to determine, for example, the extent of inequality in a community, state, or nation. If the nation fails to fund education, social programs, and safety-net programs, it decreases the chances that low-income people can improve their lot. If the nation gives affluent individuals tax breaks, it increases the odds that they will retain their dominant economic position. If a state possesses inferior vocational and job-training programs, low-income individuals will find it difficult to improve their economic standing.

Policies are vertically distributed at the federal, state, and local government; community; and agency or organizational levels. The *federal government* funds myriad entitlements, such as Social Security, Medicare, and Medicaid. It funds many means-tested programs like SNAP (food stamps) and the Supplemental Security Income (SSI) program. It funds the Earned Income Tax Credit (EITC) that gives tax rebates to many families. It funds hundreds of smaller programs through its annual budget, such as health prevention programs, Head Start, and block grant programs that give funds to states for mental health, childcare, and many additional programs. The U.S. Justice Department and the federal Equal Employment and Occupational Commission (EEOC) monitor violations of civil rights and take corrective action. The federal government funds the bulk of the American welfare state because its resources from the federal tax system and other kinds of taxation far exceed the resources of the states.

State governments often share the cost of public education with the federal government, covering only 10% of the cost themselves. They also share the costs of the nation's huge correctional system, including prisons, parole departments, and local police—save for federal prisons and federal law enforcement through the Federal Bureau of Investigation (FBI) and other federal police functions. States often fund many public health programs. They often inspect health facilities, such as hospitals, clinics, and nursing homes. States have been given many additional roles in overseeing the health system under the ACA. (Considerable variation exists between states regarding which policy functions reside at state versus local levels and the extent to which states and local governments share policy responsibilities and costs.) States provide direction for child welfare, mental health, public health, and other public systems of care. They often are conduits for federal resources that they supplement with their own funds. They set standards for many public services provided by counties and municipalities. State governments contribute significant resources, as well, to social programs and policies. They cofund such programs as Medicaid and other federal–state programs. They establish and fund many of their own programs, such as public health programs that provide health clinics to low-income areas and inspect food facilities for safety.

Local governments determine how land can be used in their jurisdictions through zoning and tax policies. They determine if specific social agencies, such as halfway homes for people released from state mental health facilities, can locate in specific areas. They provide police and fire services. Cities and counties raise taxes and decide how to use tax revenues, such as for police and fire services, schools, recreation programs, and social service programs. They orchestrate many housing programs. County or municipal agencies distribute welfare benefits to people under the Temporary Assistance for Needy Families (TANF) program and general assistance programs. Many counties and cities administer public systems of healthcare as well as assume important roles in child welfare, mental health, and many other social programs.

Public organizations are largely funded by local, state, and federal governments to implement programs defined by public statutes. They have considerable leeway, however, in making implementation decisions. Not-for-profit agencies, which are exempted from paying taxes by local, state, and federal governments, raise their own resources from public and private sources as well as from fees paid by consumers of their services. They select a mission that shapes what programs they will fund by grants from public agencies, consumer fees, or resources from private donors. They hire staff to implement these resources. For-profit organizations and agencies have owners or shareholders who seek profits in the marketplace. For-profit agencies provide a wide array of social services, such as childcare, nursing home care, job training, education, and other services—and sometimes receive contracts from public authorities to implement welfare, correctional, educational, and other services.

JOINING THE REFORM TRADITION OF SOCIAL WORK

Social work has a social reform tradition extending back to the formation of the social work profession. Such founders of social work as Jane Addams militantly supported an array of social reforms in the Progressive Era at the beginning of the 20th century, including housing codes to protect tenants, governmental inspection of food to avert illness, factory regulations to protect workers, and pensions for single mothers with children to avert dire poverty (Jansson, 2014; Wenocur & Reisch, 1989).

In succeeding eras, many social workers joined this reform tradition by working for policy reforms in local, state, and federal jurisdictions. Their work was bolstered by numerous theorists who developed a systems or environmental perspective on human behavior, arguing that social inequality, blighted neighborhoods, inadequate resources, unemployment, environmental pollution, discrimination, and economic uncertainty cause human suffering and contribute to clinical conditions such as depression and poor health (Germain & Gitterman, 1980; Meyer, 1970).

Honest differences of opinion often exist among social workers. We may disagree about the merits of specific policies. We may support different political candidates. We may draw upon conflicting research findings to support our preferred policies. Yet we are linked by a shared commitment to social justice even as we may differ about how best to advance it.

In this book, you will learn about scores of social policies in the eight policy sectors. You need to know about them because you will often refer clients or patients to them and would be derelict if you were not familiar with them. This book provides an empowerment and advocacy approach to social policy that facilitates your personal involvement on multiple levels. It encourages you to:

- Examine your values and personal perspectives, since they shape how you relate to controversies in American society regarding social policy
- Understand NASW's Code of Ethics as a foundational statement about ethics developed by and for social workers
- Understand and work to reduce the marginalization of many vulnerable populations in the United States and abroad by engaging in policy advocacy
- View social policy from an empowerment perspective so that you participate in it at multiple levels, including helping specific clients and patients to obtain rights, benefits, services, and opportunities to which they are entitled (micro policy advocacy) and reforming social policies in organizations, communities, and government settings (macro policy advocacy)
- Seek out information on the Internet while remembering that accuracy varies from site to site
- Learn about advocacy groups that work toward creating more just and equitable policies

LEARNING OUTCOMES

You are now equipped to:

- Identify eight policy sectors
- Identify similarities and differences between micro policy advocacy, mezzo policy advocacy, and macro policy advocacy

- Define seven core problems that cut across the eight policy sectors
- Identify provisions of the Code of Ethics of the National Association of Social Workers that require social workers to engage in policy advocacy
- Define and identify a variety of social policies as well as their location in the American welfare state
- Identify the reform tradition of the social work profession

REFERENCES

Barria, L., & Roper, S. (2010). *The development of institutions of human rights: A comparative study.* New York, NY: Macmillan.

Brislin, R. (2000). *Understanding culture's influence on behavior* (2nd ed.). Belmont, CA: Wadsworth.

Galanti, G. A. (2008). *Caring for patients from different cultures* (4th ed.). Philadelphia: University of Pennsylvania Press.

Gelb, J., & Palley, M. L. (2009). *Women and politics around the world* (Vol. 1). Santa Barbara, CA: ABC-CLIO.

Germain, C., & Gitterman, A. (1980). *The life model of social work practice.* New York, NY: Columbia University Press.

Holland, S. (2012). *Arguing About bioethics.* New York, NY: Routledge.

Jansson, B. (2014). *The reluctant welfare state.* Belmont, CA: Wadsworth.

Kao, D., & Jansson, B. (2011). Advocacy to promote culturally competent health services. In B. Jansson (Ed.), *Improving healthcare through advocacy: A guide for the health and helping professions* (pp. 179–210). Hoboken, NJ: Wiley.

Meyer, C. (1970). *Social work practice: A response to the urban crisis.* New York, NY: Free Press.

National Association of Social Workers. (n.d.). *Code of ethics of the National Association of Social Workers.* Retrieved November 18, 2014, from http://www.socialworkers.org/pubs/code/code.asp

Perkins, J., & Youdelman, M. (2008). *Summary of state law requirements: Addressing language needs in healthcare.* Los Angeles, LA: National Health Law Program.

Perkins, J., Youdelman, M., & Wong, D. (2003). *Ensuring linguistic access in healthcare settings: Legal rights and responsibilities.* Los Angeles, LA: National Health Law Program.

Piketty, T. (2014). *Capital in the twenty-first century.* Belknap Press of Harvard University Press.

Tomuschat, C. (2008). *Human rights: Between idealism and realism.* New York, NY: Oxford University.

Wenocur, S., & Reisch, M. (1989). *From charity to enterprise: The development of American social work in a market economy.* Urbana: University of Illinois Press.

Chapter 2

DECIDING WHEN TO CHALLENGE THE STATUS QUO

LEARNING OBJECTIVES

In this chapter, you will learn how to:

1. Understand how foundational beliefs often shape people's views about policies

2. Describe different ideologies, including liberal, conservative, libertarian, and radical ones

3. Identify guidelines for trying to reach common ground

4. Understand how vulnerable populations are discussed in the Code of Ethics of the National Association of Social Workers (NASW)

5. Identify 16 vulnerable populations

6. Understand the history of women's oppression in the 20th century and the current era

7. Decide when to initiate policy advocacy

   - Using ethical first-order principles
   - Using evidence-based information
   - Using pragmatic considerations

We often have to decide when to challenge the status quo, whether in our personal or professional lives. When we decide in our professional careers that specific clients possess problems that have the potential to harm their well-being, we may provide a micro policy advocacy intervention. When we perceive organizational, community, or government policies to be inimical to clients' well-being, we may provide a mezzo policy or macro policy intervention. In this chapter, we turn to how foundational beliefs, beliefs about vulnerable populations, evidence-based findings, and ethical reasoning help us to make these decisions.

ANALYZING FOUNDATIONAL BELIEFS

VIDEO LINK 2.1
Challenging the
Status Quo

Foundational beliefs shape whether and how we address specific social problems at the micro, mezzo, or macro policy levels. These foundational beliefs flow from our personal experiences, culture, religious affiliations, ideology, and research findings.

Personal experiences from our upbringing, our parents' beliefs, our social class, our religious background, and our personal problems powerfully shape our decisions about whether and when to engage in policy advocacy. People who contract specific diseases or mental illnesses, for example, often engage in policy advocacy to help their victims. People who have seen or experienced family violence as children sometimes become advocates for children later in their lives. Children with parents who engage in social action often participate in it as adults.

We should not exaggerate the effects of personal experiences, however. Some affluent individuals, such as Franklin Delano Roosevelt, become advocates for low-income people even when they saw such people mostly as servants or laborers in their childhoods. Conversely, some people do not engage in social action even when they have been exposed to social reform as children.

Our *culture* shapes how we perceive specific social problems. Specific cultures stigmatize specific conditions. Consider, for instance, the widespread disdain for people on welfare in the United States, the shunning of individuals with mental health problems in many Asian nations, and prejudice against people who are gay or lesbian in many nations. Conversely, cultural beliefs sometimes induce sympathy toward people with specific social problems, such as toward children who suffer serious illnesses and veterans with trauma from their military service in the United States. We should not exaggerate the effects of culture, because considerable diversity exists within specific cultures. While many Americans believe welfare recipients are responsible for their dependency, many other Americans implicate environmental causes, such as unemployment and low wages.

Religious affiliations can powerfully shape our policy views. Take the case of the Religious Society of Friends (Quakers), whose members assumed leading roles in supporting the rights of Native Americans, African Americans, and women in the 19th century—and the rights of immigrants and prisoners in the 20th century. One statement of their social and civic responsibility, from a document handed out during an Orange Grove meeting in Pasadena, California, read as follows: "Poverty within a wealthy society is unjust, cruel, and often linked to skin color, gender, and language. We must examine our own privilege and role in the economic order that deepens this disparity." It invites members to ask, "Am I persistent in my efforts to promote constructive change? . . . How do we attend to suffering of others in our local community, in our state and nation, and in the world community?" (For further discussion of Quakers' social justice philosophy, see Pacific Yearly Meeting, 2001.) Members of some evangelical groups hew to a more conservative ideology.

POLICY ADVOCACY LEARNING CHALLENGE 2.1

Discuss with others how your religious background or affiliations have shaped your views about social policy. In what ways are your views consonant *or* dissonant with the NASW's Code of Ethics? Can you identify religious views that are not consonant with this Code? Why do you think some people of faith have views like these? Why are other people, like the late Senator Ted Kennedy, convinced that the New Testament mandates policies akin to his liberal views? (When asked why he was such a dedicated advocate for vulnerable populations, he impatiently asked his questioner, "Haven't you *read* the New Testament?")

Ideology powerfully shapes our views of the external world. Sharp divisions have long existed in the United States between conservatives and liberals about the causes of many social problems, as well as how to address them. Members of the so-called Tea Party, for example, disagree with most Democrats on myriad social issues. Contenders for the Republican presidential nomination often castigated the views and policy choices of President Barack Obama in the spring and summer of 2012. President Obama and Republican presidential nominee Mitt Romney took turns denouncing each other in strongly ideological terms during the presidential campaign of 2012.

ANALYZING IDEOLOGY IN A POLARIZED NATION

Polarization has increased in the United States during recent decades as the Democratic Party has become more liberal and the Republican Party has moved further to the right due to several factors. Many congressional districts have been revised by states so that they contain fewer moderates and more people who affiliate themselves with the Democratic or Republican Party. As Republican strategists have successfully brought evangelical voters into their party from the early 1980s onward, it has incorporated their views on many social issues, such as abortion, contraception, and gay marriage. When many conservative Southerners migrated to the Republican Party from the Democratic Party from the mid- 1960s through the 1980s, they made it more conservative and the Democratic Party more liberal. Polarization is reflected in radio and television talk shows when conservative commentators, such as Rush Limbaugh, clash with liberal commentators, such as Rachel Maddow on MSNBC. It is also reflected by gridlock in Congress.

At least four ideologies currently dominate political discourse in the United States. Democrats have mostly rallied behind *liberal* ideology and Republicans behind *conservative* ideology. Far smaller groups favor *libertarianism*, as explicated by Republican congressman Ron Paul, and *radicalism*, promoted by members of the Occupy Movement that began on Wall Street and spread to other cities in the fall of 2011 and into 2012. We now discuss how these ideologies influence people's sense of what is right and wrong.

Divergent Core Values

Conservatives prioritize such values as freedom (or liberty), localism in social policy, and individualism. They want to reward people who are successful by minimizing their taxes and providing them with tax incentives, such as low taxes on capital gains and stock dividends. Libertarians rally around liberty and individualism. They want minimal taxes on all citizens, contending that this would be possible if the functions of government were drastically reduced. Liberals want liberty to be tempered by many social programs and progressive taxation that promotes greater equality than conservatives favor. They favor considerable roles for federal and state governments in repairing infrastructure, funding public schools, funding entitlements, and funding social programs. They want affluent Americans to pay higher taxes than they currently do. Radicals place greater emphasis on equality and social justice than conservatives, libertarians, or liberals. The Occupy Movement wanted much higher taxes on affluent Americans as well as tighter regulations on banks and corporations.

What We Believe the Social Problems Are

Social problems are human constructs. People perceive specific actions or behaviors in the external world, or specific conditions such as poverty. They attach positive, neutral, or negative meanings to these actions, behaviors, or conditions. They describe them as social problems if they believe they have negative repercussions for people who possess or exhibit them, for their families or friends, for their communities, or for the broader society—or if they violate social norms.

Conservatives are less likely than liberals and radicals to believe that inequality is a serious problem, often believing that successful individuals should be financially rewarded and less affluent individuals should be encouraged to work harder. They are less likely to want to commit resources to social programs. They are more likely to emphasize social issues like restricting abortion, gay marriage, and use of marijuana. Libertarians want to curtail government, not only opposing a substantial domestic government agenda but also advocating cutting taxes. They want government to refrain from shaping lifestyle choices such as use of drugs.

Liberals have provided the impetus for enactment of many American social programs and civil rights measures in the New Deal, the Great Society, and the presidency of Barack Obama. Radicals favor major redistribution of resources from wealthy and powerful interests to people currently in the lower and middle classes.

Beliefs About Levels of Government

Conservatives favor diminution of federal power, preferring to transfer many federal policy roles to state and local governments. They want to increase the role of private charity in American society while reducing public expenditures markedly. Libertarians wish to reduce the role of federal, state, and local governments even further. They want the federal government to focus on providing necessary *domestic* defense while drastically curtailing military spending for wars abroad. Liberals favor far greater spending by the federal government than conservatives or libertarians. Radicals favor spending and tax policies that will markedly decrease economic inequality.

Beliefs About Private Markets and Regulation of Corporations

Conservatives believe private markets weed out inefficient businesses while rewarding other ones. They often oppose regulation of corporations, such as the Dodd-Frank banking regulations enacted by President Obama. Libertarians also believe that private markets produce positive results if government leaves them alone. American liberals view private markets favorably but want them to be regulated to prevent them from providing low wages, harsh working conditions, and toxic waste. They strongly favor the Dodd-Frank banking regulations, environmental regulations, and work safety protections. They often favor increasing the power of trade unions. Radicals believe corporate officials often enhance profits at the expense of workers and the public. They criticize the undue power of corporate lobbyists in federal and state capitols. They believe existing regulations of business are too lenient.

Views of the Safety Net and Human Nature

Conservatives often believe that low-income people "game" safety-net programs, such as Temporary Assistance for Needy Families (TANF), the Supplemental Nutrition Assistance Program (SNAP), and Section 8 housing subsidies, when they do not truly need them. They often favor cutting the level of benefits these programs provide and placing restrictions on their use. They favor placing safety-net programs under the control of local and state governments while minimizing or ending federal oversight and funding. Libertarians, too, believe that many people illicitly seek benefits and that benefits deter them from working hard. Liberals favor most safety-net programs. They agree that some fraudulent use occurs, but believe most recipients are honest and seek assistance for genuine problems, such as poverty, lack of sufficient food for themselves and their children, inability to afford housing costs, and inability to obtain or afford health insurance. They often want to increase benefits and services provided by social programs. They favor retention of entitlement status for Medicaid and SNAP so that their funding automatically increases annually to the level of claimed benefits rather than requiring them to compete for resources in annual budget battles in local, state, and federal governments. Radicals want safety-net and entitlement programs to be expanded. These expansions would be funded, they contend, by marked increases in taxes on affluent Americans and on corporations.

POLICY ADVOCACY LEARNING CHALLENGE 2.2

Take any important social issue in contemporary America. Discuss how conservatives, libertarians, liberals, and radicals would differ with respect to:

1. Whether it is an important issue
2. How it is caused
3. How it might be addressed or resolved

What strengths and weaknesses do you believe exist in each of these perspectives? Do the views of any of these groups appear to conflict with the NASW's Code of Ethics—and, if so, how?

Divisions Within Ideological Groups

Conservatives, liberals, and radicals often do not agree with members in their own groups. Moderate Republicans often want relatively more public spending, more government regulations, and less military spending than more conservative Republicans, even if their ranks have been greatly diminished in Congress. Jeb Bush, the former Republican governor of Florida and the brother of former President George W. Bush, "questioned the [Republican] party's approach to immigration, deficit reduction and partisanship, saying that his father, former President George Bush and [President] Reagan would struggle with 'an orthodoxy that doesn't allow for disagreement'" (Rutenberg, 2012). Conservatives drawn from fundamentalist churches often prioritize social issues such as contraception, abortion, and gay marriage more than other conservatives, such as Presidents Ronald Reagan and George H. W. Bush.

Some Democrats are more conservative than others, such as so-called Blue Dog Democrats in the House of Representatives who often pull rank and vote with Republicans in Congress on issues of social spending, bank regulations, and healthcare programs.

Radicals often differ from one another, as evidenced by internal struggles within the Occupy Movement about policies and strategy (Eckholm, 2012).

Forty percent of voters considered themselves to be "independent" in 2012—although most of them leaned toward a specific party—leaving about 10% to 15% of voters to decide the outcome of the presidential election of 2012 when they veered toward contender Barack Obama and away from Mitt Romney (Lauter, 2012).

SEEKING COMMON GROUND WITHOUT ABDICATING THE CODE OF ETHICS

Here are some rules that may often help us to have respectful dialogue in academic and other settings in a polarized nation, yet not concede values expressed in the Ethical Code of NASW.

- *Guideline 1.* Acknowledge that some policy issues are complex in nature, since they involve ethical and scientific dimensions, so they do not lend themselves to consensus, even among reasonable people who share the same ideology, much less among people who have conflicting ideologies.
- *Guideline 2.* Identify commonalities if they can be found, such as goals like reducing poverty, improving health, cutting the rate of suicide, and cutting healthcare costs.
- *Guideline 3.* Don't "write off" specific solutions, but listen respectfully to those that participants identify.
- *Guideline 4.* Identify specific research information about the effectiveness, cost, and other likely outcomes of specific remedies to the problem at stake.

Discuss whether this information is accurate by identifying who produced it and with what research methodology. Discuss whether researchers agree about the likely outcomes of specific remedies. Acknowledge flaws in existing research to the extent that they exist. When existing data are insufficient, state why a specific solution appears more meritorious than others based on human behavior or other theory.

- *Guideline 5.* Engage in respectful debate that does not negatively characterize opponents' personal character, morality, or intentions, but rather focuses on specific problems, possible solutions, ethical issues associated with specific solutions, and research information about the cost and effectiveness of the solutions.
- *Guideline 6.* Ascertain if compromises are possible that "split differences" between contending factions, even if this often requires considerable time.
- *Guideline 7.* Do not assume that policy advocacy is not feasible because different people have different values and points of view. By withdrawing from policy arenas, you increase the likelihood that opposing groups will prevail.
- *Guideline 8.* Do not violate the NASW's Code of Ethics by conceding its key points to people who do not honor its provisions. Conflict is often necessary when others hold views that violate the Code of Ethics. As a social worker in training, you are obliged to support the rights, opportunities, benefits, and services that enhance the well-being of vulnerable populations.

IDENTIFYING "VULNERABLE POPULATIONS" IN THE CODE OF ETHICS

Recall that the NASW's Code of Ethics (see Chapter 1) not only identifies the existence of vulnerable populations, but also says,

> Social workers should act to expand choice and opportunity for all people, with special regard for vulnerable, disadvantaged, oppressed, and exploited people and groups. Social workers should act to prevent and eliminate domination of, exploitation of, and discrimination against any person, group, or class on the basis of race, ethnicity, national origin, color, sex, sexual orientation, age, marital status, political belief, religion, or mental or physical disability.

The Code also uses the adjectives "disadvantaged, oppressed and exploited" to describe vulnerable populations.

The Code's language could lead social workers to believe that people with different ideologies mostly acknowledge that these and other populations *are* vulnerable, as well as disadvantaged, oppressed, and exploited. These terms are not in the lexicon of many conservatives and libertarians, however, for reasons we have discussed. They often believe that virtually everyone can be successful if he or she works hard enough. In their view, many people suffer poverty and other problems *not* primarily because of external adverse factors, such as discrimination or other external factors, but because they possess personal shortcomings. Some conservatives do not like terms like "vulnerable populations" or adjectives like "disadvantaged," "oppressed," and "exploited."

An exploration of American history reveals that conservatives have often opposed, or sought to cut, domestic policies to help vulnerable populations. Ronald Reagan and former president George H. W. Bush, Sr. opposed the Civil Rights Acts of 1964 and 1965. Many conservatives have opposed civil rights legislation for women, gays and lesbians, immigrants, poor people, and other populations during the past 50 years, and many are still doing so. These policies led substantial majorities of voting members of some vulnerable populations, including women, African Americans, Latino/as, Asian Americans, Native Americans, low-income people, and gays and lesbians, to vote for Democrats in the presidential elections of 2008 and 2012.

We need to be careful, however, not to stereotype Democrats or Republicans excessively. Democrats have sometimes taken positions that were harmful to specific vulnerable populations, such as President Bill Clinton's support for the policy of "don't ask, don't tell" for gay personnel in the military. Republicans have supported rights for specific vulnerable populations, such as President George H. W. Bush's support of the Americans with Disabilities Act of 1990 that required corporations and units of government to honor the rights of disabled individuals. Some Republicans and Democrats, including President George Bush, Republican senator John McCain, and Democratic senator Ted Kennedy, supported comprehensive immigration reform in 2007 and 2008 that was defeated in Congress.

IDENTIFYING 16 VULNERABLE POPULATIONS

To merit the term *vulnerable* a population must be subject to or experience the following:

- Considerable discrimination in interpersonal relationships, families, and communities
- Considerable exposure to verbal and/or physical assaults
- Considerable denial of opportunities in education and employment
- Considerable economic deprivation

- Health and mental health deficits, including low self-esteem, that partly stem from their marginalized condition
- Considerable opposition to programs and policies meant to improve its economic status and legal status

The population must have been subjected to or experienced these events or health or mental health deficits over an extended historical period so that prejudice, discrimination, and other indicators of vulnerability are deeply embedded in culture, social relationships, and the economic system. At least 17 populations qualify as vulnerable ones using these criteria, including:

- *African Americans, Latino/as, Asian Americans, and Native Americans*, who have been subjected not only to overt racism in personal interactions with employers, teachers, physicians, the police, and people in other professions, but also to policy discrimination as reflected in schools, training programs, housing, and community amenities that give poorer services or fewer resources to members of these groups than they give to Caucasian populations. Latino/as, African Americans, and Native Americans have been subjected to harsher sentences that whites in the criminal justice system.
- *Women, older people, and people with disabilities*, who are often expected to assume relatively dependent roles in society, either in places of employment or in the broader society. They are often denied access to certain kinds of jobs, to promotions, and to roles within decision-making bodies because of widespread belief that they are incapable of moving beyond residual or lower-level roles within society. Women have additional burdens stemming from efforts to control their reproductive choices, such as whether to have an abortion or even to have access to contraception.
- *Children*, who must often rely on society for basic amenities, such as financial assistance, health care, dental care, and adequate housing, but are often given inadequate governmental support because they lack political clout.
- *LGBTQQ people, criminal offenders, homeless people, and juvenile delinquents*, who are subject to discrimination because they are widely viewed as violating important social norms, such as sexual norms and social norms.
- *Jewish Americans, some Asian Americans, and some white ethnic Americans* are denied resources and services because many Americans believe they have no or few social problems.
- *Low-income groups*, who often lack sufficient resources, well-paying employment, or stable employment. Lack of resources, in turn, precludes them from some life options that are available to more affluent individuals, such as safe neighborhoods, adequate housing, and economic security.

- *Veterans* often suffer discrimination in employment and have a combination of problems in the wake of their military service—including mental and physical trauma, low income, homelessness, and family violence.

Many members of vulnerable populations are able to contend with the social and economic barriers that they confront. They create advocacy groups. They develop political organizations that marshal support for public officials who enact policies that address their economic, legal, and social needs. They develop self-help organizations that allow them to share economic resources.

Many individuals are members of two or more of these vulnerable populations. Consider, for example, African Americans who are disabled due to their participation in the Vietnam War, people with mental illness in each of the vulnerable populations, and female heads of households who live under federal poverty levels. People with membership in multiple vulnerable populations often confront greater barriers or challenges than people with membership in only one of them.

Each vulnerable population possesses many subgroups. Members of these subgroups may have different views and positions on many issues. Racial populations contain relatively affluent, middle-class, working-class, and low-income subgroups. They may live in different communities, such as low-income African Americans who live in inner-city areas as compared to affluent African Americans who live in suburban areas. Émigrés from Vietnam, Cambodia, and Thailand in the 1970s and 1980s are, on average, less affluent than Asian Americans whose ancestors emigrated from Japan. People with criminal records include those who have committed homicides and people who have committed so-called white-collar crimes. Disabled individuals include those with physical disabilities and those with mental disabilities.

Intermarriage has somewhat blurred distinctions between white, African American, Latino/a, Native American, and Asian populations. A leading analyst of this trend, Richard Rodriguez (2002), argues, "All things brown in time." He disputes the concept that Latino/as are a racial group, noting that "there are many cultures in Latin America" as well as many variations in physical characteristics such as skin color. He notes the emergence of new terms, such as "Blexicans" to describe people of Latino and African American descent and "Hinjews" for people of East Indian and Jewish descent. He predicts that the U.S. Census will soon not even use racial categories, as more and more people find them to be inapplicable.

Rodriguez's argument may be ahead of its time, however, because many people still describe themselves as belonging to a specific racial group, live in areas and attend schools dominated by it, are perceived by others as coming from it, and experience discrimination in employment and other places based on it. Nor has the time come to declare that people of color have merged into the general population with respect to their income, employment, and education, even though many of them have made extraordinary gains in recent decades, as evidenced by a growing middle and upper class in Latino/a and African American populations.

Members of subgroups sometimes find it difficult to work together to change policies. Women of color sometimes conflicted with white women during the women's movement in the 1970s. Affluent Latino/as and African Americans may not relate to economic and social barriers confronted by low-income members of their groups—or to one another.

POLICY ADVOCACY LEARNING CHALLENGE 2.3

Identifying Subgroups Within Vulnerable Populations

Take any of the 16 vulnerable populations. Identify several subgroups within one of them. What kinds of social policies are needed by each of them? Do tensions exist between the subgroups that make it difficult for them to work together to achieve reforms?

Each of the vulnerable populations is represented in political venues by advocacy groups, such as the National Association of Colored Persons (NAACP) for African Americans, the Mexican American Legal Defense Fund (MALDEF) for Latino/as, the National Organization for Women (NOW), the National Alliance on Mental Illness (NAMI), the Children's Defense Fund (CDF), and the Center for Budget and Policy Priorities (CBPP) for low- and moderate-income individuals.

Locate additional advocacy groups that work to improve policies for specific vulnerable populations on the Internet.

ANALYZING THE OPPRESSION OF WOMEN IN THE CONTEMPORARY PERIOD

Each of the groups that we have described as "vulnerable" has experienced a long history of discrimination in the United States. Examine, for instance, five incidents in contemporary America related to women:

1. *Incident 1.* The Komen Foundation, a widely respected organization that funds breast cancer awareness, treatment, and research, had given grants to Planned Parenthood for its cancer testing for many years, but abruptly announced it would stop funding it in the spring of 2012. A massive protest ensued as women used Facebook and other social media to attack this decision. Some protesters alleged that the foundation had been influenced by evangelicals to protest the

contraception and abortion services of Planned Parenthood. The Komen Foundation apologized for cutting off Planned Parenthood and resumed its grants to the organization. The foundation became embroiled in internal conflicts, however, as three top executives resigned amid reports that Catholic bishops had pressured Komen to rescind the grant and Komen's local affiliates in Texas, Arizona, and Louisiana reported shortfalls in fundraising campaigns.

2. *Incident 2.* Catholic bishops protested the inclusion of mandatory coverage of women's contraception services in the Affordable Care Act—legislation that mandated that insurance companies fund specific preventive services found by researchers to be effective. They contended that the government infringed on the separation of church and state by requiring Catholic hospitals and universities to fund contraception when it violated Catholics' religious views. President Obama forged a compromise that held that private health insurance used by these hospitals and universities should fund contraceptive services—not the Catholic institutions themselves. When Republicans sided with the bishops, Democrats charged that Republicans opposed funding of contraception due to their insensitivity to women's health needs.

3. *Incident 3.* Democrats invited Sandra Fluke, a Georgetown University law student, to testify before a House subcommittee in favor of the government mandate to fund women's contraceptive services. When the Republican leadership refused to allow her to testify, Democrats invited her to testify before a group of Democratic representatives, where she contended that contraception is a women's health issue that should be funded by private health insurance or by government programs like Medicaid for several reasons. Many low-income women cannot afford physician visits and pills or other contraceptive devices. Many women need contraception for health reasons, such as the timing of having children or for medical reasons that would make pregnancy harmful at particular points in their lives. Rush Limbaugh, the outspoken Republican radio commentator, entered the fray by contending over the next five days that female birth control is tantamount to to promiscuity and sex for hire—and calling Fluke a "slut" and a "prostitute" and asking her to provide the public with a videotape of herself engaging in sexual relations, since the public would pay for her contraceptives through their health insurance premiums. Some Republicans condemned his language, but Mitt Romney, the front-runner for the Republican presidential nomination, remained silent. President Obama telephoned Fluke to congratulate her for stating her opinions in a public venue.

4. *Incident 4.* The U.S. Senate began proceedings in the spring of 2012 to reauthorize the Violence Against Women Act that Congress had enacted in

1994—legislation that provides funds for police departments and agencies to aid victims of domestic violence and to prosecute domestic violence offenders. It had been reauthorized with bipartisan support on prior occasions, but conservative senators announced their opposition on grounds that the legislation would be expanded to include Indian tribes, rural areas, and same-sex couples. It would also allow more battered illegal immigrants to obtain temporary visas, expand the definition of definition of violence against women to include stalking, and train court personnel to help families with domestic violence. Many Republicans contended that Democratic senators used the issue to entice women to vote for Democrats in the congressional and presidential elections of 2012. Democratic senators retorted, "Republican opposition falls into a larger picture of insensitivity toward women that has progressed from abortion rights to contraception to preventive health care coverage—and now to domestic violence." Republican senator Li Murkowski from Alaska warned her Republican colleagues that their party risked being successfully portrayed as anti-woman by Democrats (Swers, 2012). The Violence Against Women Act was eventually enacted in 2013, possibly because some Republicans changed their minds when they saw that women had voted for President Obama in the presidential election of 2012 by a large margin.

5. *Incident 5.* Two Republican senators opposed restrictions on abortion that outraged many members of both political parties during the presidential election of 2012. Senator Todd Aiken (R.-Mo.) contended that only women who had been subjected to "legitimate rape" needed help in preventing or terminating pregnancy. Senator Richard Mourdock (R.-Ind.) argued that women do not need help in terminating pregnancies when they have been raped because their bodies reject sperm under these circumstances. Partly because of these statements, Democrats won both of these senatorial races and retained control of the U.S. Senate.

POLICY ADVOCACY LEARNING CHALLENGE 2.4

Are Women a Vulnerable Population?

Take the criteria that we listed earlier in this chapter that allow us to describe specific populations as vulnerable. Using materials from this historical overview, as well as additional information you possess, answer these questions:

- Are women a vulnerable population?
- Are specific subgroups within the overall population of women *particularly* vulnerable—and, if so, which ones?

- Is *any* subgroup of the overall population of women *not* vulnerable? If so, why?
- Has the United States made progress addressing causes of women's vulnerability in the last 50 years?
- Do the five 2012 incidents in the historical overview above suggest that progress has been uneven?
- Are Republicans generally more insensitive to women's issues and needs than Democrats? If so, why?
- Take another vulnerable population, such as African Americans, Native Americans, Latino/as, immigrants, Asian Americans, or LGBT persons. Can you identify recent incidents that illustrate policies and incidents that reflect how the broader society marginalizes them?

We also know that members of vulnerable populations are subjected to negative stereotypes that can negatively impact them in their jobs, in their schools, and in their communities. Take the example of Jeremy Lim, an Asian American graduate of Harvard University who suddenly became a star for the New York Knicks in the National Basketball Association before continuing his career with the Houston Rockets. Reporters and spectators worked hard to come up with derogatory phrases. A CNN reporter was fired for writing this headline: "Chink in Armor."

POLICY ADVOCACY LEARNING CHALLENGE 2.5

Confronting Negative Stereotypes and Myths

1. As an exercise, consider the 16 vulnerable populations. Imagine yourself as a member of one of the populations of which you are not a member. Imagine yourself applying for a job. Ask what stereotypes an employer might possess about you that would lead him or her to refrain from hiring you for a relatively high-level position. For example, veterans returning from Iraq and Afghanistan *often* confront assumptions that they have brain trauma and mental problems that would make them inferior employees.
2. Locate research or other materials that *refute* the stereotype. For example, find research or evidence that veterans who return from Iraq and Afghanistan are often high-performing employees.

UNDERSTANDING WHY SOCIAL POLICIES ARE NEEDED FOR EVERYONE AND FOR VULNERABLE POPULATIONS

Our discussion of vulnerable populations raises two broader issues: Why do people in the broader society need social policies, and why do members of vulnerable populations particularly need them?

Imagine American society—or any society—with virtually no social programs, regulations, or civil rights. Let's make several assumptions about this imaginary society. Assume that its economy is organized in a capitalist fashion where its citizens work in corporate or other business settings—and where people are expected to meet their needs through wages, investments, and savings. Also assume that all who live in this society are expected to purchase their medical care, their housing, their education, and their social services with personal assets. Assume, as well, that no civil rights laws exist to protect specific groups or individuals that might be subject to violent acts, discrimination in places of work, or other forms of discrimination in schools, communities, medical services, commerce, or social services. Assume, as well, that people purchase their own cars as their principle means of transportation. Assume that they fund their retirements exclusively from their savings. Also assume that this imaginary society possesses no regulations over businesses, landlords, drug companies, or medical providers. Nor does the society possess police, fire, and public health programs.

Life in such an imaginary society would be uncertain and difficult. Minus a police force, people would be subject to violent acts and theft. Minus fire departments, their homes and businesses would be threatened as small fires became conflagrations. Minus public health departments to regulate restaurants and markets, sewage disposal, and refuse—as well as inoculate people against diseases—communities would encounter devastating epidemics. If government did not build and maintain roads, bridges, and airports, people could not travel to work or other destinations. Minus any public transportation, the nation would experience gridlock on those roads that did exist. People lacking the resources to purchase cars would be mostly unable to work if no system of public transportation existed—or to get to health facilities, grocery stores, drug stores, and other destinations essential to their well-being.

Even if we gave government some minimal police, fire, and public health functions—and allowed it to construct highways, bridges, and other physical amenities—life would still be brutish and uncertain for many people. With no minimum-wage requirements, employers could pay employees whatever the market would bear regardless of the impact on workers, such as wages comparable to those in developing nations, for example, $2.50 per hour. Workers would find it difficult to form trade unions to pressure employers to raise their wages because employers could fire or otherwise intimidate union organizers, as occurred prior to enactment of the Wagner Act in 1936 that required secret elections to determine if workers wanted to join a union. If the United States currently possesses tens of millions of people who subsist under or near official poverty lines because minimum-wage jobs pay them at such low levels, imagine how many more individuals would face this economic crunch if government had *no* minimum wage. The plight of workers would be made harsher, moreover, because government—under our minimalist assumption—would not require or help to fund some fringe benefits that many workers currently receive. Many American corporations currently fund their employees' health insurance because they receive huge tax incentives from the federal government to do so—incentives that do not exist in our imaginary society. Nor would employers provide workers' compensation to fund healthcare for workers who were injured at work. Not required to heed work safety requirements currently established by the Occupational Safety and Health Administration (OSHA) or similar agencies in many states, many employers would *not* purchase machines with safety features, *not* reduce pollution at the work site, and *not* curtail workers' exposure to toxic chemicals—omissions that would endanger the lives of many employees through death or illness. With no regulations prohibiting the use of child labor, many employers would hire children even for physically taxing work. Not prohibited from making employees work long hours, some employers would fire workers who were unwilling to work as much as 14 hours per day. Imagine, too, how uncertain people's lives would be if no safety-net programs existed such as those that currently provide food, healthcare, housing, preschool education, income, and other basic needs to tens of millions of Americans. Many Americans cannot currently purchase these necessities because they have lost their work due to downsizing or recessions, possess injuries and poor health, are unable to find work, or receive extraordinarily low wages. We can surmise that many people would have had to resort to begging or theft to survive in our imaginary society had they encountered the Great Recession from 2007 to 2009 and beyond.

Life would be difficult, too, for tens of millions of retirees. Roughly half of people who reach age 65 do not own their own homes and lack significant savings—and many of them have significant credit card debt. Unable to afford rent, many of them would be forced to live on the streets unless relatives or charities came to their assistance.

All persons in the United States benefit from social policies, but the vulnerable need policies to help them meet their basic human needs and protect their rights.

POLICY ADVOCACY LEARNING CHALLENGE 2.6

Identifying Policies to Help Vulnerable Populations

As an exercise, take any of the following statements and ask yourself what kinds of policies would be helpful to the specific vulnerable population mentioned.

Poverty

The American poverty rate was 12.67% in 2006—or almost 1 percentage point higher than in 2001. It rose to 15.1% by 2010—the highest level since 1992.

Homelessness

About 744,000 people are homeless on any given night in the U.S.—and between 2.5 million and 3.5 million people experience homelessness over the course of a year.

Lack of Medical Insurance

The number of Americans who lack health insurance rose to 47 million in 2006—or 15.8% of the population. Included in this number are 8.7 million children—or 11.7% of all children.

Failed Transitions From Foster Care

About 20,000 of the nation's 500,000 foster children "graduate" from foster care each year at age 18—only to encounter a difficult transition into life in the community. About 30% of America's homeless people were once in foster care.

Lack of Reentry Help

Seventy percent of the 650,000 people released annually from state and federal prisons will commit new crimes within three years. The vast majority of them receive no reentry help before they leave prison.

Low Wages

About one in five (or 41 million) people fall into a "hardship gap" where their earnings, when combined with work benefits (such as health insurance and child care), together with assistance from programs such as SNAP and the Earned Income Tax Credit, do *not* meet their basic needs. (See Albelda & Boushey, 2007.)

Feminization of Poverty

If the poverty rate for all women 18 years and older was 12.7% in 2004, the poverty rate for women in households with no spouse present was 24.8%. Many of these female heads of household hold two or more jobs and still cannot reach, or barely reach, above-poverty levels.

Economic Victimization of Immigrants

More than 55 million immigrants have settled in the United States since its founding, yet every wave of immigrants has encountered hostility. The roughly 12 million undocumented immigrants in the United States are no exception. American corporations, food growers and processors, contractors, restaurants, and hotels depend on their labor, yet Americans grant them few rights. Congress has repeatedly failed to enact legislation to clarify their rights, most recently in 2007. Immigrants work for minimum wage—and, in some cases, even less when employers' reimbursement of them is not monitored by the Department of Labor. Many immigrants do not even receive some or all of their pay when fraudulent employers believe they will not dare to go to authorities for fear of being deported.

Lack of Upward Mobility

Americans have prided themselves on the ability of low-income people to be upwardly mobile. Generations of Americans have contended that people have only to work hard to enter the middle or even upper reaches of their society. Has not this been the script for tens of millions of Americans from the colonial period onward? Have not many of the great corporate leaders—including most recently Steve Jobs— become highly successful entrepreneurs? This American dream has recently been tarnished by five large studies in recent years that have revealed that the United States has lower rates of mobility than some European nations and Canada (DeParle, 2012). One research project discovered that 42% of males raised in the bottom fifth of incomes stayed there as adults, compared to only 25% in Denmark and 30% in Britain. Research by the Pew Charitable Trusts found that 62% of males and females raised in the top fifth of incomes *stay* in the top two fifths—and 65% born in the bottom fifth stay in the bottom two fifths. Another study found that 22% of Americans raised in the bottom tenth of the income distribution stay there as adults, compared with only 16% of Canadians (DeParle, 2012).

On a more positive note, researchers discovered more mobility by individuals raised in the middle fifth of the income distribution as compared to the highly "sticky" top and bottom rungs, where people tend to stay where they are raised.

Tensions between the rich and poor were also increasing in 2011 and 2012. A Pew Research Center study found that "conflict between rich and poor now eclipses racial strain and friction between immigrants and the native-born as the greatest source of tension in American society" (Morin, 2012). Two thirds of Americans (or a larger number than in any poll since 1992) believe there are "strong conflicts between rich

(Continued)

(Continued)

and poor in the United States" (Tavernise, 2012) This belief is common among independents (68%), Democrats (73%), and persons earning from $40,000 to $75,000 annually (71%). When polled in 2009, only 47% of the last group had held this belief (Tavernise, 2012).

Criminalizing Poor People on the Street

According to the National Law Center on Homelessness and Poverty (n.d.), many jurisdictions enacted ordinances that criminalized poor people during the Great Recession of 2007 to 2009 and beyond. These ordinances included bans on begging; restrictions on lying, sitting, or sleeping on sidewalks or loitering in the streets; and authorizations to raid shelters at night to find men with outstanding warrants. Some cities made it a crime to share food with people in public places, even as a federal judge declared it to be unconstitutional in Orlando, Florida (Ehrenreich, 2009).

Different Police Standards for People of Color

An incident in 2012 reminded Congressman John Lewis, an African American leader in the civil rights movement, of the racial violence of the 1950s and 1960s. Trayvon Martin, a high school student in Sanford, Florida, was shot to death on February 26, 2012, by George Zimmerman, a white person who served as a neighborhood watch captain. Zimmerman had called 911 to report a suspicious person—and had been told by police not to follow Martin, but to leave the matter to local police, who would soon arrive. Zimmerman followed Martin. Zimmerman claimed he was attacked by Martin, who bloodied his nose, threw him to the ground, and beat him. Zimmerman says he opened fire on the unarmed Martin for self-defense, as allowed under a Florida statute called "Stand your ground." Local police did not question him at the scene, collect evidence, take photographs, or even ask him what happened. They did not take him into custody as a suspect in a homicide, so he remained free a month later. They took no steps to establish the identity of the slain teenager—not even calling numbers on his cell phone—so his parents did not learn he had died for three days. The case became national as the press came to learn these details. African Americans protested across the nation that Zimmerman had not been arrested pending trial. They doubted that local police would investigate the case fairly because they had not investigated cases of homicides against other black youth in the area in recent years. Many people wondered if the police would have taken a different course of action and launched a more thorough investigation if the alleged murderer had been an African American and the victim a white person. The decision by a jury to acquit Zimmerman during summer 2013 appeared to justify the fears of many people and brought renewed energy to the movement to repeal "Stand your ground" statutes in Florida and elsewhere.

No Restrictions on the Interrogation of Immigrants

Immigration statutes enacted in various states in 2010, 2011, and 2012 gave police the right to detain and interrogate anyone who they believed *might* be an undocumented person. These statutes gave no criterion that police would use in making this determination. Would not this legislation greatly increase the apprehension of Latino/as, including citizens?

Restriction of Black Voting

Conservatives launched an ambitious effort to cut the voting rates of low-income individuals (who were likely to vote for Democratic candidates) in many jurisdictions in 2011 and 2012. They enacted state ordinances to require voters to show identification photographs at polls as a requirement for voting. They knew that this seemingly innocuous policy would reduce voting rates in low-income areas because considerable numbers of low-income people do not have documents with photographs. Many of them do not have licenses because they do not own cars or passports. Conservatives claimed that the measure would cut voter fraud, but they lacked evidence that fraud was a significant problem in the United States. Enactment of laws to restrict voting continued into 2013 and 2014 in the wake of a ruling by the U.S. Supreme Court that they did not violate the federal Voting Rights Act.

DECIDING WHEN TO INITIATE POLICY ADVOCACY

We have argued that social workers' Code of Ethics requires them to engage in policy advocacy. They must decide whether to initiate micro, mezzo, or macro policy advocacy *in specific situations.*

Let's recall that we define micro policy advocacy as helping clients obtain services, rights, and benefits that they would (likely) not otherwise receive and that would advance their well-being. Micro policy advocacy is provided to clients and can include referrals, provided that social workers ascertain that their clients actually received assistance from the person or agency to which they were referred. We defined mezzo policy advocacy as seeking to change dysfunctional policies in institutions and communities that may create the need for micro policy advocacy in the first place. We used the same definition for macro policy advocacy, except that it is directed at policies at the governmental level.

Social workers must decide at the outset whether the well-being of specific clients is threatened at a sufficient level to warrant micro policy advocacy—and whether specific policies are sufficiently dysfunctional to warrant mezzo or macro policy advocacy. They make this decision by considering ethical first-order principles and evidence-based research.

Using Ethical First-Order Principles

Social workers engage in policy advocacy when specific clients (micro policy advocacy) and groups of clients (mezzo and macro policy advocacy) find their ethical rights violated. A social worker who engages in micro policy advocacy can assert that a patient has not been given sufficient information about available medical options to treat her condition—a violation of *self-determination.* Or she can assert that this patient has been given lesser or different services than a male patient with a similar condition—a violation of *fairness.* Or she can assert that the patient's medical information has become known to others without the patient's consent—a violation of *confidentiality.* Or she can assert that she has not been given accurate information, such as possible side effects or other complications that might ensue from a particular treatment—a violation of *honesty.* Social workers can assert that certain policies violate the principle of *social justice* when a person receives no or poor services because she or he is a member of a vulnerable population.

A social worker might initiate advocacy at the organizational, community, or government levels when she believes that one or more existing policies violate these ethical principles with respect to specific groups or vulnerable populations. Advocates have initiated innumerable projects at the mezzo and macro levels to enhance the civil rights of many vulnerable populations during recent decades, including for African Americans, Asian Americans, Latino/as, Native Americans, women, and people with mental and substance abuse problems in local jurisdictions, states, and the federal government.

Using Evidence-Based Research

Social workers use evidence-based research to decide whether to provide *micro policy advocacy* to specific clients who do not receive specific benefits, services, opportunities, and rights. Assume, for example, that a woman who is released from prison for minor drug infractions fails to receive any of the following services or benefits: job training, counseling, help to surmount substance abuse, childcare, SNAP, or Medicaid. A social worker might engage in micro policy advocacy to help this woman obtain one or more of these services or benefits when she discovers that specific research findings suggest that her well-being *will be* improved. She might find research that specifically examines the impact of services and benefits on released female prisoners. She might also rely on research that discusses how these benefits, services, rights, and opportunities improve the well-being of broader vulnerable populations, including released prisoners, women, low-income populations, and people with substance abuse.

Social workers can also use evidence-based research when deciding whether to provide *mezzo or macro policy advocacy.* Assume that the social worker discovers research that shows that released prisoners (male and female) are more likely to gain employment if they are not required to divulge that they have been imprisoned for a nonviolent offense. The social worker would then determine who has the policy authority to require these women to divulge their imprisonment in a specific local jurisdiction or state—and then engage in mezzo policy advocacy if the authority is vested in a municipal or county agency, or macro policy advocacy if it is vested in a state agency or legislature.

When evidence-based research does not exist or does not focus on a specific population, such as released female prisoners with relatively minor drug offenses, social workers can engage in policy advocacy if it is reasonable to assume that specific clients or populations *will* benefit from access to specific services, benefits, opportunities, and rights. Perhaps they will find qualitative research findings, such as from fellow social workers who have observed positive results for their clients when they receive access to these benefits. Perhaps they will observe positive results for *other* kinds of clients or populations who have received them.

Specific policies may help specific clients or populations, but be so costly that they are not economically feasible to implement. Assume, for example, that a substance abuse program has been shown to be effective, but only at a cost of $30,000 per enrollee—a cost that may exceed likely funding from public sources. A social worker might seek a less costly alternative that demonstrates considerable success.

Pragmatic Considerations

It takes time and effort to engage in advocacy at the micro, mezzo, and macro levels. Social workers have to triage specific clients to ascertain if they suffer sufficient harm to warrant engagement in micro policy advocacy. They have to triage specific policies to decide whether they are sufficiently dysfunctional and harmful to groups or populations to warrant engagement in mezzo and macro policy advocacy.

They must sometimes gauge the difficulty of obtaining policy successes by obtaining information with knowledgeable persons. It may be impossible to enroll a specific client in a needed program, for example, if it is already oversubscribed due to lack of sufficient funding. Some policies in mezzo and macro venues may be difficult to change because they are supported by powerful interest groups.

It is important not to rationalize *not* engaging in advocacy, however, when important ethical or evidence-based research suggest that clients will otherwise suffer serious harm. Social workers can sometimes find allies who can assist them or through whom they can work, such as existing advocacy organizations that are identified in each of the eight policy sectors addressed in Chapters 7 through 14.

Social workers' decisions about whether and when to engage in policy advocacy are powerfully shaped by the organizational context in which they work. Social workers are probably more likely to engage in advocacy in organizations that have a culture of teamwork; in which they are encouraged and expected, by their peers, supervisors, and higher administrators, to provide advocacy; in which they experience a shared ethical commitment to advocacy; and in which they are given tangible support for providing advocacy in their job descriptions and expectations.

Social workers must sometimes be advocates *for* advocacy in their work settings to the extent that a shared commitment does not currently exist there. In Chapters 4, 5, and 6, we discuss how social workers can develop organizational supports for micro policy advocacy, mezzo policy advocacy, and macro policy advocacy

PUTTING IT ALL TOGETHER

In this chapter, we have discussed a pivotal decision that policy advocates must make: whether and when to engage in policy advocacy in the first place. The Code of Ethics of social workers, as well as the codes of ethics of nurses, physicians, and other helping professions, *requires* them to engage in advocacy but does not specify *when* they should initiate this intervention. We have argued that ethical first-order principles, evidence-based research, and pragmatic considerations shape whether and when we engage in micro, mezzo, and macro policy advocacy. We have discussed how social workers must sometimes be advocates *for* advocacy in their work settings.

LEARNING OUTCOMES

You are now equipped to:

- Identify foundational beliefs that shape people's views about social policy, including ideology, self-interest, and culture
- State basic beliefs of people with different ideologies
- Enumerate guidelines for attempting to reach common ground
- Identify how vulnerable populations are discussed in the NASW's Code of Ethics

- Define why certain populations are "vulnerable" and identify many vulnerable populations
- Analyze contemporary experiences of women to identify factors that make them a vulnerable population
- Identify many reasons why social policies are needed in American society
- Identify three factors that shape whether and when social workers engage in policy advocacy: ethical first-order principles, evidence-based research, and pragmatic considerations

REFERENCES

Albelda, R., & Boushey, H., with E. Chimienti, R. Ray, & B. Zipperer. (2007, October 10). *Bridging the gaps: A picture of how work supports* work *in ten states.* Retrieved November 11, 2014, from http://www.bridgingthegaps.org/publications/nationalreport.pdf

DeParle, J. (2012, January 4). Harder for Americans to rise from lower rungs. *New York Times.* Retrieved from http://www.nytimes.com/

Eckholm, E. (2012, February 11). Occupy Movement regroups, preparing for its next phase. *New York Times.* Retrieved from http://www.nytimes.com/

Ehrenreich, B. (2009, August 8). Is it now a crime to be poor? *New York Times.* Retrieved from http://www.nytimes.com

Lauter, D. (2012, March 15). The election's crucial wild card. *Los Angeles Times,* pp. A1, A12.

Morin, R. (2012). Rising share of Americans see conflict between rich and poor. *Pew Research Social and Demographic Trends.* Retrieved November 24, 2014, from www.pewsocialtrends.org

National Law Center on Homelessness and Poverty. (n.d.). *No safe place: The criminalization of homelessness in U.S. cities.* Retrieved November 24, 2014, from www.nichp.ort/reports

Pacific Yearly Meeting. (2001). *Faith and Practice* (pp. 52–53). Pasadena, CA: Author.

Rodgriguez, R. (2002). *Brown: The last discovery of America.* New York, NY: Viking.

Rutenberg, J. (2012, June 11). Jeb Bush questions G.O.P.'s shift to the right. *New York Times,* p. 1.

Swers, M. (2013). *Representing women's interests in a polarized congress.* In S. Thomas & C. Wilcox (Eds.) *Women and elective office: Past, present, and future.* (3rd ed.) New York: Oxford University Press, 176.

Tavernise, S. (2012, January 11). Survey finds rising perception of class tension. *New York Times.* Retrieved from http://www.nytimes.com/

Ware, S. (1985). Women and the New Deal. In Harvard Sitcoff, ed., *Fifty Years Later: The New Deal Evaluated.* Philadelphia, PA: Temple University Press.

Woloch, N. (1984). *Women and the American experience.* New York, NY: Knopf.

Chapter 3

Using a Policy Advocacy Framework

LEARNING OBJECTIVES

In this chapter, you will learn how to:

1. Use a multilevel policy advocacy framework (Figure 3.1)

2. Provide policy advocacy at three levels

3. Identify differences between policy advocacy and clinical counseling

4. Develop Red Flag Alerts in specific settings

5. Develop Red Flag Alerts at the three levels of policy advocacy

Policy advocacy is a *skilled* intervention, whether it takes place at the level of individuals (micro policy advocacy), at the level of organizations and communities (mezzo policy advocacy), or at the level of governments (macro policy advocacy). We discuss each level in this chapter. We discuss each of them in more depth in Chapters 4, 5, and 6, respectively. We illustrate each of them in the eight policy sector chapters.

USING A MULTILEVEL POLICY ADVOCACY FRAMEWORK

A multilevel policy advocacy framework is presented in Figure 3.1, which portrays micro, mezzo, and macro policy advocacy. Advocates at each of these levels:

- engage in eight challenges, which are portrayed around the outer edge of the circle
- contend with a policy context that sometimes assists them (assets) and sometimes provides roadblocks (constraints), which are portrayed outside the circle
- use political, interactional, value-clarifying, and analytic skills as they implement each of these eight tasks
- help people individually (micro policy advocacy) or collectively (mezzo policy advocacy and macro policy advocacy) surmount the seven core challenges discussed in Chapter 1, including by advocating for ethical rights, human rights, and economic justice; improving the quality of social programs; making social programs more culturally responsive; increasing preventive strategies to decrease social problems; improving access to social programs; increasing the scope and effectiveness of mental health programs; and making social programs more relevant to households

Figure 3.1   A multilevel policy advocacy framework

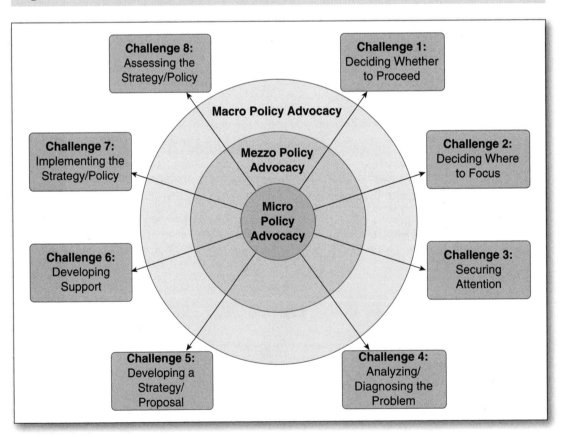

Advocates at the micro, mezzo, and macro levels undertake eight tasks, including determining whether to proceed (Challenge 1), determining where to focus (Challenge 2), obtaining recognition that a client has an unresolved problem from other staff in an agency (micro policy advocacy) or securing decision makers' attention for a policy issue or problem (mezzo or macro policy advocacy; Challenge 3), analyzing or diagnosing why a client has an unresolved problem (micro policy advocacy) or why a dysfunctional policy has developed (mezzo or macro policy advocacy; Challenge 4), developing a strategy to address a client's unresolved problem (micro policy advocacy) or a proposal to address a policy-related problem (mezzo or macro policy advocacy; Challenge 5), developing support for their strategy to resolve a client's unresolved problem (micro policy advocacy) or to enact a policy proposal (mezzo or macro policy advocacy; Challenge 6), implementing their strategy (micro policy advocacy) or their enacted proposal (mezzo or macro policy advocacy; Challenge 7), and assessing whether their implemented strategy (micro policy advocacy) or enacted policy has been effective (mezzo or macro policy advocacy; Challenge 8).

Advocates use four kinds of skills as they undertake these challenges—skills that we discuss in more detail in Chapters 4, 5, and 6:

- *Value-clarifying skills* to determine whether to initiate an advocacy intervention in the first place and to conduct their advocacy ethically, such as by not using deceptive or dishonest tactics whenever possible. They should empower individuals to be their own advocates whenever possible, while realizing that some people need some or considerable assistance.
- *Political or influential skills* to surmount the disinclination of specific individuals to agree with specific policy advocacy initiatives at the micro, mezzo, or macro level. Resistance to changes sought by advocates can be mild or intense, as illustrated by the opposition of many conservatives to President Obama's Affordable Care Act (ACA)—and subsequent attempts by many attorney generals to overturn portions of the legislation in 2010 and 2011, as well as involvement by the U.S. Supreme Court. Obama, in turn, countered with use of his own political skills.
- *Analytic skills* to analyze situations and issues to decide what remedies will improve the well-being of specific individuals, such as appealing the denial of eligibility to a program by a government official during micro policy advocacy, or developing policy proposals during mezzo and macro policy advocacy.
- *Interactional skills* to communicate effectively to persuade others to take specific actions. Advocates must decipher the motivations of other people so that they can speak to their concerns, decrease their anger, and appeal to their values. They must work in and with task groups often formed during advocacy projects.

PROVIDING POLICY ADVOCACY AT THREE LEVELS

VIDEO LINK 3.1
Engaging in Policy
Advocacy

Advocacy interventions occur at the micro, mezzo, and macro levels. Let's discuss each of these levels. Social workers engage in *micro policy advocacy* when they advocate for specific individuals or families to help them obtain services, rights, opportunities, and benefits that they would (likely) not otherwise receive and that would advance their well-being. This kind of advocacy is given to *specific clients and families*, as the following three examples illustrate:

- Parents with an autistic child are concerned about the adverse effects of medication on their child, but fear antagonizing the mental health professional who has helped their child. A micro policy advocate helps them understand that they have specific rights as consumers of service—and that getting a second opinion is their legal right, as is consulting other parents with similar concerns.
- A woman with a physical disability is not given workplace accommodations for her condition. A micro policy advocate refers her to a public interest attorney who specializes in cases related to the rights of disabled individuals.
- A woman mistreats her elderly husband with dementia by giving him inadequate nutrition and medical care. (The elderly man and his wife have no living relatives.) A micro policy advocate informs the woman of her husband's legal rights and, when no improvement occurs, refers the case to an agency that investigates cases of elder abuse.

We define micro policy advocacy as interventions to help clients obtain services, rights, and benefits that they would (likely) not otherwise receive and that would advance their well-being. We discuss it more fully in Chapter 4.

Social workers engage in *mezzo policy advocacy at the organizational level* when they seek to change dysfunctional policies in agencies and communities that may create the need for micro policy advocacy in the first place and that impede the provision of needed services, benefits, and opportunities, as well as the protection of clients' rights. These dysfunctional policies can include standard operating procedures, budgets, mission statements and organizational culture, eligibility requirements, selection of staff, allocation and training of staff, evaluation procedures, planning mechanisms, official organizational policies, and informal policies. We illustrate mezzo policy advocacy with the following two examples:

- A woman does not receive translation services to allow her to understand her transactions with a service provider, so a mezzo policy advocate informs the physician that she is required by federal law to provide translation services.

- Because a health clinic does not use a team approach when helping people with diabetes, patients fail to receive integrated services needed for their well-being, including physical therapy, occupational therapy, counseling, preventive services, and medical assistance A mezzo policy advocate brings evidence-based literature to her supervisor, providing data showing that team-based treatment of diabetes is more effective than traditional care delivered by multiple physicians who do not communicate with one another. Her supervisor, in terms, takes that recommendation to higher levels of the health clinic with the goal of obtaining high-level support for the team approach.

Social workers engage in *mezzo policy advocacy at the community level* when they seek to change dysfunctional policies in specific communities. Such policies might include funding, zoning, and land-use planning decisions; the policies of community-based public agencies; and policies that address the allocation and training of first responders in police and other agencies, community social and other services, housing inspections, and repair of infrastructure. We illustrate mezzo policy advocacy at the community level with the following two examples:

- A city has no regulations that limit the number of fast-food outlets in specific neighborhoods, leading to their disproportionate location in low-income areas. Alarmed about high rates of obesity in these low-income areas, an advocate works to allow the city to establish limits on placement of fast-food outlets in low-income areas.
- The well-being of many low-income people is jeopardized by the failure of a specific city to monitor and enforce housing regulations for their apartments. An advocate establishes a community coalition to pressure the city council and mayor to replace the current director of the city's housing agency, who, they believe, receives kickbacks from some landlords.

We discuss mezzo policy advocacy in more detail in Chapter 5.

Social workers engage in *macro policy advocacy* when they seek to change dysfunctional policies in government that may create the need for micro policy advocacy and mezzo policy advocacy in the first place and that impede the provision of needed services, benefits, and opportunities as well as the protection of clients' rights. These dysfunctional policies can include unwise budget priorities and allocations, statutes, regulations, administrative decisions, court rulings, and planning decisions. Macro policy advocates work to change policies and decisions in local, state, and federal governments. We illustrate macro policy advocacy with the following examples:

- A social worker who is the chief lobbyist for Planned Parenthood of Utah lobbies the Utah legislature to enact legislative measures to protect women's reproductive rights, including a law that protects their right to end pregnancies under certain conditions.
- A social worker develops a coalition to raise the rates paid to foster parents with infants to a level sufficient to reimburse the full costs of this care (the current level reimburses them for only half of this care).
- A coalition of mental health advocates secures the enactment of a proposition on the statewide ballot that sets aside a large and guaranteed sum of money each year for the treatment of people with mental health problems in the state.
- A state chapter of the National Association of Social Workers (NASW) endorses candidates who endorse the chapter's policy and budget priorities— and gives them resources to help fund their campaigns.

We discuss macro policy advocacy in more detail in Chapter 6.

IDENTIFYING DIFFERENCES BETWEEN ADVOCACY AND CLINICAL COUNSELING

It is useful to contrast advocacy with clinical or counseling practice in social work. Clinicians do not usually view themselves as advocates because they focus on helping clients improve their mental condition *within* the counseling relationship by addressing personal emotions, beliefs, and actions. By contrast, advocates help individuals, families, and communities deal with *external providers, institutions, laws, and policies.* Clinicians often seek *internal changes* in their clients, such as by helping them resolve conflicts, develop personal strategies, and surmount fears. Advocates, by contrast, focus on ways to persuade, entice, or coerce *external entities* to give needed amenities to specific individuals, families, or populations. Clinicians do not usually view themselves as *representing* clients or populations as they deal with service providers or governments, since they often focus on transactions and verbal interchange with clients themselves. Advocates often work for or on behalf of clients or populations. Advocates also often help individuals, families, or populations to obtain skills that enable them to advocate for themselves at the micro, mezzo, or macro levels.

LINKING THREE LEVELS OF ADVOCACY: THE CASE OF PREGNANT TEENS AND TEEN MOTHERS

Social workers sometimes move between micro, mezzo, and macro advocacy, as illustrated by strategies that social workers have used or could use to improve educational and other services for teenage women who become pregnant.

POLICY ADVOCACY LEARNING CHALLENGE 3.1

Providing Micro Policy Advocacy for a Pregnant Teenager

According to California Women's Law Center, California has the second highest rate of teen pregnancy in the nation (www.cwlc.org), and although many school-based programs aimed at addressing teen pregnancy have been successful in reducing early childbearing, schools have often neglected the rights of teens who are pregnant or choose to parent.

My placement of internship is at an urban hospital. A part of my duty as a social work intern at the hospital is to meet with moms who are 17 years old and under to assess their needs and offer them support and resources. When I intervene and assess teen pregnancy, I normally ask the moms questions related to their relationship with the father of the baby, their family background, their support system, their emotional status, their substance abuse history, their education, current resources that they are receiving, and so forth.

Before my internship, I did not have much interest in teen pregnancy and was not aware of the seriousness of the situation. Surprisingly, there are at least three to five teen pregnant patients per week coming to the hospital for labor and delivery. Not all, but a great number of them, are Latinas from low-income family. Many of them and/or their parents are undocumented immigrants, have low education, and work two to three different jobs to support their family.

Even more surprisingly, many teen moms report that they were not aware of their pregnancy until they were four to five months pregnant. Others who have sexually transmitted infections (STIs) report that their schools did not teach them about any risks factors associated with unprotected sexual activities, contraceptive use or methods, or preventive care in general. Not only that, but many teen moms also report that they did not seek help or obtain prenatal care because of their family's legal status and their own confidentiality needs.

Among many stories of these teen moms, one in particular caught my attention. Annette is a very cute, smart, and dedicated 16-year-old teen mom. During teen pregnancy assessment, she reported to me that she usually gets up at 6:30 every morning and catches two buses to go to a continuation school because of her current situation; her tummy started showing, and her "normal" school not only did not provide her any support, but also suggested that she go to a special school for pregnant teens. Sometimes Annette misses continuation school because it is a burden and tiring for her to wake up early in the morning and catch two buses to go to the school. She went on to say that a girl from her school was also transferred to the continuation school just days before her graduation, apparently to spare the school the embarrassment of having a pregnant girl stroll across the stage in cap and gown

(Continued)

(Continued)

before hundreds of onlookers. This report was very alarming to me. The decision of these teens to leave their old school to attend a special program for pregnant and parenting teens was virtually automatic for them.

When I asked Annette about her education plan after recovery from labor and delivery, she replied as follows: "I'm planning to go back to the continuation school because of my current situation, but I wish I could return to my 'normal' school, because at a regular high school you learn more." Even though she believed the parenting classes were good at the continuation school, she worried she was not learning the right things. Annette stated that a lot of the girls at the continuation school were scared about passing the high school exit exam. One of the pregnant teens had taken the test earlier that week, and she did not understand much of what was on it. Annette told me, "They don't teach you the kind of math they give you on the test. We're not going to pass that."

Identifying a Micro Advocacy Situation

Even though both federal and state laws guarantee pregnant and parenting teens equal rights and opportunities in all public and private educational institutions (www.cwlc.org), apparently some schools still pressure or force pregnant and parenting teens to leave regular high schools for some kind of continuation school. These teens lose their legal right not only to an equal education but also to the goodies that go with it: college entrance assistance, advanced-placement classes, and the experience of being at a high school with kids who are not pregnant or being punished for school infractions.

Alternative schools, such as the ones most pregnant girls are being sent to, are by law voluntary (www.cwlc.org), but many girls and parents do not seem to know this. Furthermore, Title IX of the federal Education Amendments of 1972 and the California Education Code outlaw all forms of discrimination by public schools on the basis of sex (FindLaw, n.d.), which can be applied to pregnant teens.

I think there is a general lack of respect for pregnant and parenting teens in many schools. They have discriminated against pregnant and parenting teens by not allowing them to have the equal rights and opportunities available to them. They have not given them proper information and options and have failed to provide comprehensive sex education to prevent pregnancy. Even Annette, who appears to be a bright student, reports that she did not know about risk factors, the importance of contraceptive use, and how to access reproductive health care services.

If schools keep discriminating against pregnant and parenting teens, they are sending the message that pregnancy is a bad thing. Some girls may resort to abortion so that they do not embarrass or disappoint their school and family. Others may end up with serious health problems because of the lack of support and preventive care. In my opinion, a pregnant teen is no worse a role model than the teen who is sexually active and just not getting pregnant. Getting pregnant does not make someone any different from anybody else who is having sex. It is a visual reminder that this can happen to anyone, and it can be a practical lesson to others. It is important to provide all students with equal rights, more support, preventive health care, and, most important of all, comprehensive sex education.

Interacting With the Patient and Diagnosing Causes

Even though Annette's biggest concern was about her education, I found several other problems and barriers in her life. She was the oldest daughter among three siblings and took the responsibility to help her mother with house chores because her mother worked two jobs, even on weekends, to support the family. Her mother was a single mom, an undocumented immigrant from Mexico who spoke very limited English and did not have any other family members or relatives in the United States whom she could rely on. Fortunately, Annette's two younger siblings were old enough to take care of themselves.

Annette dedicated herself to her schooling and activities because she did not want to become like her mother. Her goal was to study hard, go to a college, get a stable job with benefits, and make a lot of money. However, her goal and dream started fading when she found out she was pregnant. She did not tell anybody at school because she knew that she would be sent to a special school for pregnant teens. She knew about the school "policy" because of her experience with a girl who had been sent to a continuation school days before her graduation. Also, Annette was afraid to ask for federal or community assistance and support to receive prenatal care because of her family's legal status. She was afraid that her family might get deported to Mexico if she received federal assistance such as Medicaid.

Annette's luck with hiding her pregnancy did not last long. Her tummy started showing and became noticeable enough for anybody to tell that she was pregnant. A school counselor called her and her mother to have a private conference with them. The counselor suggested that Annette leave the school for a continuation school for teen moms. She told them about benefits Annette could get from the continuation school, but she did not explain to them that it was just an option for her. Annette and her mother thought it was the school's policy and that they had to follow it.

Developing a Strategy

Annette had many barriers in her life, but she also had a big asset that helped her to overcome in her situation. This asset was her intelligence and desire to pursue higher education. My foremost desired outcome for Annette was for her to claim her right

(Continued)

(Continued)

to go back to her normal high school to receive regular education. Also, I hoped she could find childcare for her baby through community programs, because she did not have any family members who could assist her with childcare while she went to a normal school. Then, my goal was to encourage her to attend parenting and family planning classes as well as to receive comprehensive sexual education. This way she would be able to get assistance and support while attending normal school and learn to take responsibility for her actions.

As a mandated reporter, my obligation was to include Child Protective Services (CPS) in my advocacy interventions procedure. I discussed Annette's case with the CPS worker and asked the worker to follow up on her and her baby's safety and care. The CPS worker stated that she would investigate Annette's home and school situation, and in the event of any type of abuse or neglect, she would follow up and provide Annette with additional support and resources.

After the report had been made, I educated Annette about the different resources available to her. I reassured her that she and her family would not get deported to Mexico just because she was receiving federal and community assistance and services. After the reassurance, I carefully explained the CPS report as well as the role of CPS and the services they offered. Then, with Annette's consent, I called a Bridges Program, a community resource program located in the hospital building, to help her and her baby receive Medicaid for medical insurance; the Special Supplemental Nutrition Program for Women, Infants, and Children (WIC), which would supply nutritious food for her and her baby; additional formula; diapers; and an infant car seat for the baby. Also, I sent a referral to public health nurse (PHN) services so that they could follow up with Annette on a regular basis regarding baby care, parenting, and health education after hospital discharge.

Furthermore, I encouraged Annette to contact the community Teen Mothers Resource Center, which provides teen moms with case management, financial assistance, teen moms support groups, childcare, parenting classes, and so forth, regardless of one's legal status. I also provided her with information on the California Women's Law Center, along with information about her civil rights in a California school. I encouraged her and her mother to advocate for her rights and services in school. I advised to call the Women's Law Center or visit the Internet sources for additional information about her rights in school.

Implementing the Strategy

Most of the advocacy interventions for Annette were skillfully implemented. CPS responded to my call and confirmed they would investigate and follow up on her case. The Bridges Program and PHN services were put in place to provide her and her baby with support, education, and resources. Also, she and her mother received information about community services and the California Women's Law Center, and they were eager to follow my advice.

All the above information and resources assisted Annette with her basic needs and empowered her to fight for her rights. Unfortunately, I was not able to see my foremost desired outcome, which was for her to be able to attend a normal school after recovery, because of my internship setting and protocols. My interventions for her were the work of planting seeds. I just hope that she was able to find her rights in school with the help of CPS and other services.

Policy, Program, and Community Reforms

Studies repeatedly show that insufficient education helps perpetuate the cycle of poverty and teen pregnancy. The "No Time for Complacency" report (Constantine & Nevarez, 2006) released by Berkeley's Public Health Institute states that teen moms exhibit poorer psychological functioning, lower levels of educational attainment and high school completion, more single parenthood, and less stable employment. Furthermore, a study reports that babies born to teens are more likely to have health troubles, exhibit poor school performance, and become parents themselves when they are teens (National Campaign to Prevent Teen Pregnancy, 2004).

After reading this case example, address the following questions:

- Which of the seven core problems was the social worker addressing in this case advocacy intervention?
- What contextual factors were liabilities that she had to deal with and surmount?
- What contextual factors were assets she could use to facilitate her work?
- Which of the eight challenges in the micro advocacy framework did she undertake?
- Which of the four skills did she use?

POLICY ADVOCACY LEARNING CHALLENGE 3.2

Moving Toward Mezzo Policy
Advocacy to Help Pregnant High School Students

Social workers engage in mezzo policy practice to help pregnant high school students when they seek to change policies and procedures in specific high schools or school districts. Despite the importance of teen education and equal education requirements of Title IX, many guidance counselors still informally counsel pregnant students to

(Continued)

(Continued)

leave their high school for alternative schools, without providing them assistance or resources and telling them they have the option to stay put. Official school policies could be established that prohibit encouraging pregnant students to leave high schools for alternative schools.

Sex education can be improved in specific schools or school districts by developing or using models that have been proven to be effective in preventing or delaying teen pregnancy. Do specific policy and program deficiencies impede *preventive* strategies, such as sex education programs that discuss not only abstinence, but also birth control strategies? Do school have nurses on the premises who distribute condoms? Do schools inform teenagers that they can consult medical staff if they have unprotected sexual encounters to see if they wish to use medications to avert pregnancy? Are schools linked to Planned Parenthood so that students can obtain information about their options?

Address the following questions with respect to mezzo policy advocacy with teenagers in schools:

- Do social workers *frequently* engage in micro policy advocacy for pregnant adolescents to help them obtain their rights, suggesting *systemic defects* in organizational policies, such as prejudice by school staff against this population or a lack of quality education programs geared to the needs of this population?
- Do pregnant adolescents drop out of a specific school due to hostile treatment by a specific teacher or guidance counselor or due to defective policies in a specific school (organizational factors), in the school district (community factors), or in the state department of education (government factors)—or some combination of these factors?
- Did deficiencies in the policy and regulatory context contribute to the problem, such as a lack of guidelines from the school district, the state department of education, or the federal department of education to protect the teens' rights to education?
- Do budgets of specific schools or school districts prioritize services for pregnant teenagers—or sex education or nurses in schools?
- Are pregnant students of color treated differently in specific schools or school districts than Caucasian pregnant students? Are low-income pregnant students treated differently than more affluent pregnant students?
- Do schools keep data on the educational paths of pregnant teens?
- Do specific schools give pregnant adolescents special accommodations, allowing them to be tardy or absent when obtaining medical care?
- What policies have specific schools or school districts developed to help young women remain in school after they have given birth, such as assistance with childcare, supportive counseling, and special accommodations?

POLICY ADVOCACY LEARNING CHALLENGE 3.3

Moving Toward Macro Policy
Advocacy to Help Pregnant High School Students

The United States has the highest rates of teen pregnancies of any industrialized nation, even though the pregnancy rate has markedly declined for teens ages 15 to 19. Only one third of teen mothers finish high school, and only 1.5% have a college degree by age 30.

Public schools differ markedly in their policies regarding pregnant teen mothers, partly because of the absence of clear state laws or federal policies. Some of them send them to continuation schools during their pregnancy, where they are separated from their friends, and do not invite them back to their regular school after they have given birth. Continuation schools are of uncertain quality, partly because their standards are not well defined by state law. State laws are often unclear about whether adolescents can remain in continuation schools even after giving birth. Various laws forbid schools from expelling teen mothers, but they receive little policy guidance otherwise. Little case law enforces or guides the provision of educational services for teen mothers in many localities and states. Some evidence suggests, as well, that African American and low-income pregnant adolescents are treated more harshly than white and affluent adolescents. The laws and policies of some states do not require schools to provide sexual education. Many schools ignore the importance of preventive health education and comprehensive sex education. Many states do not require schools to keep data on the educational trajectories of teen mothers prior to giving birth or after they give birth.

Nor is it clear to what extent some states fund special programs for pregnant teens and teen mothers. While some teens can count on support from their parents and relatives, others lack such support—and may particularly need financial assistance from schools for medical care, childcare, counseling, and other provisions.

Nor is it clear what budgetary and policy roles exist for school districts as compared to state educational agencies and policies. Some state officials may wish to cede responsibility to school districts that lack resources and staff to help pregnant teens and teen mothers.

Advocates need to consider, as well, whether and under what circumstances pregnant teens can seek termination of their pregnancies. What laws in their states impact these decisions—and do these laws need to be reformed? What positions do Planned Parenthood and other advocacy groups take on this issue in specific states?

These kinds of *systemic policy factors* can be addressed only through **macro policy advocacy.**

Identify some dysfunctional policies in your locality, region, or state that might be addressed through macro policy advocacy by social workers working with teenagers in schools or other settings.

Our discussion suggests that advocacy at micro, mezzo, and macro levels can be linked. Discuss how a social worker might move between micro policy advocacy, mezzo policy advocacy and macro policy advocacy.

DEVELOPING RED FLAG ALERTS

We now return to the seven core problems that we discussed in Chapter 1 that provide the reason why social workers engage in advocacy at three levels in the first place. We need to move beyond general descriptions of these seven core problems to identify specific manifestations or examples of them so that we can anticipate them.

Let's illustrate the way social workers can develop Red Flag Alerts by taking an example of a recent research project I conducted with a research team. We wanted to know to what extent social workers, nurses, and medical residents engage in micro policy advocacy, mezzo policy advocacy, and macro policy advocacy in acute care hospitals.. We generated a list of 33 specific manifestations of the seven core problems by consulting medical research and by enlisting the help of a panel of healthcare experts that included nurses, social workers, a physician, and a patient (see Table 3.1).

Table 3.1   Twenty-Nine Manifestations of the Seven Core Problems in Acute-Care Hospitals

CORE PROBLEM 1: ETHICAL RIGHTS **Patients' ethical rights may be at risk in the following areas:**
1. Informed consent for medical intervention
2. Accurate medical information (e.g., risks, diagnosis, prognosis, discussion of treatment planning and timeline)
3. Confidential medical information
4. Advance directives
5. Competence to make medical decisions
CORE PROBLEM 2: QUALITY OF CARE **Patients' quality of care may be at risk in the following areas:**
1. Lack of evidence-based healthcare
2. Medical errors
3. Whether to have specific diagnostic tests
4. Fragmented care
5. Nonbeneficial treatment
CORE PROBLEM 3: CULTURAL CONTENT OF CARE **Cultural content of care may be lacking in the following areas:**
1. Information in patients' preferred language

2. Communication with patients with limited literacy or health knowledge

3. Religious, spiritual, and cultural practices

4. Use of complementary and alternative medicine

CORE PROBLEM 4: PREVENTIVE TREATMENT
Preventive treatment may be lacking in the following areas:

1. Wellness exams

2. At-risk factors not addressed (e.g., smoking, obesity, lifestyle, substance abuse)

3. Chronic disease care

4. Immunizations

CORE PROBLEM 5: AFFORDABILITY OR ACCESS TO CARE
Affordability or access to care may be problematic in the following areas:

1. Financing necessary healthcare and medications

2. Use of publicly funded programs

3. Coverage from private insurance companies

CORE PROBLEM 6: MENTAL HEALTH CONDITIONS
Care for mental health conditions may be lacking in the following areas:

1. Screening for specific mental health conditions

2. Treatment of mental health conditions while hospitalized

3. Follow-up treatment for mental health conditions after discharge

4. Medications for mental health conditions

5. Mental distress stemming from health conditions

6. Availability of individual counseling and/or group therapy

7. Availability of support groups

CORE PROBLEM 7: COMMUNITY-BASED HEALTHCARE
Community-based healthcare may be lacking in the following areas:

1. Discharge planning

2. Transitions between community-based levels of care

3. Referrals to services in communities

4. Reaching out to referral sources on behalf of the patient, such as coordinating services, providing a warm handoff, and monitoring or assessing services

5. Assessment of home, community, and work environments

Once we had identified specific manifestations of the seven core problems, we then asked roughly 100 social workers, 100 nurses, and 100 medical residents in eight acute-care hospitals to indicate the extent to which they had engaged in micro policy advocacy for their patients with respect to those problems during the prior two months. We discovered that many of these health professionals had engaged in micro policy advocacy regarding these specific manifestations of the seven core problems, even though considerable variation existed between them in terms of level of advocacy. We had successfully identified Red Flag Alerts that could help these health professionals anticipate these specific manifestations of the seven core problems in the hospitals where they worked. They could now look for them and, when possible, help patients solve these specific problems.

We also asked these providers to indicate the extent to which they engaged in mezzo policy advocacy and macro policy advocacy. They reported far less of these kinds of policy advocacy as compared to micro policy advocacy, possibly because their work focuses on helping specific patients with the kinds of problems listed in Table 3.1.

POLICY ADVOCACY LEARNING CHALLENGE 3.4

Identifying Red Flag Alerts in Specific Settings

Take any setting that provides human services with which you are familiar, whether your field agency or where you have volunteered or worked. Select any of the seven core problems that we discussed in Chapter I and that are listed in Table 3.1. Try to develop a list of one specific manifestation of each of the seven core problems listed in Table 3.1. Then ask a professional who works in the setting you have identified to discuss with you the extent to which these seven manifestations are relatively common in the setting. Also ask this professional to augment your list with several additional problems, and perhaps to delete one or more of the problems that you have identified.

Discuss the following questions:

- Is it possible to develop specific Red Flag Alerts in the setting that you have chosen?
- Would these Red Flag Alerts facilitate the use of micro policy advocacy by social workers in this setting?
- To what extent did you use research findings, ethical principles, or pragmatic factors to develop these Red Flag Alerts?

DEVELOPING RED FLAG ALERTS AT THREE LEVELS

We have discussed how specific Red Flag Alerts can be developed in specific agencies. It is also possible to identify specific manifestations of one of the seven core problems that could require advocacy at micro, mezzo, and macro levels. Let's use an example drawn from schools. Assume that you have read extensive research literature documenting that many children are overmedicated for specific mental problems like autism, attention deficit hyperactivity disorder (ADHD), and behavioral problems. You could make this a micro policy Red Flag Alert falling under the sixth core problem (failure to address mental problems of clients): "Children may be overmedicated for behavioral or mental health problems, including autism, attention deficit hyperactivity disorder (ADHD), or behavioral problems." Were you to work in a mental health or education setting, you would be alert to this issue and might launch a micro policy advocacy intervention to help the child's parents obtain second opinions to ascertain if their child *is* overmedicated.

You could transform this micro Red Flag Alert into a mezzo Red Flag Alert or a macro Red Flag Alert by placing it in an organizational, community, or government context. Assume that *many* children may be overmedicated in a large school system. The micro Red Flag Alert can be changed to a mezzo Red Flag Alert: "Many schoolchildren who have been diagnosed with autism, ADHD, or behavioral problems have been overmedicated with respect to type of medication, number of medications, and dosage." A social worker could consider launching a mezzo policy advocacy intervention, such as:

- Developing training programs to teach teachers, social workers, school counselors, school speech therapists, and other staff in a school district to recognize signs of overmedication
- Developing guidelines in the state's board of education regarding overmedication of children

A social worker could contact a children's advocacy group in Washington, DC, to see if specific regulations by the Food and Drug Administration (FDA) could be developed to regulate the use of medications with children under a specific age— much as the federal government is now attempting to limit prescriptions of pain medications that currently lead to preventable deaths. Of the 22,114 deaths related to pharmaceutical overdose in 2012, 16,007 involved opioid analgesics, also called opioid pain relievers or prescription painkillers (Centers for Disease Control and Prevention, n.d.). This could be a macro Red Flag Alert: "Many schoolchildren are overmedicated for autism, ADHD, or behavioral problems due to lack of federal regulations about the use of medications for these problems in children under a specific age."

POLICY ADVOCACY LEARNING CHALLENGE 3.5

Locating Information About Specific Social Problems

Other manifestations of the seven core problems can be obtained by consulting the Internet, such as by typing problems into online search sites such as Google Search, Google Advanced Search or Google Scholar, or Microsoft's Bing. Assume, for example, that you wonder if you are likely to encounter malnutrition among schoolchildren in a particular low-income neighborhood. You can find information about malnutrition among low-income children generally or in specific regions. This information may not accurately predict or measure malnutrition in a specific geographic area or a specific school district, so you would need to interview or contact researchers with geographic-specific knowledge about childhood malnutrition.

Take a stab at obtaining information about one of the following problems—and deciding if it should be designated a Red Flag Alert. Identify where social workers might encounter individuals with these problems by sector and geographic area, as well as by the type of agency or hospital where they work.

- The extent to which veterans receive services for brain trauma or for mental problems
- The extent to which homeless people receive affordable housing
- The extent to which sufficient services are given to truants in schools
- The extent to which released prisoners receive assistance with finding employment

We use the term *connected policy interventions* to describe linked policy interventions. Social workers can begin with micro, mezzo, or macro policy intervention and then consider progressing to other levels. Assume, for example, that a local child welfare department receives many reports from neighbors, school officials, and others that they suspect that specific children have been abused or neglected by their parent or parents. Also assume that a social worker discovers that many of these children, as well as their families, possess serious mental health and substance abuse problems, even though child abuse and neglect are not discovered—and finds that her perceptions are supported by evidence-based research. Yet she finds that these children and their families receive no assistance from child welfare workers once they do not find evidence of abuse or neglect. The social worker may begin with a single child or family and work to get them supportive services from community agencies (a micro policy advocacy intervention), and then decide that the child welfare department should develop a policy to facilitate these referrals for many or all of these children (a mezzo policy advocacy intervention). Or perhaps the social worker could inquire whether child welfare regulations at the state level sufficiently mandate the provision of preventive services for children who are referred to child welfare departments, allowing her to determine whether she and others should launch a macro policy advocacy intervention to modify these regulations.

We will refer in this book to:

- Micro policy advocacy interventions
- Mezzo policy advocacy interventions
- Macro policy advocacy interventions
- Connected policy advocacy interventions

LEARNING OUTCOMES

You are now equipped to:

- Provide advocacy at the micro, mezzo, and macro levels
- Identify similarities and differences between these levels of advocacy
- Identify differences between policy advocacy and clinical counseling
- Develop Red Flag Alerts in specific settings
- Develop Red Flag Alerts at the three levels of policy advocacy in specific settings

REFERENCES

Centers for Disease Control and Prevention. (n.d.). *Prescription drug overdose in the United States: Fact sheet.* Retrieved January 7, 2015, from http://www.cdc.gov/homeandrecreational safety/overdose/facts.html

Constantine, N. A., & Nevarez, C. R. (2006). *No time for complacency: Teen births in California.* Berkeley's Public Health Institute.

FindLaw. (n.d.). *Gender discrimination in education.* Retrieved January 7, 2015, from http://civilrights.findlaw.com/discrimination/gender-discrimination-in-education.html

National Campaign to Prevent Teen Pregnancy. (2004). *Teen pregnancy—so what?* Retrieved March 10, 2008, from http://www.teenpregnancy.org

Chapter 4

ENGAGING IN MICRO POLICY ADVOCACY

DEFINING MICRO POLICY ADVOCACY

Curiously, social work curricula often fail to provide students with skills to advocate for specific clients or consumers of service—an omission that is addressed in this textbook through "micro policy advocacy." Micro policy advocacy helps clients or consumers obtain services, rights, opportunities, and benefits that they would (likely) not otherwise receive and that would advance their well-being.

Micro policy advocacy can be provided directly to patients or through referrals, provided that micro policy advocates ascertain that their clients or consumers of service actually received assistance.

Micro policy advocates engage in eight challenges (see Figure 3.1). They decide whether to proceed (Challenge 1). They decide where to focus (Challenge 2). They obtain recognition that a client has an unresolved problem from other staff in an agency (Challenge 3). They analyze or diagnose why the client has the unresolved problem (Challenge 4). They develop a strategy to address the client's unresolved problem (Challenge 5). They obtain support for their strategy to help resolve the client's unresolved problem (Challenge 6). They implement their strategy (Challenge 7). They assess whether their implemented strategy or policy has been successful (Challenge 8).

Advocates may decide to progress from micro policy advocacy to mezzo or macro policy advocacy if they decide that a client's unresolved problem is shared by other clients or individuals and is caused by dysfunctional policies of agencies or communities (mezzo policy advocacy) or by dysfunctional policies in government settings (macro policy advocacy).

A PRELIMINARY CHALLENGE: READING THE CONTEXT

VIDEO LINK 4.1
Micro Policy
Advocacy: Human
Trafficking

Like mezzo policy advocates and macro policy advocates, micro policy advocates must be acutely aware of the context in which they are helping specific individuals and families, including both opportunities and constraints. The context includes policies, procedures, court rulings, funding sources, personnel, economic factors, and any other factor that shapes how social workers engage and work with clients and families. Our discussion will clarify why we use the term "micro *policy* advocacy" in this chapter as well as in the eight chapters devoted to specific sectors. Social workers and their clients are surrounded by policy and policy-related factors—and social workers have to help their clients navigate these factors so that they receive their benefits to the fullest extent possible.

These contextual factors vary with different agencies and with different policy sectors. Social workers who work in mental health clinics, hospitals, schools, corrections, child welfare agencies, and programs assisting seniors must be aware of those unique and cross-cutting policies that shape their work with clients and families.

Micro policy advocates need a strategic view of the organizations where they work so that they can identify (or find) *assets* that will facilitate their micro policy advocacy with specific consumers, while not neglecting those contextual *liabilities* that will make it more difficult. For example, individuals with insurance policies that exclude specific services or require considerable out-of-pocket payments may not be able to surmount them when an advocate seeks to help them contend with their health costs (a liability). An advocate who wishes to help an uninsured patient *not* be transferred from a private to a public hospital before she is medically stabilized can cite federal regulations that prohibit such transfers (an asset).

The context contains many "streams" that flow into and through specific agencies from external sources. Each of these streams may contain assets or liabilities for advocates in specific situations, including:

- Court rulings that require health staff to take certain actions and to avoid other actions, such as those concerning when to withdraw food, medications, and/or hydration from a dying person
- Statutes (or legislation) that require specific actions, services, or accountability by health organizations and their staff
- Civil rights legislation that prohibits providers from violating specific rights of specific populations, such as requirements for ease of movement by individuals with disabilities as specified by the Americans with Disabilities Act (ADA), or requirements that agencies provide translation services to people with limited English proficiency (LEP)
- Flows of revenues to clients and agencies from private insurance companies, employers, Medicare, Medicaid, the Children's Health Insurance Program (CHIP), contracts that many nonprofit agencies have with public agencies, and scores of public programs
- Potential sanctions or adverse publicity that specific organizations might confront, such as allegations that specific child welfare agencies fail to sufficiently protect children's well-being in foster care placements
- Competition from other agencies in a specific policy sector, such as between nonprofit agencies, between for-profit agencies, or between public and nonpublic agencies
- Accreditation standards established by accrediting agencies in each sector
- Regulations of specific local, state, and federal departments, such as those that require schools to mainstream developmentally disabled children
- Legal litigation and inquiries of public interest attorneys and private attorneys
- Monitoring and oversight of public clinics and clinics by public authorities and funders in specific cities, counties, and states
- External advocacy groups that help consumers contest specific decisions or policies of mental health, education, and other agencies
- Resources and regulations of publicly funded programs from which consumers may be able to receive assistance, including Medicare, Medicaid, CHIP, the Supplemental Nutrition Assistance Program (SNAP), Supplemental

Security Income (SSI), insurance exchanges established by the Affordable Care Act in many states, Social Security benefits, unemployment insurance, rent subsidies, and scores of additional programs

- Specific findings in professional literature or from private or governmental sources that are widely viewed as being based on empirical research
- Policies and procedures of specific agencies

The context also includes many streams from internal sources within specific organizations that can be assets or liabilities in specific instances of case advocacy, including:

- Budgets and their relative surpluses or deficits in specific health settings that establish what agency programs and functions receive priority
- Mission statements that state the priorities and goals of a provider
- Organizational culture as it favors specific activities while discouraging others—including case advocacy and policy advocacy
- Specific units that engage in advocacy or advocacy-related work, such as departments of compliance, risk management departments, bioethics committees, institutional review boards (IRBs), patient representatives or advocates, social work departments, care managers, and financial departments
- Specific officials, administrators, professionals, or staff who have expertise and clout in specific areas and programs, such as social workers in child welfare agencies

These internal factors can also be assets or liabilities in specific policy advocacy situations. Budget deficits may lead to cuts in services that can diminish the size of specific programs needed to provide services to specific consumers (a liability), but budget surpluses or increased funding from external sources can increase services (an asset).

Advocates have to update their knowledge to be effective. Laws and regulations frequently change. New and revised evidence-based practice frequently emerges. Ethical standards change. Budget priorities of agencies often change rapidly. Policy and service preferences of the funders of services in specific agencies often change.

I place URLs for Internet sites with a reputation for accuracy at strategic places throughout this book to facilitate this updating process. These include websites of governmental agencies, advocacy groups, and self-help groups. Policies by public agencies shift as they are modified by government agencies, regulatory bodies, and legislatures.

CHALLENGE 1: DECIDING WHETHER TO PROCEED

Social workers must ask themselves whether specific consumers might suffer harm if they do not provide them with micro policy advocacy. These individuals may include members of vulnerable populations, people with high-threshold problems, people with multiple problems, people not receiving any care or only partial or delayed care, people with overlooked problems, people caught in a revolving door, people enmeshed in destructive relationships, people in physical or psychological jeopardy, people who are unable to self-advocate or to receive advocacy from others, people who are bewildered by systems of care, and people who are currently harming themselves.

Membership in a Vulnerable Population

Vulnerable populations include consumers whose predisposing or intrinsic characteristics often expose them to one or more of the seven problems (Anderson, 1995). They include consumers with distinctive racial or ethnic characteristics, such as African Americans, Latino/as, Asian Americans, and Native Americans, as well as specific immigrant populations from the Middle East, Africa, Eastern Europe, Russia, and Asia. They include documented and undocumented immigrants as well as individuals with uncertain immigration status. They include women. They include consumers in different age groups, such as children and adolescents, as well as elderly people. They include consumers with specific sexual orientations, including the LGBTQQ population. They include consumers with stigmatized health conditions, including people with HIV/AIDS or other sexually transmitted disease (STDs), and victims and perpetrators of family violence and rape. They include people with stigmatized forms of mental illness, such as schizophrenia and clinical depression. They include people with addictions. They include people with eating disorders. They include people with reduced mental capacity, including people with dementia, Alzheimer's disease, and developmental disabilities.

Vulnerable populations include people with enabling factors that often expose them to one or more of the seven problems (Anderson, 1995). They include consumers who lack medical insurance or who are underinsured. They include rural and inner-city consumers who live in areas with shortages of medical services. They include consumers with LEP. They include low-income consumers. They include consumers with chronic diseases such as chronic obstructive pulmonary disease, congestive heart failure, heart disease, arthritis, degenerative muscle and nerve diseases (e.g., muscular dystrophy, Lou Gehrig's disease), cerebral palsy, and genetic disorders (e.g., Huntington's disease). They include consumers with life-threatening diseases including some kinds of cancer and chronic diseases. They include people with limited literacy. Many individuals who are members of two or more of these vulnerable populations are at particular risk.

Micro policy advocates should prioritize services to people with limited income because they often possess multiple health, economic, mental health, employment, housing, disabling, and other conditions that, taken together, make it difficult for them to navigate the service systems in the eight sectors. They often have lower literacy skills that compromise their ability to understand written documents. They are more likely to encounter negative responses from highly educated professionals. Background factors, such as evictions, loss of employment, poor housing, and exposure to violence in their neighborhoods, make it difficult for them to engage and use services. They are more likely to have high-threshold and multiple problems and to have other characteristics of people who need priority in social workers' micro policy advocacy.

Clients With High-Threshold Problems

Clients particularly need micro policy advocacy when any of the seven core problems reach a high threshold that endangers their well-being or their ethical rights. Remember, however, that ethical issues that seem low-threshold may be important to specific consumers (Daley, 2001). Advocates can make this determination by using the following kinds of information to ascertain that care is divergent from evidence-based findings or from ethical standards, including informed consent:

- Information from specific consumers
- Notations in medical records
- Direct observations
- Feedback from other professionals
- Feedback from family members

Clients With Multiple Problems

Many clients are plagued by more than one of the seven core problems that we discussed in Chapter 1. Often, advocates should provide micro policy advocacy to clients with two or more of these problems. Some clients possess multiple, interacting problems that, together, place them in jeopardy—but receive care for only one of them. Clients who are obese, diabetic, depressed, and lack insurance, for example, are likely to need micro policy advocacy to develop strategies for obtaining multifaceted care for their multiple problems.

Clients Receiving No Care, Partial Care, or Delayed Care

Some clients do not receive any care for a specific problem. Perhaps they lack transportation. Perhaps they lack childcare so they cannot use needed services. Perhaps their lives have been disrupted by evictions from their places of residence. Perhaps they lack resources to pay the fees associated with specific services. People of color sometimes do not seek attention for HIV/AIDS, for example, because it is stigmatized in their communities.

Clients may be deterred from seeking assistance when they find their treatments or assistance excessively delayed. They may be caught in long lines in public clinics. Perhaps they are placed on waiting lists.

Clients With Overlooked Problems

Many clients receive assistance for a presenting problem, but find that their other problems are not addressed by specific agencies. For example, a disabled person may receive care for her physical limitations but no attention for her anxiety or depression.

Clients Caught in a Revolving Door

Some clients repeatedly return to service providers. A considerable portion of medical and social services are devoted to helping the "worried well," that is, to people who do not have serious problems, but who want reassurance, attention, or companionship from providers. Some clients come to specific mental health facilities repeatedly for the same condition, such as alcoholism, substance abuse, or attempted suicide. Advocates may need to help them receive preventive, counseling, or other services to address causes of this repetition.

Clients Enmeshed in Destructive Relationships

People who experience destructive relationships often need micro policy advocacy. Advocates are often required to inform authorities when specific consumers, such as women, children, or elderly individuals, are subject to violent acts from family members or others.

Clients in Physical or Psychological Jeopardy

Social workers and other professionals sometimes engage in micro policy advocacy when they fear that specific consumers will otherwise die or suffer grievous physical injury. For example, a nurse in a public clinic in the Bronx in New York City took it upon herself to locate consumers who had recently received biopsies revealing aggressive and advanced cancer, but had not returned for follow-up visits.

She persuaded many of them to return for treatment that they might not otherwise have received—and possibly saved some of their lives (Perez-Pena, 2005).

Clients Unable to Self-Advocate or to Receive Advocacy From Others

Some clients are able to advocate for themselves because they are highly skilled at navigating the service and health systems and have read about their conditions or searched the Internet diligently. They may have already received a second opinion from experts and already received advice from other people who have experienced their condition. They are appropriately assertive, skilled communicators, and persistent. They keep records. They know about emerging treatments and tests. They are not traumatized by adverse diagnoses. Social workers may decide that these individuals are able to advocate for themselves with no or minimal assistance from them. They should prioritize micro policy advocacy for consumers who lack these skills and knowledge, particularly when they possess serious problems that could threaten their well-being and their ethical rights.

Some consumers have supportive families and friends who help them self-advocate or become surrogate advocates when they lack the skills, knowledge, or ability to advocate for themselves. Healthcare professionals need to consider providing advocacy when consumers do not have these supports.

Often, in the case of comatose individuals, people with limited cognitive function, or people under sedation or heavy medication, healthcare professionals should obtain the concurrence of family members or friends before engaging in micro policy advocacy.

Clients Bewildered by Bureaucratic and Policy Complexity

Social workers often provide services in complex bureaucratic and policy systems. Welfare, education, correctional, health, and many other service organizations are complex institutions with multiple professions, administrative staff, internal units, and linkages with myriad external organizations. Their staff use complicated jargon. It is not surprising that many clients find it difficult to understand them or to navigate within them, particularly when they have complex or serious problems and when they contend with medical and other professional jargon. Many providers are not good communicators.

Skilled micro policy advocates can better decide who needs advocacy by viewing these institutions from the bottom up as their clients do. They can bring simple improvements to their care, such as scheduling visits so that consumers do not lose their privacy when professionals flow through their rooms at nonstop and unpredictable intervals. They can interpret procedures for them, help them locate places, facilitate family members' visits, and learn to detect clients' confusion and angst. Clients and families need this kind of assistance in each of the eight policy sectors we discuss in this book.

Clients Who Endanger Themselves

Micro policy advocates usually focus on factors that preclude clients from receiving needed services or that violate their rights. In some cases, however, they provide "reverse advocacy" that focuses on clients' self-destructive behaviors like smoking, substance abuse, lack of exercise, or poor diet—topics often not discussed by health and other professionals who do not want to antagonize or confront them.

Micro policy advocates can point consumers in new directions tactfully. They can ask, for example, whether anyone has informed them of support groups, Internet sites, or counseling assistance that might prove helpful in reducing their smoking, excessive use of alcohol, or other self-destructive behaviors. They can ask if they have received data that examine their health prognosis if they do not curtail or eliminate specific destructive behaviors.

CHALLENGE 2: DECIDING WHERE TO FOCUS

Advocates identify relevant policies, regulations, and organizational factors. They identify individuals, programs, regulations, laws, resources, organizations, and services that are relevant to helping a client surmount an unresolved problem. Assume, for example, that a child needs a preventive preschool program, but Head Start is oversubscribed in his geographic area and his parents lack resources to pay fees for private nursery schools. Also assume his parent is disabled and cannot help him travel to other areas. A micro policy advocate might find it difficult to help this child, but might nonetheless be able to locate scholarships or reduced fees to allow this child to gain entrée to a church-based or other program in this area—or might find resources to empower the child's mother to help him with reading or other activities that parallel those provided in Head Start. By contrast, an advocate would have a simpler task if the local Head Start program was not oversubscribed.

The context includes key contacts of social workers. Perhaps they know a specific worker in a program who can be trusted to help a client gain access. Perhaps they can counsel a client *not* to see a specific intake worker who has proven relatively hostile to similar clients in the past—unlike another intake worker.

Social workers need a *strategic view* to help their clients navigate not only the programs, staff, and resources of their own agencies, but also those in the vicinity. Assume, for example, that a woman with a prison record wants to have it legally expunged from the records she gives to potential employers because she knows it may lead to her inability to secure work, since many employers will discriminate against her *no matter* her actual talents and reliability. A social worker would need to know how to link this person to a legal aid attorney or other resource to help her resolve this issue.

Social workers empower people to develop context-reading and navigational skills. They help them use the Internet. They engage them in role-playing to help them develop questions and interviewing skills. They help them to become appropriately assertive. They give them strategic advice.

CHALLENGE 3: OBTAINING RECOGNITION THAT A CLIENT HAS AN IMPORTANT UNRESOLVED PROBLEM

Micro policy advocates devise strategies for placing their clients' unresolved problems on the agendas of other people so that those individuals will provide assistance in resolving them. The advocate locates people who have the authority and motivation to help individuals with unresolved problems. They find fellow professionals at the service delivery level. They involve specific supervisors or higher-level administrators when needed.

Micro policy advocates often help to assemble a team that works together to help a client resolve a problem. It may include professionals, family members, and friends. Assume, for example, that a senior citizen needs help making his home more accommodating to his physical and mental problems, such as by moving a bedroom downstairs, placing ramps over outside steps, remodeling the bathroom to include a downstairs shower, and removing impediments that could make him fall. The team might include a spouse, an adult child, a contractor, a financial adviser, and a professional from a senior center. The advocate helps to convince each of these people that the issue is sufficiently important to be placed on their agendas because, absent these modifications, this senior citizen could suffer a life-threatening facture or brain injury from a fall.

In simpler cases, the advocate may need to convince only a single person to place an issue high on his or her agenda. She might convince the senior's gerontologist to contact the executive director of a senior center funded by the Older Americans Act to assume leadership in helping this senior citizen. Advocates often involve family members and friends in their micro advocacy because their concurrence and cooperation is often needed. Without the help and encouragement of his spouse and children, for example, this senior citizen might be so overwhelmed at the thought of remodeling his home that he fails to take action.

Social workers can sometimes use shortcuts. They can convince other professionals to provide micro case advocacy for and with a specific individual—what I call "advocacy punting" (Jansson, 2011, p. 33)—because they have greater expertise or may already have the trust of a particular client. They can empower specific clients to self-advocate if they have the skills and motivation to be their own advocates.

CHALLENGE 4: ANALYZING OR DIAGNOSING WHY A CLIENT HAS AN UNRESOLVED PROBLEM

Before they can devise strategy, social workers must diagnose why a client experiences one or more unresolved problems from the seven core problems that we discussed in Chapter 1.

Developing Narratives

Micro policy advocates often develop narratives of specific transactions between specific clients and their interactions with other professionals and staff. They construct an account of events, service transactions, motives or beliefs, the nature of communications, and key actions (Steiner, 2005). They obtain evidence from records, direct observations, feedback from other professionals, and feedback from family members, as well as their prior experiences in specific service settings

Advocates should understand some challenges in constructing accurate narratives. They cannot assume that reports or perceptions of specific participants are necessarily accurate, such as those of teachers, mental health professionals, or physicians. For example, a physician may report in the medical record that he had an extended discussion with a client where he covered the plusses and minuses of specific treatment options, but the actual discussion may have been relatively brief and may have covered treatment options only tangentially because the physician was already committed to a specific diagnosis and course of treatment.

Clients, too, may exaggerate, distort, or even falsify events and communications. When given serious diagnoses, for example, some clients may be sufficiently traumatized that they cannot process information accurately, so they may wrongly believe they were given (or not given) specific information. A few people may even deliberately falsify information to advance their claims for workers' compensation or to lay the groundwork for malpractice litigation.

The narrative should lead to an informed opinion about why a specific consumer needs case advocacy. Here are some recurring causes:

- Prejudice
- Negative responses to client behaviors
- Narrow mindsets
- Flawed transactions and communications between specific consumers and specific medical staff
- Poor ethical reasoning
- Inadequate use of evidence-based medicine
- Bureaucratic and organizational malfunctioning
- Flawed policies and procedures
- Lack of team practice
- Lack of knowledge
- Lack of policy guidance
- Causation by multiple factors

Prejudice

Advocates need to be alert to prejudicial treatment of specific clients in specific sectors. They need skills not only in recognizing when prejudicial treatment exists, but also in helping specific consumers surmount it. Prejudice can take the form of overt prejudice, such as excluding specific people from services, but it has been greatly reduced by the enactment of federal and state civil rights laws. Considerable evidence suggests, however, that more subtle forms of prejudice exist, such as making some people wait longer than others, discouraging some people from using specific services when they need them, and providing some people better-quality care than others (Institute of Medicine [IOM], 2003).

POLICY ADVOCACY LEARNING CHALLENGE 4.1

Identifying Types of Prejudice

Identify some kinds of prejudice displayed by professionals and staff who work in other sectors, such as the education, safety-net, mental health, child welfare, gerontology, and immigration sectors. Could you provide micro policy advocacy to people who experience this prejudice?

Negative Responses to Client Behaviors

Some professionals and staff may be biased against clients who are not "good" clients, such as those who are excessively compliant and noncommunicative, do not ask important questions, do not seek alternatives, and do not educate themselves about their specific problems. Unless their providers take the time to elicit their ideas and level of information, they often do not receive full explanations. Social workers should not let bothersome actions and behaviors distract them from the ethical goal of offering a person optimal care.

Narrow Mindsets

Professionals sometimes have excessively narrow perspectives. Many counselors focus on clients' psychological state sufficiently that they ignore realities and life pressures that they experience, such as insufficient resources, lack of job training, and poor housing. Some physicians rely excessively on *technological remedies*. They may not refer patients with mood disorders or other mental conditions for counseling—or they may simply give them medications without referring them to mental health experts. They may not consider implications of specific surgeries or medications for consumers' employability or lifestyles. They may not warn consumers of side effects of specific treatments that might have led them not to agree to them.

Many providers are *excessively specialized*, not able to see beyond the confines of their practices and specialties. For example, older people may see an array of specialists who treat them for separate conditions but are unaware that others have given them medications that adversely interact with ones that they have prescribed. Specialists often do not communicate with clients' primary physicians, who often do not follow their care even when they receive surgery and other treatments in hospitals. Many of them do not refer consumers with mental health problems to psychiatrists, psychologists, or social workers.

Professionals sometimes suffer from excessive *insularity* that leads them *not* to link their services to clients' households and communities, even when their clients might benefit from community-based mental health services, job-training services, alternative medicine, welfare programs, childcare services, schools, rehabilitation services, services for seniors, services for disabled people, independent-living programs, and physical therapy programs—to name only a few of them.

Inadequate Communication

Consumers often do not receive information from providers sufficient to enable them to make intelligent choices, as in the case of a psychiatrist who fails to inform a patient about the side effects of specific medications. They often receive information that they cannot understand because it uses terms and concepts beyond their grasp. People with LEP often cannot understand English sufficiently to comprehend mental health, medical, educational, and other options discussed with them. Providers often fail to listen to consumers.

Lack of Ethical Reasoning Skills

Some professionals possess inadequate ethical reasoning skills. They may believe they have given consumers sufficient information to make informed choices, even when they have not. They may believe they have protected confidential information, only to divulge it to family members and others without seeking the consumer's permission. They may believe that they have honored the ethical value of honesty but failed to warn clients about the likely side effects of treatments and medications.

Lack of Knowledge of Relevant Research

Some providers are unaware of recent empirical data that suggest that specific consumers would likely benefit from specific helping strategies. Despite in-service training and continuing education, many providers are not current with existing research (IOM, 2008).

Unwillingness to Consider New Approaches

Some providers may be aware of specific evidence-based findings pertinent to the care of specific consumers, but not want to change their customary approach. Berwick (2003) contends that "innovators" constitute a relatively small portion of the workforce of most organizations, with many of the other staff not implementing innovations—or waiting until they see others who have adopted innovations, even years later.

Misinterpretation of Research

Professionals sometimes interpret research incorrectly. Perhaps they think it is more definitive than it is. Perhaps they do not realize that it applies to a specific population, but is untested or not successful with other populations. Perhaps they do not realize that some interventions bring short-term improvements that do not last.

Bureaucratic and Organizational Malfunctioning

Social workers deliver services in relatively complex organizational settings. These settings possess not only bureaucratic structures, but rules, protocols, budgets, and cultures that profoundly influence their provision of services. Clients, too, must navigate these bureaucracies, which often appear confusing to them.

Failure to Follow a Preferred Sequence of Events

Errors can often be reduced if providers follow a specific sequence of actions when treating certain clients. Researchers have discovered, for example, that rates of injuries and deaths in intensive care units are markedly reduced when health professionals follow a sequence of actions (Gawande, 2010). A patient may not otherwise be given a test, medication, or treatment at the correct time—or at all. If there is no sequence of events to follow, a consumer may receive the wrong test result or even the wrong surgical procedure. Pharmacists may not have been able to read a physician's handwriting, leading to an incorrect medication. Nurses may fail to give proper medications.

POLICY ADVOCACY LEARNING EXERCISE 4.2

Assume that an elderly person with early-stage dementia and some disorientation receives help from a professional in a mental health clinic. Assume as well that the professional focuses primarily on relieving the presenting symptoms, such as with medications provided by a consulting psychiatrist.

1. What key questions might the professional have asked during this visit that might have led to better services? These questions may be about, for example, the home situation, the presence of other family members, the possible dangers the client might encounter in her or his environment, the client's diet, and other medications that the elderly person currently receives.
2. Does this failure to ask questions parallel failure to follow a preferred sequence of events in intensive care units?

Lack of Team Practice

Many people with chronic diseases, substance abuse problems, and serious mental problems benefit from team practice that couples medical assistance, "talking therapies," and other professional assistance such as physical therapy, nutritional counseling, and occupational therapy. Many elderly people benefit from team practice. Many barriers frustrate team practice, however. Insurance companies and health plans often do not fund it. Some physicians do not want to share their patients—or their medical information—with other professionals. Many mental health clinics lack resources to hire or to contract with members of multiple professions.

Lack of Knowledge

Clients suffer violations of their rights or nonoptimal care because specific professionals lack knowledge of specific regulations, protocols, and standards. Perhaps they did not participate in briefings or in-service training. Perhaps they received inaccurate information from other staff. Perhaps they are unaware of specific accreditation standards. Perhaps they possess a mistaken view that their professional status makes them not subject to policies and procedures, and they are not aware of specific court rulings and regulations or of relatively new policies. They may not realize that they could be subject to litigation and legal sanctions if they fail to adhere to specific regulations and laws.

Lack of Policy Guidance

Policies and procedures may not even exist in some situations—or may be excessively vague. Assume, for example, that child welfare staff in a particular jurisdiction conduct an investigation to see if a specific child has been abused or neglected. Not finding evidence to support this finding, they terminate the investigation—but fail to refer the child and her family to supportive services after they document serious mental problems of the child and one of her parents.

POLICY ADVOCACY LEARNING CHALLENGE 4.3

When Does a Social Worker Move From Micro to Mezzo Policy Advocacy?

Should a social worker, when encountering the preceding situation, move from micro policy advocacy to mezzo policy advocacy to develop a policy that defines the child welfare agency's obligation to children and their parents even when they do not find evidence of abuse or neglect?

Causation by Multiple Factors

Many factors, operating in tandem, often compromise the care of specific patients or lead to violation of their ethical rights. Perhaps a consumer is subject to prejudice, receives inadequate communication, and runs into bureaucratic snafus. The work of micro policy advocates is often made more complex as the number of causal factors increases.

CHALLENGE 5: DEVELOPING A STRATEGY TO ADDRESS A CLIENT'S UNRESOLVED PROBLEM

Social workers can accomplish the strategizing task by dividing it into steps, including deciding who will provide advocacy services at the outset, setting goals and time frames, identifying assets and liabilities, assessing motivations of decision makers, allocating responsibility as the advocacy intervention proceeds, developing a sequence of actions, and developing specific actions.

Step 1: Deciding Who Will Provide Advocacy Services at the Outset

Even when triaging suggests that specific consumers possess indicators for micro policy advocacy, healthcare professionals cannot always provide it for legitimate reasons. They sometimes can find advocacy shortcuts, as well.

Social workers often encounter daunting workloads when their regular work is combined with paperwork and other bureaucratic requirements. The urgency of their regular work may sometimes trump case advocacy because micro policy advocacy takes time, particularly in complex situations.

Social workers sometimes decide that positive outcomes are highly unlikely in specific instances. Perhaps they have attempted policy advocacy on prior occasions with a particular consumer with no success, or a consumer does not want advocacy, or they cannot gain access to specific consumers who might otherwise benefit from it.

Micro policy advocates often question the status quo, such as the failure of mental health staff to obtain informed consent, follow evidence-based practices, or attend to consumers' depression or anxiety. They may decide that they would encounter excessive risk if they injected themselves into certain situations, jeopardizing their ability to engage in micro policy advocacy in future situations.

Social workers need to beware, however, of using rationalizations to refrain from engaging in micro policy advocacy, such as deciding they do not have time to do it or that they might experience adverse repercussions. They need to remember that they have an ethical obligation to increase consumers' well-being and to protect their ethical rights even when it is inconvenient or expedient not to engage in it. They may also wrongly conclude that they will suffer repercussions or wrongly decide that case advocacy takes a lot of time.

Social workers should also realize that they can use legitimate shortcuts and avoidance even in those situations where they cannot devote much time to micro policy advocacy or fear repercussion. They can try to convince other professionals to provide advocacy to a particular client—what is called "advocacy punting." These staff may have more time in particular situations, more expertise relevant to a specific consumer, or "better standing" with a particular professional or staff member—and they may be better able to fit advocacy into their workloads at a particular moment.

They may also diminish the likelihood of adverse repercussions to themselves by empowering specific consumers to self-advocate. Consumers possess considerable power in advocacy situations based on their right to self-determination and their ability to seek another provider if they are dissatisfied with their current services. Micro policy advocates can empower consumers by referring them to the Internet, educating them, coaching them, and engaging in role plays with them.

Step 2: Establishing a Goal and a Time Frame

Micro policy advocacy requires the development of a goal, a subgoal, and a time frame. Goals that contain these three components become actionable ones that can be monitored to see if consumers have actually achieved them. The goals can be illustrated by using the seven core problems that consumers often confront in human services:

- *Overarching goal:* Surmount a financing problem as it adversely affects a consumer's medical care. *Subgoal:* Gain eligibility to Medicaid to allow financing of specific tests, medications, or procedures. *Time frame:* Obtain eligibility within two weeks and receive charitable care in the interim.
- *Overarching goal:* Surmount a possible threat to a consumer's quality of care. *Subgoal:* Help a consumer obtain a second opinion. *Time frame:* Obtain it within three weeks so the consumer can better decide what course to take.
- *Overarching goal:* Obtain specific preventive services. *Subgoal:* Have a diabetic consumer receive a consultation from a nutrition consultant. *Time frame:* Obtain it within one month.
- *Overarching goal:* Obtain culturally relevant care. *Subgoal:* Obtain the services of a certified translator in Vietnamese. *Time frame:* Obtain the translator within one hour.
- *Overarching goal:* Obtain an appointment to relevant resources outside a specific agency. *Subgoal:* Obtain an appointment at a local welfare office to make applications for SNAP (food stamps) and to obtain information for filing for an Earned Income Tax Credit (EITC). *Time frame:* Obtain the appointment within two days.
- *Overarching goal:* Address excessive anxiety, depression, or other mental issues. *Subgoal:* Have a suicidal consumer in the emergency room get an appointment with a mental health provider at a mental health agency. *Time frame:* Obtain it within three days, using medications as well as daily phone calls in the interim.
- *Overarching goal:* Protect the ethical rights of a consumer. *Subgoal:* Obtain separate consultations for a client for palliative care and hospice rather than regular care. *Time frame:* Obtain two consultations within five hours.

Micro policy advocates may decide to accomplish two or more goals in the same time frame, such as helping a consumer surmount a financial issue *and* obtain quality services—both within two weeks. They may decide to accomplish these two goals sequentially, beginning with one of them and progressing to another after the first has been achieved.

Step 3: Identifying Assets and Liabilities

It is sometimes useful to make a list of assets and liabilities in the context—and their locations outside or within the site of a micro policy intervention. Assume, for example, that a social worker wants to help a client get into a smoking cessation program. Also assume that the client is uninsured and Latino—and has early-stage emphysema. Also assume that the physician who has treated him has made no effort to get him into such a program. Assets and liabilities are summarized in Table 4.1.

Even with her limited information, the advocate finds that the context contains both favorable and unfavorable factors—suggesting that a positive outcome is possible. Clinics do exist. Other physicians in the hospitals have referred consumers to them. State subsidies do exist. Empirical evidence supportive of smoking cessation is strong. Yet liabilities also exist. This physician has not made prior referrals. She believes that this patient is less likely to join a smoking cessation program if the physician does not refer him to it, because he has told her that "my smoking must not be that important because my physician did not discuss it with me."

She realizes, too, that she does not know some important facts. Do culturally competent and accessible services exist for this client? Does a smoking cessation clinic exist near her home? Does it have evening or weekend hours and a short wait list? What costs would he bear because he has no health insurance? By listing the assets and liabilities, she concludes that a favorable outcome is possible.

Table 4.1 Evaluating the Context

	Assets	Liabilities
External	1. Evidence-based research exists 2. State-subsidized clinics at community sites exist	1. No referral system in place
Internal	1. Other physicians have referred people to smoking cessation programs 2. Accreditation standards require referrals for people with lung disease	1. Client's physician hasn't made referrals in the past

Step 4: Assessing the Motivations of Decision Makers

Advocates' effectiveness often hinges on their ability to assess the motivations of specific decision makers. Why did the client's physician *not* refer this person to a smoking clinic even though he has early-stage lung disease? Did he fear offending him? Was he not aware that smoking cessation programs exist? How likely was it that the client could be persuaded to get help from the smoking cessation program even without the physician's referral? Do subsidies from the state to the clinic allow significant or full financing of services from this clinic? Micro policy advocates need to factor into their strategies ways to address these motivations effectively to increase the chances that decision makers will change directions and take different actions that enhance clients' well-being.

Step 5: Allocating Responsibility

Social workers must decide who takes responsibility for advocacy intervention. Different possibilities exist. They can become the prime movers in an advocacy intervention, such as with comatose consumers, consumers with limited cognitive function, consumers with serious mental disorders, or consumers overwhelmed by their health condition or by external realities. Some clients may expect them to be the prime mover under these circumstances.

Social workers can empower consumers to advocate for themselves. They provide them with knowledge about resources, health conditions, treatment options, and relevant research, whether by giving them written materials or by helping them to use the Internet if they do not already have sufficient Internet skills. They may coach them, such as by helping them to develop questions to ask medical staff. They may help them to be appropriately assertive, giving them suggestions about how to ask questions or communicate with medical staff to increase the likelihood of successful outcomes. They may engage in role plays with them where they assume the role of the medical staff.

Even when empowering consumers, social workers may wish to keep in touch with specific consumers to see if they have taken key actions. They may discover, for example, that certain clients fail to follow through with specific actions. Perhaps other life events intrude so that they cannot advocate for themselves.

Social workers can partner with consumers as well as other medical staff in a team arrangement. They can decide who does what and by when—and select someone to be the lead person who keeps track of progress. In partnering arrangements, a lead person tracks the implementation of the strategy—and troubleshoots when key actions are not taken.

Social workers can initiate a team approach where a number of professionals and family members participate in an action system. Perhaps a nurse works with a consumer to obtain an appointment for a second opinion *as* a social worker helps him get an appointment in a community-based agency and *as* the consumer agrees to adhere to specific medications and to keep the appointments. Perhaps progress on these three actions is monitored online, by telephone, or through a case conference to be held at a specified time. Considerable research suggests that people with chronic diseases need to be helped by a team to obtain a full range of interventions not available to them under solo practice. For example, diabetics need help in monitoring their weight, living a healthy lifestyle, and monitoring their insulin as well as occupational therapy, counseling, and participation in support groups.

Professionals can shift their roles as events unfold. Perhaps someone begins as the prime mover but discovers a family member or friend who is willing and able to take more responsibility. Perhaps a client who had wanted to take responsibility for self-advocacy wants some assistance.

Step 6: Developing a Sequence of Actions

Advocates plan a tentative sequence of communications, fact finding, contacts, and meetings at the outset of their work—with some contingencies included in it. In the case of the Latino with lung disease who will not join a smoking cessation clinic unless his physician "prescribes" it and signs a referral form to a specific smoking cessation clinic, she decides to implement the following sequence of actions:

- She will conduct some research for the client, such as finding a smoking cessation clinic near his residence that has evening and weekend hours, provides free services, and has Spanish-speaking staff.
- She will ask the client to take this information to his physician and ask for a medical referral to this clinic—and to let her know if he has received it.
- *Contingency.* If he does not receive the referral, she will work with the physician's nurse to get the referral from another physician in the clinic that serves people with lung disease.
- She will ask the client to get an appointment at the clinic—telling him to see a specific Spanish-speaking staff person whom she has contacted by telephone—and she will ask him to leave a message on her cell phone to let her know whether he kept his appointment.
- *Contingency:* She will place in his medical record a notation that he failed to keep his appointment if she learns this from the clinic staff person—and suggest further discussions with him about how his smoking could greatly increase the progression of his lung disease.

Different kinds of sequences exist. The simplest of them involves a single action by an advocate who helps a person who lacks skills or ability to self-advocate. Perhaps she asks a physician to make a medical referral for counseling that she can present to a hospital-based psychiatrist. A more complex sequence of action takes place when an advocate empowers a client to get this referral from his physician. The advocate works with the client at two points in time: coaching him to get the referral from his physician and coaching him to get an appointment with the psychiatrist. An even more complex sequence of action occurs when the advocate initiates a team approach that involves a physician, a social worker, a psychologist, and an occupational therapist. Suppose that the social worker assumes the lead role in helping a client with serious mental illness. She initiates a case conference to help a consumer receive medications (from the physician), counseling (from the psychologist), and job readiness and job search skills training (from the occupational therapist). She monitors the client's progress and orchestrates another case conference in three months.

Sequences also vary by the extent to which they include contingencies and question marks. Contingencies take place when case advocates anticipate two (or more) possible courses of action depending on the outcome of a particular meeting or event, as illustrated by the referral to a smoking cessation program where two contingencies were identified. Question marks can be placed on a sequence of actions where the case advocate does not know what specific actions might be needed after a certain point in the sequence. Perhaps a client will have numerous options—and the advocate does not know what they will be until an interview, case conference, diagnosis, or medical procedure is complete.

Step 7: Selecting Specific Actions

Social workers possess a smorgasbord of actions that they can take during their micro policy advocacy.

Using Technology

Social workers can use technology to facilitate their advocacy in several ways. They can use spreadsheets to identify the goals, subgoals, and timelines of an advocacy intervention. They can select specific activities, as well as who does them and by when. If they evolve a team approach where different people agree to perform specific actions, they can enter them into the spreadsheet and record when they are completed. They can email spreadsheets that show what activities have been accomplished and which ones have not. For simpler advocacy plans, they can resort to email or texts between the lead person and those clients who have Internet access.

Empowering Consumers

Advocates can empower consumers in many ways. They can show them Internet sources that may be useful to them—and give them some instruction about how to distinguish between accurate and inaccurate information.

Advocates can refer clients to support groups that meet within a hospital or clinic or that hold meetings in community-based organizations, schools, and religious organizations. The members of support groups often give clients invaluable information as well as emotional support. They often encourage members to be appropriately assertive.

They can direct clients to reliable sources of data about specific institutions and providers on the Internet.

Advocates can help clients develop a list of questions *before* they see providers. They might ask about treatment options and the side effects that could accompany them. They can obtain information about the skills and experience of the staff that might help particular clients. They can inform them about their ethical rights, such as disclosure of information, so that they can make informed choices. Advocates can give consumers hotlines, as well as names of advocacy groups outside their hospitals or clinics, to help them contest decisions by insurance companies or managed-care plans about the coverage and financing of specific medical procedures, tests, and medications.

Advocates can empower specific consumers by coaching them to prepare for specific encounters with agency staff. They can encourage them to be appropriately assertive. They can give them a list of specific questions they might wish to ask. They can encourage them to have a spouse, family member, or friend accompany them.

Arranging Case and Family Conferences

Social workers can arrange case conferences that include the staff at an agency and a client to discuss available services and their likely cost.

If a retirement facility is disinclined to admit an elderly person because of his medical condition, an advocate can orchestrate a case conference to discuss why he was rejected—and to see if the decision can be reversed.

Case conferences can be used to arbitrate or settle disputes between a client and an agency, such as over the cost of services, the effectiveness of services, or any other issue. Denial of errors in hospitals and clinics harms not only the institution by increasing malpractice lawsuits, but often has a devastating impact on consumers and their families (Delbanco & Bell, 2007). Clients sometimes need a place where they can voice their criticisms of the services that they received even if they do not seek redress.

Family conferences can usefully expose different points of view so that they can be factored into the decision-making process. Disagreements can be brought into the open so that they can be resolved.

Locating External Advocates

Some consumers will believe that they cannot seek redress unless they use external advocates, whether advocacy groups, government personnel who regulate and oversee healthcare in a specific jurisdiction, private attorneys, or public-interest attorneys such as those in legal aid organizations.

Many advocacy organizations advocate for specific consumers. Some of them mediate among insurance companies, medical administrators, and consumers to solve specific reimbursement or coverage issues—often successfully. Others request that specific clients gain services or resources to which they are entitled, such as translation services, equipment funded by Medicare for older persons, and referrals to home health agencies before they are discharged.

Other advocacy organizations seek to educate consumers about services and resources that they can obtain on discharge, such as support groups for people with breast cancer, diabetes, and many other health conditions. They sometimes visit clients in hospitals before they are discharged.

Many organizations possess internal arbitration mechanisms so that aggrieved consumers can seek redress without taking legal action. Many managed-care organizations require enrollees to sign agreements that require them to use arbitration rather than courts to seek redress.

Many private attorneys represent clients. They may threaten or take legal action against specific medical staff or specific hospitals or clinics, insurance companies, health plans, and managed-care organizations. Public-interest attorneys often represent people who lack the resources to obtain private attorneys.

Making Referrals

Advocates become involved in referrals when they believe that consumers will not otherwise receive them. They can coach consumers to call for appointments on repeated occasions, often early in the morning, in hopes of getting an appointment through a cancellation. Advocates can increase the odds that specific people will receive prompt service by making direct contact with intake staff—and by getting to know them professionally.

Some clients do not keep appointments even when they have serious problems. Advocates may sometimes email or phone specific clients to increase the odds that they keep the appointment—and then help them, or urge them, to reschedule them if they miss them.

Finding Resources

Clients often need to obtain eligibility to specific programs. Advocates not only inform clients of these programs and their guidelines, but also help them prevent adverse decisions by educating them about their requirements. They inform them about requirements that they receive eligibility information in their own language—or with special materials that are developed for people with limited literacy. They inform them that they have the right to appeal eligibility decisions.

Using Intermediaries

Social workers often use intermediaries as advocates for their clients, such as their supervisors, highly placed nurses, administrators, or physicians. These intermediaries often have clout, information, and resources that may be helpful to a client. Perhaps a client needs a referral to palliative care or hospice—and a social worker knows that a specific nurse has oversight responsibilities for these programs. This nurse can easily initiate an action system for the client to get expedited information to her, such as having personnel from these programs visit the client soon after she calls them.

Honoring Clients' Wishes

Clients often find that some of their wishes are not honored or are marginalized by staff in a particular agency, clinic, or hospital. Advocates can acknowledge that clients and patients have the ethical right to decide what services to use, as long as they are mentally competent.

Citing Regulations, Protocols, and Ethical Guidelines

Advocates can take several actions when they observe apparent violations of regulations or court rulings by other professionals, such as a specific court ruling that requires that clients give their "informed consent" to a mental health treatment. They can remind or inform people about these regulations or court rulings. They can ask, "Are we following guidelines that mandate us to . . . ?" Or, "Have we heard what course of treatment the patient desires?" They can discuss possible penalties that providers can encounter if they violate specific regulations. They can report violations to an intermediary, such as an administrator. They can report them to a relevant department, such as the compliance or risk management department. They can inform clients where they can find specific regulations.

Steering Clients

Social workers sometimes steer consumers to specific programs and professionals because they believe they offer outstanding services—and steer them away from programs and professionals that they believe offer inferior services.

CHALLENGES 6, 7, AND 8: IMPLEMENTING AND ASSESSING MICRO POLICY STRATEGY

A micro policy advocate may assist a client in developing strategy, but the advocate and the client will succeed only if it receives support from those officials who confer resources, opportunities, benefits, or rights to a specific client. They need to implement this strategy with skill. Micro policy advocates and clients assess specific advocacy interventions to determine their relative success in improving the well-being of specific clients. If they are not successful, they may provide another advocacy intervention, possibly relying on a different strategy.

LEARNING MICRO POLICY ADVOCACY SKILLS

During this chapter, we have discussed various skills that are integral to micro policy advocacy—skills that have been identified by a panel of 300 social workers, nurses, and medical residents as important to advocacy at the level of individual patients, but that also apply to micro policy advocacy in other settings (Jansson, article forthcoming on data from the federally funded project "Improving Healthcare Outcomes Through Advocacy"). Curiously, these specific skills are not usually covered in foundation-level practice and behavior classes in social work schools that give relatively scant attention to "case advocacy," a term often used in social work to describe advocacy at the level of individual clients (see, e.g., the marginal discussion of case advocacy in such widely used texts on social work practice as Hepworth, Rooney, Larsen, Dewberry Rooney, & Strom-Gottfried, 2005). Use Table 4.2 to rank your current level of skill with respect to this list of skills. Have they been covered in your direct practice courses or other courses? See if you can actually use and hone them in your professional work.

Table 4.2   Sixteen Micro Policy Advocacy Skills Identified by 300 Health Professionals

Please rate the extent you have the following skills from 1 (not at all) to 5 (high level).

1. I have the skill to assess why specific clients have unresolved problems.

2. I have the skill to develop alternative strategies to help clients resolve specific problems.

3. I have the skill to use influence to persuade others to help specific clients.

4. I have the skill to use appropriate assertiveness to help specific clients obtain assistance from others.

5. I have the skill to use intermediaries to facilitate micro policy advocacy.

6. I have the skill to negotiate and bargain on behalf of specific clients.

7. I have the skill to resolve conflicts that arise during micro policy advocacy

8. I have the skill to empower clients to advocate for themselves.

9. I have the skill to coach clients to advocate for themselves.

10. I have the skill to advocate clients' wishes with other professionals.

11. I have the skill to call specific unresolved problems to the attention of other professionals.

12. I have the skill to decide which unresolved problems warrant immediate attention and to prioritize them.

13. I have the skill to faithfully represent clients' wishes when they cannot advocate for themselves.

14. I have the skill to question plans or actions of other professionals to improve clinical outcomes and avoid adverse events.

15. I have the skill to network with other professionals to facilitate micro policy advocacy.

16. I have the skill to refer clients to community resources.

LEARN HOW A SOCIAL WORKER ENGAGED IN MICRO POLICY ADVOCACY

Read this case study of micro policy advocacy and then address the questions at the end of the case.

POLICY ADVOCACY LEARNING EXERCISE 4.4

Engaging in Micro Policy Advocacy: Why Is It Particularly Needed by and for Low-Income People of Color?

Jim Smith is a 45-year-old African American male from South Los Angeles. He is also a member of the poor working class and is uninsured. Jim has been married for the past 11 years to his high school sweetheart, Ava, and they live in a small, two-bedroom home. Jim is well known in his community as the neighborhood mechanic. For the past 20 years, Jim has generated his income by fixing the cars of his neighbors and others they refer to him. His wife, Ava, has spent the past eight years as a full-time lead cashier for Walmart. The Smiths barely generate enough money to pay all their bills, but they are content with their life. They are most pleased about having their own home, which

(Continued)

(Continued)

they hope to pay off in the next six years. Jim's other accomplishment is six years of sobriety following a crack addiction that robbed him of his early adult years.

Yet the last three years have been extremely difficult for the Smiths. In 2006, the couple lost their 14-year-old son, Tom, to gang violence. While walking home from school, he got caught in gunfire between two rival gangs, was shot in the head, and died instantly. Both parents were devastated by the loss of their son. Jim has taken Tom's death the hardest because he blames himself. He thinks he failed as a father because he did not protect his son from the gang violence in his community as his father did for him. But Jim will not admit this to anyone, not even to himself. Instead, he has spent the past three years building up a "thick skin" that allows him to avoid his feelings and avoid talking to anyone, including his wife, about his deepest thoughts. In fact, his wife frequently refers to him as being indifferent to everyone and everything around him. In addition, Jim's health has diminished. Jim relapsed six months after his son's death and began smoking crack cocaine again.

Jim has been uninsured most of his life. His wife's job offers various health insurance plans, but due to the high costs, they decided it would work better for their budget if they paid for insurance only for their daughter Lily and their son. Jim intentionally decided to pay for healthcare only as needed. Whenever Jim has felt sick and needed medical attention in the past, he has first attempted to receive service at a small community clinic near his house. However, if the clinic is closed or can't offer free care, Jim's next resort is the emergency room at a public hospital. Jim has felt most comfortable going to nearby health facilities because he is able to receive help there primarily from African American doctors. Jim has a strong prejudice against white and foreign doctors; he doesn't think that they understand his culture and that they look down on black people.

Jim sometimes uses a small community clinic that offers primary care to poor Los Angeles residents. Most of the clinic's patients receive Medicaid, and a smaller number are part of the working poor, like Jim, who do not qualify for Medicaid but also do not make enough money to pay for health insurance. Because the clinic has had difficulty surviving, it has had to cut down on its psychosocial services, including free transportation and social service programs, in order to continue providing medical care to its patients.

What is more, during the same year that Jim lost his son, the clinic made a dramatic cut in its mental health services. Jim's last visit to this clinic was three months after his son's death. He was complaining of frequent headaches and dizziness. Medical tests ruled out any chronic illnesses, and Jim was found to be in fair health with the exception of the beginning signs of high blood pressure. Jim's doctor was also troubled by his flat affect, but due to time constraints, the doctor did not address this matter with Jim. Instead, he prescribed Jim medication for his blood pressure, gave him a handout on how to reduce it, and hurriedly moved on to his 10th patient for that morning. Jim's depression symptoms went unaddressed and untreated. No follow-up care was planned. Moreover, due to fiscal problems, the clinic was forced to close permanently toward the end of the year.

Several months after closure of the clinic, Jim's depression worsened. He was very unreliable in fixing people's cars, stayed in bed most of the time, and showed little interest in doing anything, and his wife began to suspect his relapse due to his leaving the house at odd hours at night. What is more, Jim did not comply with the medication given to him before the clinic closed. Jim's wife pleaded with him to go to an emergency room for a medical evaluation, but it wasn't until he fainted in the shower that he agreed to the visit.

A medical evaluation at the emergency room discovered that Jim was suffering from hypertension and a major depressive disorder. The attending psychiatrist connected Jim to the hospital's mental health program for depression as well as drug abuse counseling. Despite the financial and emotional strain that Jim's wife was experiencing, she was very supportive of him and made sure he made it to his appointments. Jim was also doing well through the services offered to him through a public hospital. Unfortunately, the inevitable announcement that it would soon be closing was a significant stumbling block for Jim's recovery. Many of the services and medical staff that Jim had built a relationship with were closed and reassigned to other hospitals, respectively. Jim was referred to yet another public hospital because it was nearest to him. Nevertheless, because Jim did not perceive it as a part of the "black community," he resisted going to it.

Accordingly, Jim spent the next six months ignoring his health problems again. His depression had fortunately improved to where he had energy to work. Similarly, although Jim's drug usage did not end completely, he was able to contain his indulgence to the weekends only. His wife continued to worry about him and the direction their marriage was headed. For the last two years she has become the sole breadwinner in addition to wiping out their savings account to help pay for their bills. And when she thought things couldn't get any, worse they did. Jim had been complaining again of feeling fatigued and having headaches. The left side of his body was extremely weak, and he occasionally dripped blood out of his nose when he sneezed. His wife took him to the public hospital, where he learned that he had experienced a stroke.

Jim's experience at the public hospital was unforgettable. He had to endure a long wait. His wife took him in to the emergency room on a Thursday night, and he was not seen by the doctor until Friday afternoon. The first thing that the doctor, a white male, did after reviewing his medical test was tell him was that his stroke was induced by his drug usage and that he needed to stop. Jim felt scared, embarrassed, and insulted. He decided to show his emotions with anger. He was belligerent with the doctor and accused him of being insensitive and ignorant of the problems of black people. The doctor decided not to argue with the patient. He admitted Jim to the hospital for further evaluation and marked him off as being just like the other drug

(Continued)

(Continued)

addicts with poor coping skills whom he had treated in the past. The doctor also referred him to be seen by a social worker.

Jim was ambivalent about meeting with the social worker, but he was also not consciously aware of how eager he was to vent his frustrations to someone. He took 35 minutes alone to share some of his grievances and losses, starting with his son, his severed relationships with his past healthcare providers, and his decreased level of functioning as a result of his stroke. He also spoke about his marital problems and drug usage. The social worker actively listened to Jim and offered him emotional support. He came down hard on himself for first not taking care of his son and second for not taking care of himself.

The social worker guided Jim in putting his experiences in the past three years into a different perspective. She helped him to differentiate between what he had control over and what was out of his control. For example, the social worker used Jim's past success of six years' sobriety to argue that he did have the power to quit using drugs. On the other hand, she also explored his lack of control over the closures of his previous healthcare sites. Afterward, Jim concluded that if he had been able to keep a longer relationship with his healthcare providers for regular follow-up visits, his health would not have diminished so severely and so quickly. He also regretted not buying health insurance, although he was still in a predicament where he could not afford it. The social worker decided to investigate whether Jim might qualify for SSI and Medicaid as a disabled person. The social worker talked to Jim's doctor, who stated that the patient's left side had a poor prognosis. Furthermore, the doctor estimated that his full recovery to where he could began fixing cars again could take six months to a year or longer.

Consequently, the doctor's prognosis meant that Jim might qualify for SSI and accordingly Medicaid as well. Therefore, the social worker directed Jim's wife to the nearest public aid office, where she could begin filling out an application for her husband. The social worker also convinced Jim's doctor to fill out the necessary paperwork to provide proof of his disability. Jim's wife is one of his biggest assets, yet the social worker could sense her physical and emotional fatigue and provided her with supportive counseling as well. Ava spoke of her frustrations with her husband's indifference toward her, his inability to help pay their bills, and her grief in relation to the loss of her son. The social worker encouraged Ava to take advantage of the counseling services offered to her through her insurance plans for both individual and couple's counseling.

In addition, the social worker helped Ava to file for paid leave from her job through the Family and Medical Leave Act of 1993. The Family Leave Act of 1993 allows eligible workers to take approximately six weeks off from work to care for a child or family member and receive 55% of their salary. The application requires documentation similar to that provided on Jim's SSI application in terms of showing the extent of his disability and its duration. The social worker once again spoke with the doctor to get the appropriate medical documentation needed for Ava's application and directed her to a number to call to request the application.

The social worker also attempted to address Jim's drug problem using motivational interviewing. Within this psychotherapy model, the social worker helped him to clarify his ambivalence toward terminating his drug usage. He stated that he was aware that crack is gradually killing him and that he needs to stop. He also stated that he doesn't like how his behavior is hurting his wife. Nevertheless, a part of him does not want to stop because the drug allows him to escape his reality and live in a state of bliss for brief periods of time. He also stated that sometimes he doesn't feel he deserves to live since his son isn't alive anymore.

The social worker reflected back their conversation, highlighting Jim's love for his son and his value for being a protector over his family. The social worker also thanked him for having the courage to share his pain with her and emphasized their conversation as being part of his walk in the right direction—to facing his fears and pains and regaining some of his hope. Moreover, the social worker asked Jim what other steps he would like to take, and he stated, "I would like more counseling." Accordingly, the social worker helped Jim and Ava set up an appointment for couple's counseling through her health insurance. The social worker also provided Jim with the contact information for a Cocaine Anonymous group in his community.

Overall, Jim spent one week in the hospital. He left the hospital with a better appreciation for the doctors and staff who helped him to receive his medical treatment despite not necessarily being a part of the "black community." Jim was more motivated to comply with his follow-up care at the outpatient clinic of the public hospital. Four weeks later, Ava received notification that her request for paid leave under the Family and Medical Leave Act had been accepted. Unfortunately, one week later, Jim received notification that his SSI/Medicaid application had been denied. The Smiths immediately called the social worker from the hospital to learn what they should do next. The social worker advised them to request an appeal hearing. She also advised them to call the SSI program to learn what documentation they lacked or needed more clarity. Last, the social worker referred them to speak to a legal aid representative familiar with government programs. Jim's case is still pending, but he and his wife are taking advantage of her paid leave time to reconnect to one another and encourage each other during this rough time in their lives.

1. Discuss how this family's well-being was greatly impacted by specific policies. Make a list of these many policies.
2. Discuss how the social worker developed multiple micro policy interventions.
3. Referring to Table 4.2, identify four specific skills that the social worker used as she developed these micro policy interventions.
4. Does this case enhance your understanding of the need to discuss micro policy advocacy in social work courses?

LEARNING OUTCOMES

You are now equipped to:

- Read the context
- Engage the eight challenges of micro policy advocacy discussed in Figure 3.1
- Analyze how a social worker engages in micro policy advocacy
- Identify specific skills needed by micro policy advocates

REFERENCES

Anderson, R. (1995). Revisiting the behavioral model and access to medical care: Does it matter? *Journal of Health and Social Behavior, 36,* 1–10.

Berwick, D. (2003). Disseminating innovations in health care. *Journal of the American Medical Association, 289,* 1969–1975.

Daley, J. (2001). A 58 year old woman dissatisfied with her care. *Journal of the American Medical Association, 285,* 2629–2635.

Delbanco, T., & Bell, S. (2007). Guilty, afraid, and alive: Struggling with medical error. *New England Journal of Medicine, 22*(2), 1682–1683.

Gawande, A. (2010). *The checklist manifesto: How to get things right.* New York, NY: Henry Holt.

Hepworth, D. H., Rooney, R. H., Larsen, J., Dewberry Rooney, G., & Strom-Gottfried, K. (2005). *Direct social work practice: Theory and skills* (7th ed.). Belmont, CA: Thomson Brooks/Cole.

Institute of Medicine. (2003). *Unequal treatment: Confronting racial and ethnic disparities in healthcare.* Washington, DC: National Academy Press.

Institute of Medicine. (2008). *Knowing what works in health care.* Washington, DC: National Academy Press.

Jansson, B. (2011). *Improving healthcare through advocacy: Guidelines for professionals.* Hoboken, NJ: John Wiley & Sons.

Perez-Pena, R. (2005, October 15). At a Bronx clinic, high hurdles for Medicaid Care. *New York Times,* p. A1.

Steiner, J. F. (2005). The use of stories in clinical research and health policy. *Journal of the American Medical Association, 294*(22).

Chapter 5

ENGAGING IN MEZZO POLICY ADVOCACY

Bruce S. Jansson and Gretchen Heidemann

LEARNING OBJECTIVES

In this chapter, you will learn how to:

1. Define mezzo policy advocacy

2. Identify five skills needed by mezzo policy advocates

3. Read the context of agencies and communities

4. Decide whether to proceed in agencies and communities

5. Decide where to focus in agencies and communities

6. Obtain decision makers' recognition of an unresolved problem in agencies and communities

7. Analyze the problem in agencies and communities

8. Develop a strategy to address the problem in agencies and communities

9. Develop support for the strategy or proposal in agencies and communities

10. Implement the strategy or policy in agencies and communities

11. Address whether the implemented strategy or proposal is effective in agencies and communities

12. Analyze a case example of mezzo policy advocacy

DEFINING MEZZO POLICY ADVOCACY

One of the 10 core competencies of the Council on Social Work Education is the ability of social workers to engage, assess, intervene, and evaluate at the micro, mezzo, and macro levels of practice. Social workers are infrequently trained *how* to provide these interventions, particularly at the micro and mezzo levels. This chapter discusses mezzo-level policy advocacy as an intervention that social workers can and should provide. We define mezzo policy advocacy as that which takes place in agencies and/or communities to address unresolved problems in the seven core areas (previously discussed) faced by groups of clients or residents. Mezzo policy advocacy seeks to change aspects of or conditions within the organization or community that contribute to the origin or maintenance of unresolved client/resident problems with respect to the seven core problems.

This chapter will identify key skills that mezzo policy advocates need to be successful at in their policy reform efforts. It will discuss each of the eight challenges from the multilevel policy advocacy framework in Chapter 3 as they apply to mezzo policy advocacy. It will offer an extended case example of the community of Watts in South Central Los Angeles, where mezzo policy advocates are working to develop much-needed social services, recreational facilities, and employment opportunities.

SKILLS NEEDED FOR MEZZO POLICY ADVOCACY

VIDEO LINK 5.1
Creating Hubs in Local Communities

Mezzo policy advocates need to have a number of skills to draw on to be effective in changing policies at the organizational and community levels. Below, we describe several skills that a mezzo policy advocate should develop.

1. *Initiating.* Mezzo policy advocates need to initiate policy-changing interventions. This is a critical skill, because failure to take initiative often means that the wishes of other individuals and officials prevail *even when they lead to dysfunctional policies.* Advocates need in general to be appropriately assertive. They have to place issues on the table while not unnecessarily provoking conflict.

2. *Influencing.* Mezzo policy advocates need to be able to influence other people to work with them to change specific policies. We discuss influence, or power, resources at more length in the next chapter.

3. *Negotiating and bargaining.* Mezzo policy advocates need to be able to negotiate and bargain with agency and community leaders to achieve their policy goals. They have to decide what outcomes or policy changes they want, while realizing that policy advocates often must compromise.

4. *Mediating conflicts.* Mezzo policy advocates need to be able to mediate conflicts between various stakeholder groups. They can mediate by identifying points or issues that competing groups have in common. They can help participants identify compromises. They can use process skills in task groups and committees to facilitate positive outcomes.

5. *Communicating.* Mezzo policy advocates need to be able to communicate with concerned citizens, agency heads, community leaders, public officials, and other people who can help resolve specific issues. The communication skills of policy advocates are often different from the communication skills direct-service professionals use with their clients. Policy participants often want to analyze broader issues that impact the quality and nature of services and programs. They want data that shed light on the nature of specific issues. They want to examine policy and program options. They want to know the cost of specific proposed reforms.

A PRELIMINARY CHALLENGE: READING THE CONTEXT OF AGENCIES AND COMMUNITIES

We use the term "mezzo *policy* advocacy" because social workers and their clients are surrounded by policy and policy-related factors in the organizations and communities in which they work; and because social workers have an ethical mandate to help resolve policy-related problems in agency and community settings with and on behalf of their clients. Like micro and macro policy advocates, mezzo policy advocates must be acutely aware of the context, which includes both opportunities and constraints, as they help groups of clients in agencies or groups of community residents. Contextual factors vary with different agencies, with different communities, and with different policy sectors. Regardless of which sector they work in, social workers must be aware of the unique and cross-cutting organizational policies that shape their work with clients and families, such as organizational budgets, eligibility guidelines, and service delivery protocols. Moreover, social workers working in *any* agency and within *any* sector must be aware of community-level factors that impact their clients, such as the existence or dearth of social services or advocacy groups, the civic engagement of residents, and community demographics, such as poverty, unemployment, and crime.

In this section, we briefly discuss the policy context of agencies: their mission statements, budgets, revenue streams, organizational culture, hierarchies, and key players (or personnel). We subsequently turn our attention to the policy context of communities: their demographics, social problems, distribution of services, level of civic engagement, involvement of community leaders and advocacy groups, presence of neighborhood councils and homeowners and business associations, involvement of law enforcement, and media presence.

The Policy Context of Agencies

Policies are essential to the functioning of all agencies. Below we discuss specific types of agency policies after discussing internal versus external agency policies, and formal versus informal agency policies.

Internal and External Policies

Agencies are affected by both internal and external policies. Internal policies establish specific rules, such as intake procedures, staffing requirements, content of services, reporting mechanisms, and a general statement about the program's purposes. Some details of funded programs are left relatively vague, so that units, departments, and staff must fill the gaps with their own policies. Some policies are originally external to agencies but are then internalized or "adopted," like the policies agencies accept when they take funding from governmental programs. An agency that has a number of externally funded programs (nonprofit agencies now receive the majority of their funds from the government and from foundations) will have multiple sets, or clusters, of these adopted policies. External policies, such as court rulings, shape agency policies as well. For example, the Tarasoff Decision requires social workers to inform intended victims when a client tells the worker that he or she intends to inflict bodily injury on them.

Formal and Informal Policies

Formal agency policies include mission statements, budgets, organizational charts, and formal written policies (such as eligibility guidelines, intake procedures, and service delivery protocols as they pertain to clients, as well as human resources policies, worker safety protocols, and ethics guidelines as they pertain to staff). Agencies are also influenced by many informal policies, including organizational culture, competition and collaboration from outside agencies, and values and preferences of staff. Both formal and informal policies have the power to shape staff's actions and choices at many points in their work and deliberations. Informal policies may diverge from official written policies, but they may also fill gaps when official policy is ambiguous (Chu & Trotter, 1974).

Mission Statements

Most nonprofit agencies have a mission statement that defines their priorities and direction (Hasenfeld, 1983). While relatively broad, mission statements establish the agency's general philosophy and help guide policies and practices related to the organization's purpose.

Written Policies

Agencies typically—but not always—have written policies that pertain to a number of interorganizational activities. These include but are not limited to service delivery policies (such as intake guidelines and referral policies), ethical practice policies, human resource policies (including those addressing hiring, grievances, and dismissals), worker safety protocols, administrative policies and procedures, meeting processes, evaluation practices, and board of directors bylaws. HR and worker safety policies provide structure and security to employees. Administrative policies ensure that the organization is run fairly and efficiently. Service delivery policies help clients/consumers know which services they are entitled to, how to access those services, and how long those services will last. Bylaws ensure that the board of directors operates ethically and efficiently.

These written policies provide a powerful system of checks and balances for all stakeholders within the organization. However, many small start-up nonprofits do not have such sophisticated policies and procedures in place. Moreover, even when such policies are in place, there is no guarantee that they will be followed. Indeed, examples of nonprofit organizations "behaving badly" abound. Watchdog and consumer information organizations, such as CharityWatch (charitywatch.org), and Charity Navigator (charitynavigator.org), play an important role in informing the public about the practices of nonprofit organizations. CharityWatch publishes an annual "Hall of Shame," spotlighting organizations that have egregiously violated basic ethical principles or otherwise acted out of concert with widely regarded standards. Such watchdog groups play an important role in educating the public and holding nonprofits accountable.

Revenue Streams

The sources from which an agency receives funding can heavily impact its policies. More than $335 billion was donated to charitable organizations in 2013 (www.charitynavigator.org). Of that, 15% was received from foundations. A typical request for proposals (RFP) from a foundation requires that the organization seeking funds agrees to certain policies regarding how it can use/disperse the funds, who can be served under the funded project, and in what types of activities the organization can engage. Organizations may also receive funding from city, county, state, and federal sources. This revenue is often also heavily regulated, which can constrict the recipient organization's activities.

Budgets

Agencies' annual budgets serve as symbolic policy statements. They shape agencies' priorities by distributing resources to various programs. To fully understand an agency's policies, one must examine both its present and its previous budgets to determine the agency's priorities and how they have changed (Gummer, 1990). Because service delivery is predicated on an organization's having funding, mezzo practitioners should pay careful attention to the budgetary process of their agency so that they have a clear understanding of funding streams and expenses.

Hierarchies and Organizational Charts

Anyone who seeks to change organizational policies should develop a clear understanding of hierarchies and divisions of labor. A hierarchy is the chain of command that gives high-level executives power to create policies, hire staff, and make budgets. The division of labor divides staff into units that focus on specific tasks. While many organizational theorists have sought ways to soften hierarchy and specialization within organizations, they remain enduring, important features of many agencies.

Hierarchy and division of labor are often reflected in an agency's organizational chart. The board of directors of nongovernmental and nonprofit agencies, which usually appears at the top of the organizational chart, makes many important policy decisions. The board establishes an agency's high-level policies (i.e., its mission), hires its executive director, oversees the development of personnel policies, examines the agency's budget, and serves as the general overseer of the organization. Executive directors (presidents or CEOs) and program directors (COOs) usually have powers that enable them to shape decisions for the entire agency. They develop the agency budget and present it to the board; participate in hiring, firing, promoting, and supervising staff; and shape the personnel and service delivery policies that guide the organization. Lower-level professionals and volunteers often carry out direct services to clients. As intermediaries between management and direct-service staff, supervisors often share the perspectives of both higher- and lower-level personnel. Program directors are directly impacted by policy choices and agency budgets for their particular division within the agency.

An organizational chart can be misleading. Organizational charts do not tell us which units or programs in an organization have considerable resources, and which the top executives favor. In addition, organizational charts imply that high-level individuals make most general policy choices, but they do not tell us who has power with respect to specific issues. Many political scientists have observed that the distribution of power often varies with the issue; persons who are exceedingly powerful concerning certain issues may have little or no power regarding other issues (Dahl, 1967). The organizational chart, moreover, does not reveal patterns of friendship and trust, enmity, or social distance that can develop among staff members. Nor does it tell us about human contacts that span different units of an organization or that cut across levels of the hierarchy, including ongoing informal clusters of people who share knowledge and who support one another.

Organizational Culture

The culture of an organization is a powerful factor that shapes the behaviors of various stakeholders, including administrators, employees, and clients. Mezzo policy advocates need to be keenly aware of the organizational culture of the agency or setting in which they are working to advance their reforms. When surveying the agency in which they work, advocates may discover that it conforms to one of the main types of organizational cultures proposed by Cook (1987).

Constructive organizations have collaborative environments where members of a group work together toward positive goals (Cook, 1987). These organizations are effective (their members are able to achieve complex tasks), self-actualizing (members are able to realize their personal potential), humanistic (members help others grow and develop), and affiliative (members cooperate with and develop pleasant relationships with others). In a constructive organization, advocates will likely find colleagues who are willing to partner with them and support their advocacy efforts. They may also find that they are able to appeal to higher-level goals as motivation for decision makers to adopt their reforms.

Passive/defensive organizations, in contrast, are characterized by social norms in which members interact with others in ways that do not threaten their own security (Cook, 1987). Members of passive/defensive cultures tend to feel pressure to please others, to avoid interpersonal conflict, and to unquestioningly follow rules and procedures. Advocates in a passive/defensive organization may find that they must appeal to their colleagues' need to please in order to recruit them to support proposed reforms, since members of this type of organization tend to avoid interpersonal conflict. They may also have to work strategically to convey how their proposed reforms do not threaten the security of high-level officials.

In aggressive/defensive organizations, people tend to focus on their own individual needs at the expense of the success of the group (Cook, 1987). This culture is characterized by opposition (members tend to be critical and cynical), power (members strive for prestige and status and desire to control others), competition (members work to protect their own status by outperforming others), and perfectionism (members have extremely high standards and place excessive demands on themselves and others). In aggressive/defensive organizations, advocates may find that they have to work largely alone to advance their reforms and may have to appeal to decision makers' desire for power and perfectionism in order to get their reforms adopted.

Collaboration and Competition

The role of collaboration and competition in influencing organizational policies—from dictating which programs will remain in operation to who is eligible for services—cannot be understated. Nonprofit organizations are forced to compete for increasingly scarce public and private dollars to maintain and expand their programs and services. Foundations, which provide funding to nonprofit and community-based organizations, increasingly call on these organizations to collaborate on special projects of concern to the community rather than operate independently. This allows funders to apply their dollars toward one goal that is achievable through collaboration, rather than to spread resources among many organizations that may only address a small piece of the problem.

Values and Preferences

Informal policies can be reflected in the values and preferences of staff members and the expression and interpretation of specific policies. For example, different staff members often have diverse and subjective notions concerning their organization's mission. While an official mission may stress services to families with single heads of households, some staff may want the agency to redirect its efforts toward serving single-mother-headed households over single-father-headed households. When confronting virtually identical client problems, one staff member may provide services based on traditional psychotherapy, while another may emphasize survival skills, advocacy, and empowerment.

POLICY ADVOCACY LEARNING CHALLENGE 5.1

Mapping Agency Policies

Take any agency with which you are familiar and trace:

- Its mission statement
- Its stated values, or any unstated values that you can determine
- Its revenue stream (i.e., primary funding sources)
- Its budget priorities (i.e., how it allocates funding across its services)
- Its organizational chart, including key personnel and their duties/functions
- Its ways of collaborating and competing with outside agencies

- Any aspects of informal organizational culture that you can determine, including organizational culture type (from those described above or from any typology in the extant literature)

Now, identify *any* written policy that exists within the organization. This can include a policy related to who qualifies for services, how clients or employees file grievances, or any other written policy.

With regard to the policy you identified, discuss or respond to the following questions:

1. How is the policy shaped by the organization's mission statement?
2. How is the policy shaped by the organization's revenue streams and budgetary priorities?
3. How is the policy shaped by the organization's culture?
4. Of the above, which has the most powerful influence on the particular policy you identified?
5. If you had a desire to reform or change the particular policy you identified, how might the most powerful factor you identified in #4 above influence whether and how you proceed with your advocacy efforts?

The Policy Context of Communities

Below we discuss various factors that shape community policies and form the back-drop to any policy change intervention a mezzo policy advocate may undertake.

VIDEO LINK 5.2
Quality of Life of Minority Youth

Type of Community

Many different types of communities exist. The terms *urban*, *rural*, and *suburban* are often given to communities to describe where they exist in relation to large cities. Typically, a large amount of commercial activity occurs in urban communities, and these communities can be extremely impoverished or extremely wealthy depending on the city's tax base and revenues. Rural communities are those located far from major cities and include small towns, villages, and remote farming communities. Similar to urban communities, rural communities span the range from extremely impoverished (such as parts of Appalachia and the deep South) to those comprising mostly middle-class residents to incredibly wealthy rural communities (e.g., those in California's wine country). The major economic driver in most rural communities is agriculture. Suburban communities are those located on the out-skirts of major cities. A map of the Chicago area, for example, lists dozens of sub-urbs located in 10 counties (including some in Indiana and Wisconsin) that spread out around Chicago proper. Communities that lie on the farthest outskirts of major metropolitan areas and are composed almost entirely of houses, schools, and retail locations (and are void of major commercial activity) are sometimes referred to as the "exurbs." Other types of communities that may not fit the urban/rural/suburban typology include college towns, resort towns, and mill towns.

Demographics

Communities' demographic characteristics are described by census data, which indicate whether they are demographically heterogeneous or homogeneous. Social work advocates should use census data to inform their policy reform initiatives. Census data can be used to determine whether the community contains a dominant ethnic group or a variety of ethnicities and whether a community is predominantly low income or affluent or possesses a mix of social classes. Census data indicate whether communities are relatively integrated or racially segregated and can be used to describe the extent of poverty and unemployment, homeownership, and many other factors that are important in understanding the social problems that may exist in the community.

Land Use and Zoning

Zoning is the practice of designating land within a jurisdiction, such as a city, town, or community, for various land-use purposes, such as commercial, industrial, residential, or recreational purposes. Zoning is often used to prevent new development from interfering with existing residents or businesses, and to preserve the "character" of a community. Because zoning is sometimes used for negative purposes, such as to control the social class and the ethnic makeup of neighborhoods, knowledge of these issues can be critical for the mezzo-level advocate. Exclusionary zoning measures may artificially maintain high housing costs through land-use regulations and maximum density requirements, which can exclude lower-income and "undesirable" groups from a given community.

Presence and Distribution of Services

Communities can be described by the extent to which they possess social service agencies and community groups that meet the social welfare needs of their residents. Many communities have a very high need for certain types of services, and yet these types of services are severely lacking. In other communities, social welfare services may be abundant. Communities that suffer high rates of high school dropout, gang violence, drug and alcohol addiction, homelessness, and incarceration are often devoid of the prevention and treatment services that would alleviate these social problems.

Civic Engagement

The extent to which members of a community vote and are otherwise engaged in civic activities is a major factor shaping the policies that emerge from and impinge upon communities. An engaged and informed citizenry is more likely to be able to secure needed services, ensure safety, and promote a high quality of life within a community. Those communities in which large numbers of residents are disenfranchised are often the same communities with high rates of poverty, unemployment, homelessness, and other social problems. This is a factor in many low-income communities of color where large numbers of people have been previously incarcerated and are no longer allowed to vote, *believe* that they are unable to vote, or believe that their vote does not make a difference.

POLICY ADVOCACY LEARNING CHALLENGE 5.2

Registering Homeless, Incarcerated, and Formerly Incarcerated People to Vote

By Gretchen Heidemann

In the lead-up to the 2004 Presidential election, which pitted George W. Bush against John Kerry, I worked as a voter registration coordinator. My job was to register homeless, incarcerated, and formerly incarcerated people to vote. Many homeless individuals living on the streets believed that they were not eligible to vote because they did not have a permanent address. On the contrary, in Los Angeles County where I was working, a homeless person could list the park or underpass or intersection where they slept as their address on a voter registration application, as long as they also provided an address where they could receive mail; this could be a relative's home, a social service agency, or a post office box. I also worked with county jail officials to register eligible individuals inside Los Angeles County jails to vote. A large proportion of jail inmates are individuals who have been charged but not yet sentenced, such as those awaiting trial. The logistics were quite complicated, but we successfully established the first-ever voter registration program inside the jail that year. I also worked to register formerly incarcerated people to vote. Although laws vary by states, in many places people who have served their sentence and are no longer on parole are eligible to vote. In many cases, I had to overcome fear and mistrust; some individuals with convictions were afraid that if they completed a voter registration card, they would be sent back to prison. These were all uphill battles, but my co-workers and I believed it was important for these groups of disenfranchised citizens to participate in key decisions that would impact their lives and their communities. On election night, we rented vans and picked people up from homeless shelters and from the streets and took them to the polls to vote.

Leaders and Key Informants

When addressing specific issues in communities, such as where to place social service organizations or how to mobilize opposition to certain policies, policy advocates need to discover which community residents, leaders, politicians, and institutions have traditionally focused on their issue. Community leaders might be rabbis or pastors in local faith-based institutions, directors of social service agencies, representatives of neighborhood councils, school principals, elderly residents who have resided in the community for a long time, or any other people who know the inner workings and politics of the community. These individuals are often referred to as key informants. Many resources are available to help mezzo policy advocates identify and interview key informants, whose expertise can be invaluable in policy change efforts within communities.

RESOURCE ON KEY INFORMANT INTERVIEWS

The UCLA Center for Health Policy Research provides a clear and easy-to-follow guide to conducting key informant interviews. It can be located at:

http://healthpolicy.ucla.edu/programs/health-data/trainings/Documents/tw_cba23.pdf

---

Existing Advocacy Groups

In seeking specific reforms in communities, policy advocates often affiliate with, consult, or enlist the support of community-based advocacy groups. These groups may include civic associations and local chapters of national groups, such as the National Association for the Advancement of Colored People (NAACP). Policy practitioners sometimes form coalitions representing social agencies and community groups when they want to oppose a specific measure or establish new programs (Dluhy, 1981).

Neighborhood Councils and Watch Groups. Community residents often organize themselves into groups—either formally or informally—for various purposes. Neighborhood watch groups began developing in the late 1960s in New York as a response to the rape and murder of a young woman in a park in Queens where over a dozen witnesses did nothing to stop the incident or apprehend the perpetrator. Neighborhood watches spread throughout the country and were a powerful force in many neighborhoods in the 1970s and 1980s. Where they still exist, these groups are typically devoted to crime and vandalism prevention within neighborhoods. Members are trained *not* to intervene when they become aware of suspicious or untoward activity, but rather to contact law enforcement officials for assistance. The shooting death of Trayvon Martin, a black unarmed 17-year-old in Sanford, Florida, in February 2012 by off-duty neighborhood watch captain George Zimmerman—who was eventually acquitted of murder charges—ignited a fierce social debate about the role of neighborhood watch groups. Once viewed as a positive and protective force in communities, neighborhood watch groups are now under intense scrutiny, particularly in ethnically diverse areas where racially motivated fears are high.

Neighborhood councils, on the other hand, are typically established through local governmental entities, such as city councils. Neighborhood Councils do not govern neighborhoods and are designed to provide an advisory role to city officials on issues of concern. Neighborhood councils usually hold monthly meetings that are free and open to the public. Any community stakeholder, whether he or she be a resident, business owner, student, or member of a faith-based institution, can become a member of the neighborhood council. Councils also have elected positions, such as chair, secretary, treasurer, business representative, and area representative. In cities including Los Angeles and San Diego, California, and Tacoma, Washington, neighborhood councils play an active and sometimes powerful role in shaping policies within their communities.

Business Owners Associations. Associations of business owners are also powerful entities that work actively to shape community policy. Business owners within a community will often join local chambers of commerce or form other less formal associations to protect the business interests within the community. They may work with their local government, such as the mayor, city council, or other local representatives, to develop pro-business initiatives. Mezzo policy advocates should be aware of such entities where they exist, as they can be either powerful supporters or opponents of issues affecting the welfare of the community.

Law Enforcement Involvement. While a thorough discussion of policing and its effects on communities and their residents is beyond the scope of this chapter, advocates should be aware of the powerful impact that law enforcement can have on a community. In many poor and ethnic neighborhoods, police–resident relations are strained at best and hostile at worst. Both historic and current examples of corruption and brutality on the part of law enforcement against residents of communities abound. An extreme example of police brutality that led to a violent six-day rebellion in the community of Watts in 1965 is described at the end of this chapter.

In other communities, friendlier styles of policing known as "community policing" and "restorative justice" are being practiced. Community policing focuses on building ties and working closely with members of communities for which law enforcement officials are responsible. Actual community-policing practices vary widely from place to place. Restorative justice focuses on addressing the needs of both victims and perpetrators of crime instead of punishing the offender. Victims take an active role in the restorative justice process, while offenders are encouraged to take responsibility for their actions by apologizing, returning stolen money, or participating in community service.

Local Media. The media, including local newspapers and television and radio stations, often assumes a pivotal role in local communities as a powerful delivery mechanism for community-level information. The media can help shape policies by playing the role of whistle-blower on local businesses, agencies, or elected officials who are operating unethically. It can also help shape policies by raising awareness about social problems within a community. Mezzo community advocates should be aware of the various news outlets within their community and develop relationships with reporters who can aid their advocacy efforts.

CHALLENGE 1: DECIDING WHETHER TO PROCEED

Mezzo policy advocates engage in eight challenges (see Figure 3.1). They decide whether to proceed (Challenge 1) and where to focus (Challenge 2). They secure key agency or community leaders' attention to unresolved problems in the agency or community (Challenge 3). They analyze why the problem(s) have developed (Challenge 4). They develop a strategy or policy proposal to address the unresolved problem(s) (Challenge 5). They obtain support for their strategy or policy proposal (Challenge 6). They implement their strategy or policy (Challenge 7). Finally, they assess whether their implemented strategy or policy has been successful (Challenge 8). We discuss each of the eight challenges as they apply to agencies and communities below.

Deciding Whether to Proceed in Agencies

Mezzo policy advocates must decide whether an issue or problem within their organization merits the development of an advocacy intervention. Social workers should consider engaging in policy advocacy within their organization when they recognize that clients possess one of the seven problems discussed in Chapter 1, and when they can connect these problems to deficits in agency policies, budget, protocols, internal culture, missions, or other organizational factors. For example, a social worker in a county mental health facility might recognize that low-income clients from certain geographic areas are unable to regularly attend their appointments (a problem with access, Core Problem 5) because the agency terminated its policy of issuing bus tokens to clients in need. The social worker would need to decide whether to proceed with an agenda to reinstate the policy of bus token distribution and thereby increase access to mental health services for this vulnerable population.

Mezzo policy advocates use the ethical reasoning skills discussed in Chapter 3 to determine whether to proceed with a policy change intervention. They consider a balance of factors, including the extent to which existing policies violate first-order principles of beneficence and social justice, the extent to which they feel ethically obligated to act, the relative difficulty of changing a specific policy, and the amount of time they estimate it might take to change a specific policy.

Deciding Whether to Proceed in Communities

Mezzo policy advocates also must decide whether an issue or problem within their community merits the development of an advocacy intervention. The views of community residents may contribute to the decision to develop an advocacy intervention. These views may be evidenced at community forums, through focus groups, or by members of specific community groups or churches. However, communities are often divided about the merit of specific issues or problems, and so the mezzo policy advocate must carefully weigh the choice whether to proceed. Mezzo policy advocates working in communities, just as those working in organizations, utilize an ethical reasoning process to help them decide whether to proceed.

CHALLENGE 2: DECIDING WHERE TO FOCUS

Deciding Where to Focus in Agencies

Mezzo policy advocates can seek to change an organization's mission, service provision policies, funding sources, programs, budget priorities, strategic plans, personnel and hiring policies, relationships between units and programs, or relationships with other organizations. Given these many options, mezzo advocates have to decide where to focus and decide if they want to make incremental or larger shifts in policy. They have to decide whether they wish to change policies of specific units or policies at higher levels of an organization.

Mezzo policy advocates sometimes try to change the culture of specific agencies. They may seek multidisciplinary training (e.g., training sessions on ethics in a hospital) if they want to increase cooperation across professions in an agency. They may bring new perspectives to helping certain kinds of consumers, such as people with disabilities, by bringing in a speaker who puts less emphasis on "a medical model" in a rehabilitation program and more emphasis on empowerment.

Social workers are more likely to succeed in their mezzo policy interventions if they develop a strategic overview. This overview allows them to identify assets and liabilities in the policy and the organizational context that are relevant to their issue. Optimism about changing the organization's strategy to deal with a specific problem may increase as they identify regulations, statutes, or court rulings that suggest the need for change. They may also focus on improving outcomes for their organization, such as by increasing resource levels, increasing client satisfaction, or attaining better outcomes for clients.

Deciding Where to Focus in Communities

Assume that strong support existed for not allowing additional liquor stores and fast-food outlets in a specific community. The mezzo policy advocate would then proceed to Challenge 2, that is, helping community residents decide how to navigate community institutions that develop policies governing whether and how many commercial outlets of specific kinds are permissible in a specific community. These institutions would include:

- City planning and zoning departments that decide which kinds of commercial institutions can be placed at specific locations
- Members of the city council who ratify decisions of city planning and zoning departments
- The top government official of an urban area (i.e., the mayor)
- Specific community groups that deal with commercial interests (i.e., the local chamber of commerce or business improvement district)
- Associations of residents (i.e., homeowners associations and neighborhood councils)

Advocates to limit the placement of liquor stores and fast-food outlets in this community would have to consider the influence and resources of specific commercial interests. For example, does a specific interest group represent the commercial interests of liquor stores and fast-food outlets in particular? How powerful are they in this particular jurisdiction?

CHALLENGE 3: OBTAINING DECISION MAKERS' RECOGNITION OF AN UNRESOLVED PROBLEM

Obtaining Decision Makers' Recognition in Agencies

Policy advocates work to place issues on decision makers' agendas so that they receive priority. This includes finding a propitious time to introduce policy changes to decision makers within their organizations. They ascertain whether the problem or issue has already been discussed or whether similar or related problems have already been identified. They determine if the executive director or CEO of their organization appears amenable to a specific problem or issue and if other high-level administrators might assume a pivotal role in advancing it. They work with specific stakeholders to gain their support and identify the ways in which a policy initiative enhances the financial well-being of the organization, its image in the community, or the outcomes of its clients. They also work with people who might join a coalition or task force to address the specific issue or problem.

Timing should be considered when considering policy changes that come with a price tag. If a problem can be solved only with considerable financial resources, advocates may want to postpone introducing it during a period of budget stringency.

Obtaining Decision Makers' Recognition in Communities

Advocates place their issue on the agendas of decision makers in their community and the larger city where they are located. They decide *when* to initiate their advocacy by considering whether background events, such as elections of public officials and the economy, are favorable. They might decide to join forces with several other communities to make their issue more relevant to other members of the city council and the mayor.

They should also ascertain whether the national climate and public opinion are helpful to them. The mass media can provide a mechanism for elevating interest in their issue by giving it substantial coverage and linking it to stories of national interest. Assume that a community organization decides to proceed with their quest to limit the number of liquor stores and fast-food outlets. They may utilize the media to draw attention to the problem, form a coalition of residents and business representatives who wish to address the problem, and set appointments with members of local zoning boards, business improvement districts, and neighborhood councils.

CHALLENGE 4: ANALYZING WHY THE PROBLEM EXISTS

Analyzing Why the Problem Exists in Agencies

Social workers seeking to address unresolved problems in agencies will need to analyze why the problem exists, including by developing an understanding of the source of this problem and what the key factors are that enable its continuance. Take the example of a nonprofit organization in which a culture of discrimination against LGBTQQ clients exists. If the organization is run or funded by a faith-based entity, the advocate might find that the policy is tied to a religious belief. Alternatively, they might find that the policy was put in place many decades ago, before the gay rights movement put the issue of equality for people of all sexual orientations on the social radar. The advocate will need to develop a historical understanding of the problem by analyzing the history of inequality and oppression directed toward LGBTQQ clients. The advocate should also understand the extent to which the organization's policy is connected to a historical set of beliefs and incorrect stereotypes. Equipped with this information, the mezzo policy advocate will be much more likely to develop an effective strategy to address the problem (an example of Challenge 5).

POLICY ADVOCACY LEARNING CHALLENGE 5.3

Advocating for Lesbian Clients in a Domestic Violence Agency

By Gretchen Heidemann

I worked as a crisis hotline counselor at a shelter for battered women early in my career. Unfortunately, I became aware of actions on the part of staff that troubled me, as I noticed that lesbian women who received services at the agency were being treated unfairly. In one instance, a staff member asserted that she would not wrap Christmas gifts for the children of "those" women. In another, a staff member began attempting to proselytize lesbian clients, telling them that God viewed their behavior as sinful and that they must repent. I felt the need to advocate on behalf of the clients. I moved quickly to bring the staff's behavior to the attention of the assistant director (AD). Although the AD heard my concerns and seemed to agree that the behavior was inappropriate and unethical, she was not quick to make changes. First, the agency did not have a formal nondiscrimination policy in place. Thus, there were no immediate grounds on which to reprimand staff or to mandate them to change their behavior. Second, there were many religious and cultural factors at play. It was not a simple matter, she informed me, to ask staff members to change their behavior on a dime. In retrospect, I wish I had done my homework before approaching the AD. Had I had more knowledge about the history of the organization and about the beliefs of various members of the community, I might have had a more strategic plan in place. I might have sought out examples of agencies that were able to change both their organizational culture and written policies with regard to this issue, while also respecting the religious and cultural beliefs of staff members. As it turned out, an informal and (in my opinion) largely ineffective conversation about "treating everyone equally" took place at a staff meeting. But a formal nondiscrimination policy was never enacted within the agency (at least during my tenure there); thus staff did not feel compelled to change their behavior.

Analyzing Why the Problem Exists in Communities

A mezzo policy advocate who identifies an unresolved problem within his or her community will need to analyze why the problem exists in that community. In communities, unlike organizations, there is no mission statement to drive a set of shared beliefs and behaviors. Moreover, communities are typically part of larger entities—cities and counties—that legislate matters that influence the capacity of a community. Whereas many organizations operate as stand-alone entities with the ability to create, enforce, and change their own policies, communities must work within the complex web of citywide ordinances, county-level law enforcement and safety (i.e., fire and emergency) services, networks of business associations, and so forth. Thus, understanding why a problem exists within a community might involve looking beyond the community itself, as well as into the past to understand its historical roots.

The case description of the community of Watts at the end of this chapter highlights some of the problems that communities face. These problems cannot be understood apart from their historical context. The gangs that currently exist in Watts are an outgrowth of mutual protection societies established in the 1960s by black residents who came together to protect one another from threats from the white community. Without this critical piece of information, a mezzo community advocate in Watts would miss an opportunity to work with gang members under the assumption that mutual protection (and not just crime or drug dealing) is a primary function of gang membership. Absent such a detailed analysis, the advocate's ability to develop an effective strategy to address the problem in Challenge 5 would be stymied.

CHALLENGE 5: DEVELOPING A STRATEGY OR PROPOSAL TO ADDRESS THE PROBLEM

Developing a Strategy in Agencies

Interagency strategy should include a series of activities designed to raise awareness about the problem and inform stakeholders about the proposed policy solution and its benefits. Activities might include staff briefings, publication of reports, interagency email blasts, mobilization of stakeholder groups to support the proposed reform, and face-to-face meetings with key decision makers. Each of these activities is carefully thought out with a planned timeline or sequence of events. A mezzo policy advocate should be aware of relevant timetables within the agency (e.g., board meeting schedules, licensing inspections, major fundraisers). With this information, the effective advocate can plan his or her activities at the most auspicious moments.

Mezzo policy advocates should also look for open policy windows to advance their cause. Open policy windows are critical events such as administrative changes, a change in decision makers' ideology, a shift in public opinion, or the onset of a crisis or "focusing event" that reflects favorably upon the issue. They occur infrequently, so mezzo policy advocates should be prepared to "pounce" when such an opportunity arises.

There will be entities that oppose any effort at policy change, even within the smallest of agencies. Awareness of this opposition is key to survival. Opposition may come from insiders, such as staff members who prefer the status quo, ideologically opposed administrative officials, or clients who feel somehow vulnerable or threatened by the change. Outside opposition should be anticipated so that when it does arise there are talking points available to counter any hostility.

Developing a Strategy in Communities

Many of the strategic elements described above apply to communities as well. Let us imagine that a social worker in a mental health clinic encounters a patient who was recently released from prison. As she works with him to develop a case plan, she realizes that this client faces obstacles and challenges beyond those of her typical client. The formerly incarcerated man not only suffers from mental illness, but also is unable to secure permanent housing. Moreover, the few halfway houses that exist in the community are being threatened by an ordinance that would close their doors. The social worker might consider engaging in advocacy to stop the proposed ordinance, to develop ordinances that actually address the needs of the community, or to fund alternative reentry facilities for formerly incarcerated people. Many of the strategies described above are applicable to such a scenario.

The mezzo policy advocate wishing to change community-level policy will need to outline a series of actions, set a timetable, look for opportunities, and plan for opposition. In addition, mezzo policy advocates in communities might incorporate the use of media and social media into their strategy. The press (e.g., radio, television, newspapers) can be a powerful tool for any policy strategy. Social media is also highly desirable for a number of reasons. Advocates have complete control over its content, so they can target messages to certain audiences and disseminate information quickly. Advocates can also be very creative with their messaging, using videos, photographs, cartoons, tweets, blogs, interactive webpages, and online petitions.

RESOURCES ON THE USE OF SOCIAL MEDIA FOR ADVOCACY

National Alliance on Mental Illness: http://www.nami.org/Content/NavigationMenu/State_Advocacy/Tools_for_Leaders/Media_Tool_Kit_Using_Social_Networking_Tools.htm

American Association of University Women: http://www.aauw.org/resource/how-to-use-social-media-for-advocacy/

CHALLENGE 6: DEVELOPING SUPPORT FOR THE STRATEGY OR PROPOSAL

Developing Support for a Strategy in Agencies

Sometimes it takes only one person to advance a policy change, but often mezzo policy advocates need to secure the support of individuals and groups to accomplish their agenda. The skill of persuasion is key to developing support for a proposed policy change. A range of stakeholders including clients, frontline staff, high-level or administrative staff, executives, members of the board of directors, community residents, funders, vendors and contractors, regulatory agencies, and collaborating organizations should be sought out. Mezzo policy advocates should carefully consider the interests of the stakeholder group and consider how the proposed policy will affect each group. They might wish to interview key informants from each group to better understand the positions and interests of that group, set up meetings or activities to build relationships with members of the different groups, and carefully craft messages targeted toward each group to gain support. A policy change might have obvious implications for some, but not all, of the stakeholder groups. The advocate should think about how members of each group will benefit from the change, as well as why it is the best possible solution for the organization. Appealing to mission and vision statements, ethical principles, professional standards of practice, and shared moral or political beliefs can be powerful ways of winning support for policy proposals.

Developing Support for a Strategy in Communities

Mezzo policy advocates in communities appeal to a broad range of stakeholders. Residents; business owners and employees of businesses; consumers of community-based services; members of faith-based institutions; fire, rescue, and law enforcement officials; and many, many other groups have vested and often competing interests in community-level policies.

Gaining support for a proposed policy agenda in a community requires much of the same strategy discussed above in relation to agencies. However, the complexity and the sheer size of some communities, when all of the many stakeholders mentioned above are included, makes this challenge a daunting one for the mezzo policy advocate. In addition, residents of communities are rarely united in their beliefs about what should change and how that change should occur. Advocates must remember that it is not possible to win everyone over and that the broadest possible support for a policy is always advantageous.

CHALLENGE 7: IMPLEMENTING A STRATEGY OR POLICY TO ADDRESS THE PROBLEM IN AGENCIES AND COMMUNITIES

Mezzo policy advocacy does not end when a policy is adopted. In fact, in some ways, adoption is just the beginning. A new community ordinance, agency-wide service delivery policy, or interorganizational operating procedure is virtually useless unless it is fully implemented. Many things can happen to hinder the implementation of a new or modified policy. In an agency, high-level decision makers may become distracted or forget about the policy altogether. Those who are involved in implementation of the policy, such as frontline staff, might not fully understand their new rules or duties. A lack of funding may affect full implementation of the policy. Individuals may refuse to implement the policy or work to block its implementation.

To counter these pitfalls, mezzo policy advocates should work to establish protocols and trainings that will help ensure that staff are fully aware of their duties under the new policy. They may devise creative solutions to bring resources to the agency or community in order to fully implement the policy. In more extreme cases, they may decide to form a watchdog group to put pressure on decision makers or administrators who are responsible for overseeing the implementation.

POLICY ADVOCACY LEARNING CHALLENGE 5.4

Conducting Watchdog Activities to Ensure Implementation of Agency Policy

By Gretchen Heidemann

I interned at a homeless coalition that worked in the greater Los Angeles area to protect the rights of homeless individuals, ensure adequate resources for homeless services, and build grassroots support to end homelessness. The organization became aware that homeless people were being denied benefits entitled to them by county welfare offices through the Homeless Assistance Program. Specifically, the dozen or so welfare offices in the county were mandated, through state policy, to provide funding to homeless families for temporary shelter for up to 16 consecutive nights. We developed a protocol to hold their feet to the fire. We created a script and systematically placed phone calls to the various welfare offices, pretending to be a family in need and requesting information about the Homeless Assistance Program. We recorded whether the welfare worker responding to the call gave us correct, partially correct, or entirely incorrect information. We then wrote up a report from our data and used it to confront directors in the welfare offices where workers most frequently provided incorrect information. We pressed the directors to conduct trainings for their workers, or, at minimum, to provide detailed materials and instructions to them so that future seekers would not be denied the benefits to which they were entitled.

CHALLENGE 8: ASSESSING WHETHER THE IMPLEMENTED STRATEGY OR POLICY WAS EFFECTIVE IN AGENCIES AND COMMUNITIES

Mezzo policy advocates will want to know whether the policy they helped to pass and implement is accomplishing its intended goals. Advocates should consider using tools that will provide the data they need to determine whether or not the policy is achieving its aims. For example, they may decide to conduct in-depth interviews with agency clients who were impacted by the policy change, develop a survey to measure the extent of their satisfaction with it, or locate standardized scales if the policy is intended to have specific health, mental health, behavioral, or other measureable outcomes. It is important to understand how the policy is impacting other stakeholders and the agency or community in general. Not only do advocates seek this information to tell them whether they policy was effective, but the information they acquire when assessing the strategy will be critical if the policy is time-limited and needs to be renewed.

Some of the questions mezzo policy advocates may seek to answer when assessing the policy include:

1. How do various stakeholders perceive the policy? Subjective perceptions about the utility of the policy can be powerful tools when it comes time to renew, expand, or replicate a policy.

2. Is the policy cost-effective? Does it have any unintended financial impacts? Knowing whether the policy can be implemented without causing undue burdens on taxpayers or other revenue providers is also critical to the advocate's ability to renew, expand, or replicate it.

3. What challenges have staff faced in successfully implementing the policy? How can the lessons learned from those challenges help to ensure better implementation in the future?

4. If the policy is falling short of accomplishing its intended outcomes, what ideas do members of various stakeholder groups have about how to improve it?

Assessing policy is not a one-time activity. It is an ongoing process that involves the constant collection and analysis of data to understand the extent to which the policy is accomplishing its intended aims. Simple instruments can be developed to collect information about outcomes to help audiences understand the impact the policy is having. Some agencies may have staff or departments specifically dedicated to program evaluation that could aid in assessing policies.

A CASE EXAMPLE OF MEZZO POLICY ADVOCACY

This section presents a case study of mezzo policy advocacy in the community of Watts in Los Angeles, California. We present the history of the community and the community's current demographics. We describe the Watts Labor Community Action Committee (WLCAC), which has been working for more than 40 years to change community-level policies to make Watts a safe and thriving place to live. Much of the information contained in this description is based on an interview conducted with Tim Watkins, the current CEO of WLCAC (December 2013).

The History of Watts

During the Second Great Migration in the 1940s, large numbers of African Americans moved to the West Coast, enticed by defense industry recruitment at the start of World War II. Although Los Angeles did not practice Southern-style racial segregation, the city was divided geographically by race. Minorities were expressly banned from housing in 95% of the city. As the population of the city of Los Angeles burgeoned, demands for housing skyrocketed. Developers began building new housing in undeveloped areas south of Los Angeles. Large-scale housing projects were built during this time, along with single family homes, and by the late 1940s neighborhoods like Compton and Watts were populated by blue-collar African American families who enjoyed a middle-class lifestyle.

In the 1950s, the area became a target of racial animosity. White residents burned crosses in the yards of black families, and white gang members in neighboring communities accosted black residents who passed through their "territory." So-called "mutual protection clubs" were formed by young black residents in response to these assaults, while white families began to flee to surrounding suburbs.

Around the same time, a new Los Angeles police chief, William H. Parker, began using military-style fear and intimidation tactics in these neighborhoods, especially against young black and Latino residents. Police brutality became widespread and erupted in violence on the night of August 11, 1965. That night, 21-year-old Marquette Frye was pulled over for driving while intoxicated near his home in Watts. His mother and brother arrived on the scene, along with several backup police officers, and an argument ensued. A physical altercation led angry resident onlookers to hurl objects at police officers. After Marquette, his brother, and his mother were arrested, an angry crowd grew. Throughout the night, police attempted to break the crowd up, but were unsuccessful.

Over the next six days, a 46-square-mile area around Watts was transformed into an all-out war zone involving looting, beatings, and mass rioting. The unrest resulted in 34 deaths, 1,032 injuries, 3,438 arrests, and over $40 million in property damage. More than 2,300 members of the California Army National Guard were called in along with the LAPD and LA County Sheriff's Department, and the violence was eventually contained. Yet the frustrations of community residents over the system of racial segregation and inequality, as well as biased and oppressive treatment by law enforcement, could not be contained.

Following the Watts riots, the mutual protection clubs that had developed in the 1950s transformed into the violent street gangs known today as the Bloods and Crips. Crack cocaine began to flood the streets in the late 1970s and early 1980s, while many of the living-wage manufacturing plants that employed black workers shut down or moved operations overseas. Large numbers of residents, particularly young black men, were arrested and became trapped in a cycle of incarceration, poverty, and homelessness. Many black women were forced to raise families on their own, often relying on welfare assistance when jobs were scarce and affordable childcare nearly nonexistent.

A second wave of civil unrest occurred in the area in 1992 after an incident eerily reminiscent of that which provoked the 1965 rebellion. On March 3, 1991, a driver by the name of Rodney King and his two passengers were pulled over by the California Highway Patrol after a high-speed chase. King was suspected of being intoxicated; a drug test later proved he was not. The LAPD arrived on the scene and took the two passengers into custody. King, a parolee who knew that an arrest would send him back to prison, resisted. As they pulled him from the vehicle, five LAPD officers tasered King, kicked him in the head, and beat him with batons while he crawled on the ground. He was then tackled and cuffed. George Holliday, a resident of the community, caught the police actions on video. The video aired worldwide on nightly news stations, and national debate about police brutality against unarmed black men was ignited.

Following the incident, four of the police officers were charged with assault and excessive use of force. A lengthy trial ensued, and a jury, composed of nine whites, one black, one Latino, and one Asian, acquitted three of the officers on April 29, 1992. They could not agree on a verdict for the fourth officer.

Riots and looting began the day of the acquittal as angry mobs formed in areas of South Central Los Angeles, including the neighborhood of Watts. Innocent residents were beaten and businesses were looted and burned to the ground in rioting that lasted for six days. Fifty-three people died and more than 2,000 were injured. Worldwide media coverage of the unrest showed broad swaths of Los Angeles on fire. More than 13,500 military forces, including the Marines and the National Guard, were called in. Most of the violence subsided by early May.

Since the 1992 civil unrest, the community of Watts has seen both growth and decline in relation to the violence. Despite a peace treaty signed by rival gangs in the early 1990s, more than 500 homicides were reported in Watts between 1989 and 2005, most of them gang related. In 2006, the Watts Gang Task Force (WGTF), a coalition of residents, business owners, schools, churches, city council members, and the Los Angeles Human Relations Commission, was founded. Meeting on a weekly basis, the group focuses on building trust between residents and law enforcement and implementing initiatives to keep residents safe. The task force touts the creation of a "safe passage" program that helps students travel safely through gang territory to get to school, the reopening of a public pool that was once considered unsafe, and the creation of thousands of summer jobs for youth. Two years after its creation, WGTF reported that violent crime had decreased by 50% in Watts.

The community has transformed in other important ways as well, partially as a result of the work of the Watts Labor Community Action Committee (WLCAC). Founded around the time of the Watts Rebellion in 1965, WLCAC operates an array of social services in Watts, including a homeless shelter, a senior center, a WorkSource center, a childcare center, a gang reduction program, and several youth development programs. In addition, the organization promotes culture and tourism in Watts through its operation of a Civil Rights Museum, an art gallery, and a performing arts center. The organization also hosts the "Watts International Marketplace," an open-air market housing embroidery, silk-screening, ceramics, fine arts, glass blowing, woodworking, and photography studios. The organization is also at the forefront of policy advocacy initiatives to improve conditions throughout the community. WLCAC has worked in collaboration with other organizations to:

- Restrict the number of liquor stores operating within the community
- Remove harmful gang injunctions that profile and sweep young men of color into the criminal justice system rather than protecting the community
- Renovate the Ted Watkins Memorial Park, the only green space within the community.
- Establish a 2-acre farm where residents can grow their own food

The organization is currently working to pass a "Zero Displacement Policy" to ensure that any development or construction that occurs within the community does not displace residents. It would also ensure that housing and retail developers give priority to agencies within the community to perform the construction and that they hire workers from within the community. They are proceeding with the Zero Displacement Policy (Challenge 1) and are focusing on working with entities such as the Central Area Planning Commission and the Industrial Development Authority, which will need to give approval before the policy goes to city council for a vote (Challenge 2). They have secured the support of two important policy makers, including one city council member and the Congress member who represents the district (Challenge 3).

POLICY ADVOCACY LEARNING CHALLENGE 5.5

A Zero Displacement Policy in Watts

Consider the community of Watts, as described above and in any supplemental information you may locate. Imagine you are working with WLCAC to pass the Zero Displacement Policy. With Challenges 1 and 2 already complete as described in Figure 3.1 and Challenge 3 in progress, outline a detailed plan for completing Challenges 3 through 8 by addressing the following:

- Challenge 3: Secure attention
    Identify other decision makers whose support you should bring to the issue and the proposed policy. Even if they will not be the ones to ultimately decide

(Continued)

(Continued)

or vote on the policy, what key figures need to be aware of the issue? Are there other individuals or groups within the community or outside of it whose support you will need to secure?

- Challenge 4: Analyze why the problem exists

  Consider the high rates of poverty and unemployment that exist in Watts, as well as the current lack of living wage jobs. What historical and socioeconomic factors have contributed to this situation?

  Consider the reasons why a developer might be unconcerned about displacing residents in the process of building new commercial structures within the community. What historical fears and mistrusts might this lack of concern ignite?

  Consider why a developer might choose not to hire from within the community or why it might choose to give its contracts to agencies from outside the community. What will you do to overcome this issue?

- Challenge 5: Develop a Strategy

  Outline a strategy for getting this policy approved by the city council. How will you frame the issue? What stories will you tell and how? Who will be featured in those stories? What sorts of materials will you develop? What activities will you undertake (e.g., a press conference, one-on-one meetings, petition gathering, a community town hall)? What opportunities will you be looking for to advance your cause? Who is likely to be your opposition, and how will you address opposition?

- Challenge 6: Develop Support for the Proposal

  Identify the range of stakeholders that this issue impacts. Develop a strategy for gaining their support. What types of messages will you develop to target the different groups? For those who are already on your side, how will you further engage them to advance your agenda? For those who are on the fence, how might you bring them over to your side?

- Challenge 7: Implement the Policy

  How will you ensure efficient and successful implementation of the policy? What groups of people will be involved in implementing the policy? What types of watchdog activities might you undertake to make sure that the spirit of the policy is being honored? Will you consider engaging in whistleblowing if you see that policy makers are not fully or correctly implementing the policy?

- Challenge 8: Assess the Policy

  How will you assess whether the policy has been effective? What are the outcomes of concern to the stakeholder groups? How will you measure outcomes?

LEARNING OUTCOMES

You are now equipped to do the following:

- Define mezzo policy advocacy
- Identify key skills needed by mezzo policy advocates
- Engage in the eight challenges identified in the multilevel policy advocacy framework in Chapter 3 in agencies and organizations
- Engage in the eight challenges identified in Chapter 4 in communities
- Apply concepts from this chapter to a specific community

REFERENCES

Chu, F. D., & Trotter S. (1974). *Madness establishment: Ralph Nader's study group report on the National Institute of Health.* New York, NY: Grossman.

Cook, M. F. (1987). *New directions in human resources: A handbook.* Englewood Cliffs, NJ: Prentice Hall.

Dahl, R. (1967). *Pluralist democracy in the United States: Conflict and consent.* Chicago, IL: Rand McNally.

Dluhy, M. (1981). *Changing the system: Political advocacy for the disadvantaged.* Beverly Hills, CA: SAGE.

Gummer, B. (1990). *The politics of social administration: Managing organizational politics in social agencies.* Englewood Cliffs, NJ: Prentice Hall.

Hasenfeld, Y. (1983). *Human service organizations.* Englewood Cliffs, NJ: Prentice Hall.

Chapter 6

ENGAGING IN MACRO POLICY ADVOCACY

LEARNING OBJECTIVES

In this chapter, you will learn:

1. How to understand the context of public policies and regulations, including:
   - Who the players in the public sphere are
   - How the public sphere includes legislatures, the executive branch, elected officials, appointed officials in executive agencies, and civil servants
   - How legislatures are organized and function
   - The role of advocacy groups
   - The mindsets of public officials
   - Connections between lobbyists, legislators, and bureaucrats
   - The important role of public opinion
   - The role of regulations

2. How macro policy advocates engage the eight challenges

3. Specific policy advocacy skills that macro policy advocates need

4. How to analyze a policy advocacy vignette to identify macro policy advocacy skills and strategies

---

Social workers engage in macro policy advocacy in local, regional, state, and federal governments because laws, statutes, regulations, and administrative decisions in these settings profoundly influence the well-being of their clientele. Many gaps and omissions in existing policies can be corrected only by developing macro policy interventions in these various venues.

In this chapter, we discuss the eight challenges that social workers confront when they engage in macro policy advocacy (see Figure 3.1): (1) deciding whether to proceed, (2) deciding where to focus, (3) securing decision makers' attention, (4) analyzing why a dysfunctional policy developed, (5) developing policy proposals, (6) securing approval or enactment of a proposal, (7) implementing a policy reform, and (8) assessing an implemented policy. Even before they undertake these challenges, macro policy advocates have to understand the context.

KNOWING THE CONTEXT

Necessary Information
About the Executive Branch of Government

VIDEO LINK 6.1
Policy Practice to
Help Veterans

Macro policy advocates have to know how the public sphere is organized so that they can maneuver within it. They have to know the players in the public sphere. These include three kinds of *elected officials*—heads of government, including mayors, governors, and presidents; legislators at the local, state, and federal levels; and people elected to special bodies, such as local school boards. They include *unelected officials*, including people appointed to public office by heads of government, such as the heads of many agencies, as well as civil servants who obtain their jobs by taking exams and interviews and are charged with running government agencies at the local, state, and federal levels. They have to be familiar with *lobbyists and interest groups* that represent a wide array of corporations, unions, professions, and nongovernmental organizations (NGOs), including state and national chapters of the National Association of Social Workers (NASW). They have to understand how *regulations* are fashioned by civil servants, as compared to *statutes*, which are enacted by legislatures.

They have to understand the *legislative process* that determines how bills become laws, including the existence of two chambers, the extraordinary power of the party that has a majority in a specific chamber, and the legislative calendar that determines when a bill must become law or else its advocates will have to start anew with the next legislative session.

They have to understand the *executive branch*. The U.S. president, as well as governors and mayors, is in charge of the executive branch of government, which comprises the myriad agencies that implement government policies. These agencies are usually called *departments*, such as the Department of Health and Human Services (DHHS). They usually initiate a budget, even though the legislators make many of the final budgetary choices. This initiating role represents an important power because it allows chief executives to influence priorities within the executive branch.

Chief executives usually develop a legislative agenda to which they often refer in general terms in speeches, such as the president's State of the Union speech. They have vast resources to help them fashion this legislative agenda, including personal aides in their own office, their political appointees in the executive branch, and political allies who occupy powerful positions on legislative committees or in the party in the legislature (Holtzman, 1970). Because heads of government have a central position in government and a high profile, their legislative proposals, which members of their own party or political allies introduce into the legislature, often have an advantage over individual legislators' proposals. Even with such power, the legislative proposals of many heads of government are defeated, particularly when the opposing party holds a majority in the legislature.

Chief executives can issue executive orders, which are directives to specific units of government that don't require legislative approval, such as when President Barack Obama issued executive orders pertaining to details of the Patient Protection and Affordable Care Act of 2010 not included in the legislation.

Capitalizing on the extensive coverage the mass media usually accords them, heads of government often try to gain support for legislative measures, rally opposition against legislators who may block their policies, and educate the public about specific issues (Smith, 1988).

Finally, heads of government can veto legislation that the legislature has approved, which is an important power since legislatures often cannot muster the votes (such as the two thirds of each chamber required in the federal government) to override a veto. Some governors have line-item veto power over the budgets that legislatures have approved.

Necessary Information About Legislatures

Legislatures seem formidably complex; in fact, they are all structured rather similarly. They are usually divided into two houses, such as the House of Representatives and the Senate at the federal level, or the Senate and the Assembly at the state level, as in Wisconsin. Usually, both houses must assent to legislation or a budget before it can become operative. Many legislatures, like the U.S. Congress, convene annually, but some state legislatures convene only every two years. Moreover, the length of legislatures' sessions varies widely; Congress meets almost nonstop each year, but other legislatures convene for only several months.

The members of each house or chamber of a legislature, whether local, state, or federal, are elected by districts, whose precise shape changes over time. Districts are reapportioned as the population shifts and as the courts decide that existing district lines are unfair to specific groups, such as Latinos or African Americans. To understand specific legislators, then, we must analyze the characteristics of their constituents, whose preferences influence their positions on myriad issues. We might ask: Is the district relatively affluent or poor? Does it have a mix of ethnic and racial groups, or does a single group dominate it? Is it urban, suburban, or rural? Is it dominated by a single party or evenly divided between two parties? We can also ask whether specific legislators occupy relatively safe seats or whether they will face closely contested elections.

To understand how specific chambers of legislatures operate, we must first ask: Which party controls a majority of the legislature's members? The majority party appoints the chairs of all committees and has a majority of the members on each committee of that chamber. Moreover, the members of the majority party in each house elect the presiding officer of that chamber, such as the president of the U.S. Senate and the Speaker of the House. These high-level leaders have considerable power in determining when specific measures will be debated on the floor, in mobilizing support for or against measures, and in making important parliamentary decisions at critical junctures in floor debate. Presiding officers often have the authority to establish committees, assign members to committees, and appoint chairs of committees. In addition, they often have the power to decide where to route specific bills for deliberation. This power is critical, because a presiding officer can often kill a bill by insisting that it go through specific committees that are known to be hostile to it.

Each chamber has a second tier of powerful leaders: the floor leaders, who are also elected by caucuses and include the majority leader and the majority whip. Working in tandem with the presiding officer, these party leaders shepherd legislation through floor deliberations and decide which measures their party will support or oppose.

A third tier of leaders, the chairs of the important committees of a chamber, are members of the majority party and have considerable power over the fate of legislation in their committees.

Though at a disadvantage, a minority party often has considerable power in a specific chamber. It has its own leader, such as the U.S. House minority leader, who can mobilize support of or opposition to pieces of legislation. The minority party is allocated seats on all committees of a chamber in proportion to its share of the chamber's total membership, and its members sometimes obtain a majority vote on a committee by teaming with committee members of the majority party. Thus, in the era of Presidents Reagan and Bush, Republicans could defeat congressional legislation that the Democrats strongly favored by joining with southern Democrats, even though the Democratic Party had a majority in the House of Representatives throughout the period and controlled the Senate from November 1986 onward.

Because of their size and the myriad issues they consider, legislatures are divided into specialized committees. In the federal House of Representatives, for example, the Ways and Means Committee processes Social Security, Medicare, and tax legislation, and the Committee on Labor and Public Welfare processes social programs such as Head Start.

As we have discussed, the presiding officers of each chamber often have considerable discretion in referring measures to committees. Many pieces of legislation go to multiple committees when they pose issues that cut across committee divisions. In other cases, certain kinds of legislation are automatically referred to a specific committee. The House Ways and Means Committee and the Senate Finance Committee in the U.S. Congress, for example, always consider Social Security and Medicare legislation.

Each legislative committee has an internal structure. Its chairperson may be elected by the committee's members or appointed by the chamber's presiding officer. Committee chairs are usually powerful figures. Like presiding officers of the overall chamber, they can kill legislation by not placing it on the committee's agenda, by referring it to a hostile subcommittee, or by merely raising strong objections to it when the committee discusses it. Each legislative committee has subcommittees that specialize in certain issues, within the whole committee's purview. Subcommittee chairs also have considerable power over issues that fall within their domain.

Legislation that presiding officers refer to a committee falls into two categories. Some of it is consigned, more or less at once, to the legislative junk heap because the committee, much less the full chamber, does not consider it seriously. The subcommittees and committees take other legislation seriously and mark it up in committee deliberations; that is, they amend it in various ways.

Most legislation, then, evolves in the course of deliberations that take weeks, months, or even years, and it can be amended on the floor of the chamber when the whole chamber decides whether to amend, accept, or defeat a bill. A bill usually starts in one chamber, progresses from committees to a floor debate, and then comes to a vote. It is then referred to the other chamber, where it follows a similar course. After the second chamber enacts its own version, representatives from each chamber seek a common version, which usually requires both chambers to make concessions. If the conference committee creates a joint version, each chamber must then ratify it before it goes to the president (or governor), who then signs it into law or vetoes it. Congress can override a veto if each chamber musters a two-thirds vote. Otherwise, the legislation dies.

Some legislative deliberations are relatively straightforward; relatively few amendments are offered and legislators move quickly to a decision. Other legislative deliberations, particularly those concerning controversial issues, are marked by various parliamentary maneuvers, such as the opponents' efforts to derail the legislation. In unusual cases, opponents in the Senate will even filibuster a bill by talking nonstop to prevent a concluding vote. Filibusters are not allowed in the House.

Necessary Information About Advocacy Groups

Advocacy groups place pressure on decision makers in city councils, boards of supervisors, and state and federal legislators. They may be community groups, coalitions, think tanks, public interest groups, groups of consumers, or professional groups like the National Association of Social Workers. Some advocacy groups exist for long periods of time, while others are relatively short-lived, such as those developed to address a specific issue at a specific time. Advocacy groups vary in their size and staff: Some are relatively small, whereas others have substantial resources from foundations and other sources. Policy advocates often work with advocacy groups when they seek to change policies.

POLICY ADVOCACY LEARNING CHALLENGE 6.1

Identifying Advocacy Groups

Examine the following list of advocacy groups in the gerontology sector. Go to the websites of three of these groups. Identify their general perspectives. Are they relatively liberal, relatively conservative, or relatively "neutral" in their orientation? How would you estimate their likely power or influence—or is that impossible to determine from their website? Were you desirous of improving policies for senior citizens, might you consider getting feedback from a staff member of one or more of these groups? Now go to be web to find advocacy groups for a specific issue such as gun control, women's reproductive rights, or immigration rights.

Table 6.1   Some Advocacy Groups Seeking Greater Social Justice in the Gerontology Sector

1. AFL-CIO
2. Alliance for Retired Persons
3. American Association of Retired Persons
4. Center for Economic and Policy Research
5. Century Foundation: Social Security Network
6. Institute of America's Future
7. National Committee to Preserve Social Security and Medicare
8. New York Network for Action on Medicare and Social Security

Necessary Information About Elected Officials

Those who engage in policy practice in governmental settings need to understand the mindsets of heads of government and legislators. Imagine that you have just spent two years planning, fundraising, and campaigning to obtain your job. You have narrowly defeated a determined opponent who has already pledged to prevail in the next election, which is several years away. In response to this threat, you are likely to have reelection on your mind throughout your tenure. You will look at most issues with an eye to their effect on your reelection, and you will spend hours wondering about the general public's preferences. To deduce their views, you will study the following:

- Public opinion polls
- Recent outcomes of other elections in comparable districts
- The mail you receive
- The views of subgroups within your constituency, particularly those that you believe will support you in the next election
- The preferences of state or national organizations—for example, professional associations or groups such as the American Association of Retired Persons—that might contribute funds to your next campaign

Moreover, you will nervously eye the statements and positions of potential opponents in the next election. In some cases, you will support an issue to steal the thunder of your likely opponents, and in other cases you will openly support issues that they oppose to publicize your differences from them. In districts divided between liberals and conservatives, relatively liberal candidates often support liberal issues to solidify their support among liberals. They realize that without committed support from this constituency, they may lose to conservative opponents (Arnold, 1990).

This nonstop campaigning will make you sensitive to the political ramifications of certain choices. Some issues, such as increasing funds for city parks, will cause you little or no concern. However, issues seen as more controversial by important segments of your constituency will make you hesitate before committing yourself.

If elected officials often have their ears to the ground, they are also extraordinarily busy. Assume that you are a member of several major committees and subcommittees, each of which handles many issues on which you need to brief yourself before and during policy deliberations. As you hurriedly read technical reports and briefing papers, you simultaneously try to raise funds for your reelection bid. You make weekly trips back to your district to meet with its citizens and convene regularly with lobbyists from various interest groups. Constituents also come to your offices every day to speak with you.

You also are concerned about your relationships with your legislative and party colleagues. As a member of legislative committees and subcommittees, you know that the chairperson holds great power and can often determine which issues will receive a serious airing in the committee and which amendments will be enacted. You belong to a political party as well, which meets regularly, agrees collectively to support or oppose certain measures, and parcels out rewards and penalties, such as committee assignments and campaign funds. If you are a complete renegade, you will suffer reprisals from high officials on your legislative committees and in your party.

With such a full agenda, you need to develop shortcuts. You have to rely heavily on aides to manage the bulk of your interactions with constituents, lobbyists, and others (Richan, 1991; Smith, 1988). You are not afraid to delegate much of your work to these trusted aides, because without them you cannot function. You create a division of labor by hiring specialists in legislative matters, in handling constituent demands (such as the woman who wants help with her husband's Alzheimer's disease), in fundraising, and in public relations. In other cases, you rely heavily on lobbyists to do technical work for you, to do reconnaissance work with other legislators, to help you draft legislative proposals, and to help you write amendments to existing legislation (Smith, 1988). Early in your term, you decide that you have to develop priorities by taking some pieces of legislation seriously and only giving glancing attention to others. You decide to expend your political capital (your power resources) liberally on issues that may bring you large political dividends when you come up for reelection, or that appeal to you for other reasons.

Your decisions on specific measures will hinge on electoral considerations, personal values and life experiences, personal expertise and interests, your views of the public interest, and the political feasibility of enacting specific measures.

Our discussion of the mindsets of elected officials suggests that policy advocates need to exercise caution in making premature judgments about legislators' choices. Many factors can impel them to support or oppose a measure and to invest energy in it.

Connections Among Interest Groups, Legislators, and Bureaucrats

Important relationships exist among lobbyists, legislators, and bureaucrats. Many lobbyists, for example, are former legislators, civil servants, or political appointees. Many civil servants are former aides to legislators, with whom they maintain important relationships, such as passing them "inside information" (McIver, 1981). So-called iron triangles sometimes link civil servants, legislators, and lobbyists (or interest groups) when the legislature considers specific issues. For instance, if legislation about child abuse goes through a state legislature, several people who know each other and have worked together in the past may become active. Such collaboration may include lobbyists associated with children's advocacy groups; an association of the directors of public child welfare agencies around the state; professional associations, such as the state chapter of the National Association of Social Workers; a key civil servant in the state's welfare department; and an aide to a legislator with a long-standing interest in child abuse. Advocates need to be aware that these relationships exist and that they can be tapped for technical advice or for the support of a specific measure.

Public Opinion

Politicians, bureaucrats, and lobbyists work in an environment of uncertainty. They realize that voters can end a politician's career and can bring down an administration (Arnold, 1990). Bureaucrats are also vulnerable to public opinion because scandals or unpopular decisions can ruin political appointees' and even civil servants' careers (Lynn, 1987). Legislators often try to implement programs in ways that will please their constituents, as illustrated by politicians who oppose placing mental health facilities and prisons in their districts.

Advocates must often be persistent when seeking help from civil servants, but they must also be aware that civil servants are responsible for numerous tasks (Bell & Bell, 1982).

Regulations

Regulations powerfully shape the content of specific publicly funded programs because they define program details *not* contained in the statutes that established them. Wanting to avoid conflict that could stymie the enactment of specific legislation, legislators often prefer to delegate some policy details to regulators, that is, civil servants and government appointees. These government regulations must be published by oversight agencies before they become official so that the public can comment on them in public hearings and through written comments. When finalized, they are officially published as *administrative regulations* in the Federal Register—and can be located at www.gpoaccess.gov/fr/, where you can find them by keywords, enabling law, or issuing agency. You can find them in state venues by using Google Search. Policy advocates can propose possible new regulations by forwarding them to oversight agencies.

Legal Action

Advocates sometimes conclude that they can achieve their goals only through litigation, as illustrated by court suits against specific laws that have been enacted by many states to allow police officers to interrogate and detain individuals they believe may be undocumented based on their appearance. Advocates can inquire about public interest law firms with established reputations in specific areas of law to determine whether legal action might be an effective strategy.

HOW MACRO POLICY ADVOCATES ENGAGE THE EIGHT CHALLENGES

Now that we have discussed the context, we can turn to the way macro policy advocates contend with the eight challenges discussed in Figure 3.1 in Chapter 3.

CHALLENGE 1: DECIDING WHETHER TO PROCEED

Policy advocates initiate a policy advocacy intervention when they decide that an existing policy is flawed. It may be ethically flawed, whether because it violates ethical first-order principles or because it leads to adverse outcomes for consumers, as discussed in Chapter 3. It may be incongruent with evidence-based practices. Policy advocates sometimes initiate policy advocacy to advance the well-being of their organizations—for example, to preserve revenues essential to their operations as well as consumers' needs by opposing cuts in a specific government program. Public officials and members of political parties often support specific policies to enhance their political fortunes. Because Latinos had voted overwhelmingly for Democrats in the presidential and congressional elections of 2012, for example, many Democratic elected officials and party members were particularly desirous of obtaining major immigration reforms to consolidate their support during the Congressional elections of 2014 and the presidential election of 2016.

Policy advocates have similar motives when they decide to block specific policy initiatives. In the case of immigration reform, for example, relatively liberal policy advocates were determined to block initiatives in specific states that they regarded as anti-immigrant in nature, such as those allowing the police to stop people they suspected were not citizens because of their appearance. They often received assistance from courts, including the U.S. Supreme Court, that ruled that some of these policies were unconstitutional.

Advocates often consider practical factors. They may gauge the relative difficulty of changing a specific policy, sometimes deciding that it is futile to change a policy that is supported by powerful individuals and interests even when they believe the policy is flawed. For example, many advocates wanted to enact policies that would restrict gun ownership, outlaw possession of assault weapons, or limit the size of cartridges in the wake of the massacre of students, teachers, and administrators at Sandy Hook Elementary School in 2013 (see further discussion on page 149). They discovered, however, that the National Rifle Association (NRA) had such extraordinary power in the U.S. Congress, as well as many state legislatures, that they could not make forward progress and even lost ground in many states, which passed laws enhancing the ability of citizens to purchase guns, including assault weapons. *We have to remember that some policy goals may take even decades to enact.* Some civil rights laws, for example, were not enacted and implemented at the federal level until a century after the Civil War. Yet many surprising policy successes take place even when they seem unrealizable to advocates at a specific point in time. President Barack Obama was warned, for example, *not* to seek passage of the Affordable Care Act (ACA) by many of his top aides on grounds that it would not be politically feasible—but the rest, as they say, is history. Some policies that seem impossible to enact *can* be enacted by making compromises in them, including the ACA, which made major concessions to powerful interests, including health insurance companies, hospitals, and physicians—but their defenders argue that the ACA would not otherwise have been approved by Congress.

POLICY ADVOCACY LEARNING CHALLENGE 6.2

Analyzing the Ideology and Compromise

Take any major controversial policy proposal currently under consideration by a local, state, or federal legislature. Identify what their most ardent advocates would want, no matter their ideology, whether liberal or conservative. Then identify some concessions these advocates might consider supporting to make it more likely that it would be enacted. *Hint:* Take examples like national immigration reform, enactment of specific policies to decrease economic inequality, proposals to limit gun ownership, proposals to decriminalize drugs like marijuana, proposals to allow people with severe illnesses to legally receiving assistance to end their lives—or any other policy initiative with which you are familiar.

Discuss why policy advocates favor these policies. Discuss how they are likely to encounter people with divergent positions. See if you can identify some concessions these policy advocates might need to make to get their policies adopted.

CHALLENGE 2: DECIDING WHERE TO FOCUS

We discussed the context of public policies earlier in this chapter. Policy advocates frequently have to decide where to focus their work. Do they want to focus on local, state, or federal levels of government? Do they want to enact new legislation or to amend existing legislation? Do they seek regulatory reforms or new legislation? Which legislative committee should they approach—and which elected officials? Do they want to work with an established lobby group—and, if so, which one? Could they initiate a lawsuit to block specific legislative initiatives—and, if so, with what law firm or attorney? Do they decide to proceed with policy advocacy at the macro level or select the mezzo level?

CHALLENGE 3: SECURING DECISION MAKERS' ATTENTION

If they wish to be effective, policy advocates often must obtain the attention of decision makers such as supervisors, midlevel managers, specific physicians, or high-level administrators in clinic or hospital settings; directors of community-based agencies; elected officials in legislative settings; civil servants or political appointees in government agencies; or elected public officials.

These decision makers sometimes serve as "policy entrepreneurs" in advocating a specific policy reform. They may help to give it a title that is appealing to others. They may couple or link it with another policy or program, such as a program geared to preventing obesity among Latinos who have recently moved from normal weight to early-stage obesity. They may negotiate and bargain with clinic program and budget officials to see if they can find resources and office space for the new program. They may assemble other sponsors and supporters of the program from within the clinic and from the surrounding community—or within a legislature in the case of proposed legislation. They may seek key endorsements, such as from the American Diabetes Association or public agencies that would implement or oversee a proposed policy.

Policy advocates sometimes persevere even when they discover opposition to specific policy reforms, such as by taking an "outside-in" approach where they exert pressure on one or more decision makers. Perhaps they gain the attention of one or more advocacy groups that places external pressure on decision makers in organizational or legislative settings, such as the American Diabetes Association, which pressured principals and superintendents of public schools to provide on-site medical care for diabetic children in many states.

Policy advocates work closely with decision makers in *framing* policy proposals so that they attract support. Imagine, for example, how less appealing the preschool program known as Head Start would have been to many legislators had it been called "Kindergarten for Low-Income Children"—or how less appealing Medicare would have been had it been called "the Medical Program for Retirees." New initiatives need to be presented in ways that appeal to top managers, boards of directors, and funders in organizational settings.

Policy advocates sometimes rely on advocacy groups to sponsor and run with an issue, such as the National Association of Social Workers, the American Nursing Association, the American Public Health Association, the American Diabetes Association, the American Cancer Association, and many other interest groups in the health field. (Each of these groups has national associations located in or near Washington, DC, as well as state chapters.) These groups have lobbyists, researchers, media officials, and others with skills and experience in advocating legislation and regulations in legislatures and government agencies. Some unions assume important roles in securing policy reforms or in blocking proposals.

Policy advocates use their communication skills to persuade specific decision makers, legislators, or advocacy groups to assume leadership with respect to a specific issue. They use organizing skills to develop coalitions. They use influence-using skills to assess the feasibility of getting support for a specific policy initiative and to assess the likelihood and power of potential opponents.

Policy advocates have to decide which legislators might sponsor a specific piece of legislation. They often seek legislators with proven clout, such as the chairs of key committees or relatively high-level members of specific political parties. They often must engage in a balancing act where they seek initial support not just from die-hard supporters of specific legislation, but from legislators who hold moderate positions on a specific topic or who they believe can be persuaded to become supporters.

CHALLENGE 4: ANALYZING WHY A DYSFUNCTIONAL POLICY DEVELOPED

Macro policy advocates must often analyze who supports existing policies and why as they develop policy proposals. Take the issue of reforming gun laws in Congress in 2013 in the wake of the massacre at the Sandy Hook Elementary School in Connecticut, when a young man, armed with multiple rifles and pistols, killed many children, teachers, and the principal. Many legislators wanted to enact multifaceted legislation that would abolish cartridges that could contain many bullets, prohibit fast-firing weapons, tighten the checking of individuals' prior criminal records and whether they had been treated for mental illness, and restrict the number of bullets people could purchase. Proponents had to ask the following questions:

1. Did the gun lobby, headed by the NRA, possess such extraordinary power in Congress that working majorities for these various reforms could not be developed?

2. What interest groups existed that could counter the power of the NRA and its allies?

3. What power could the president and vice president exert?

4. Could public opinion in the districts of legislators be mobilized so that many of them would support gun reforms?

5. What specific committees in Congress would have to support gun reforms— and how were their members likely to vote?

6. Would the memory of Sandy Hook fade so that the urgency of enacting gun reforms would ebb?

Only after undertaking this kind of analysis could gun reform legislators decide what gun reforms to seek. This example illustrates how even skilled advocates often cannot quickly succeed: Not only did Congress not enact far-reaching gun controls, but *many* states loosened their gun laws. Gabby Giffords, the former congresswoman from Arizona who had suffered a serious brain injury from a gun-wielding assailant, concluded that gun reform could succeed only if its proponents continued their course for years to come. Most legislative initiatives take three or four years to bring to fruition—and some take even longer—so macro policy advocates have to be ready for protracted work. They must be persistent to realize their goal, but the sheer number of enacted policies in local, state, and federal jurisdictions attests to their many successes. Imagine a nation that lacked Medicare, Medicaid, the Supplemental Nutrition Assistance Program (SNAP), the Earned Income Tax Credit, and many facets of the Affordable Care Act, such as those that do not allow health insurance companies to cease coverage to people with preexisting conditions.

CHALLENGE 5: DEVELOPING POLICY PROPOSALS

Policy advocates develop proposals to reform specific policies. They typically identify a number of policy options for addressing a specific problem—and then compare the options to select the best one. They might compare the policy options with respect to criteria like cost, effectiveness, and political feasibility. They might then have to decide, on balance, which option is the best. In a specific state, for example, advocates of gun control decide whether to seek sweeping legislation that would outlaw all automatic weapons, including so-called assault weapons used by the military, versus legislation only limiting the size of cartridges, versus legislation denying these weapons only to people who have been incarcerated or shown to have serious mental illness. Some advocates may favor the first option but choose only to limit the size of cartridges on the grounds that the first option is not politically feasible at the present time. In jurisdictions more favorable to sweeping gun reform, such as Chicago, they might opt for a ban on all automatic weapons.

Macro policy advocates sometimes use specific analytic techni
policies in a process of *policy analysis*. They begin by identifying
tive that they wish to achieve, such as "decreasing the number of
in the general population" (Step 1). They select a *policy stre*
the policy objective, such as limiting the ability of guns in the gen
to injure or kill large numbers of people (Step 2). They identify *speci*.
options that enable them to address this problem, such as those we have iden.
fied in the preceding paragraph (Step 3). They *develop criteria* that allow them to
evaluate the merits of the specific policy options—and they determine the relative
weight or importance of each criterion (Step 4). They might decide, for example,
that the criteria are likely cost, effectiveness (in achieving the policy objective) and
political feasibility. They score each of the policy options on each of the criteria,
and then sum the scores of each policy option to determine the one that they will
prioritize in their macro policy advocacy.

We can illustrate policy analysis in Table 6.2. We list the criteria across the top of
the table—in this case, cost, effectiveness, and political feasibility. We could have
chosen different or additional criteria, such as ease of implementation or ethical
merit. (Ethical merit could include, for example, whether it is fair to keep weapons
away from people with prior mental illness or released felons when the vast majority
of them do not kill other people with guns.) We determine the weight of each criterion by giving it a score from 0 to 1.0 and make the sum of the scores of the different
criteria add up to 1, such as 0.2, 0.4, and 0.4 in Table 6.2. Here, too, we could have
made different choices, such as weighting "political feasibility" even lower in those
states where gun ownership is part of a hunting culture as compared to more urban
states. We then score each of the options by each criterion from 1 to 10—realizing
that we are making best guesses if scientific evidence does not exist. In Table 6.2, for
example, we had to guess the likely cost of each option from 1 (lowest) to 10 (highest), since it is hard to guess what the exact costs might be when we consider the
cost to the government to monitor each of the options. We then multiply the weight
of each criterion times the score we give each option—and then add the scores that
are in bold print in each cell and place the total as the overall score on the far right
of Table 6.2. As you can see, Option 2 (limiting the size of cartridges) received
the highest score at 5.8, Option 3 (limiting access to guns to mentally ill people)
received the second highest score at 5.2, and Option 1 (banning assault weapons)
received the lowest score. These scores would likely vary from state to state because
the political feasibility would vary by the culture and politics of each.

It is important not to dwell on the details of scoring rules, but on the structured,
step-by-step *analytic process* used to develop a final proposal. A specific policy
option rarely receives a perfect score, because it likely scores relatively high on
some criteria but lower on others.

ble 6.2 Policy Analysis to Compare Options for Gun Reform

Criteria Weight	Cost (0.2)	Effectiveness (0.4)	Political Feasibility (0.4)	Total Scores
OPTION 1 BAN ASSAULT WEAPONS	SCORE = 4 FINAL SCORE $(4 \times 0.2) = \textbf{0.8}$	SCORE = 6 FINAL SCORE $(6 \times 0.4) = \textbf{2.4}$	SCORE = 2 FINAL SCORE $(2 \times 0.4) = \textbf{0.8}$	**OVERALL SCORE = 4.0**
OPTION 2 LIMIT SIZE OF CARTRIDGES	SCORE = 7 FINAL SCORE $(7 \times 0.2) = \textbf{1.4}$	SCORE = 5 FINAL SCORE $(5 \times 0.4) = \textbf{2.0}$	SCORE = 6 FINAL SCORE $(6 \times 0.4) = \textbf{2.4}$	**OVERALL SCORE = 5.8**
OPTION 3 LIMIT ACCESS OF MENTALLY ILL PEOPLE TO GUNS	SCORE = 6 FINAL SCORE $(6 \times 0.2) = \textbf{1.2}$	SCORE = 2 FINAL SCORE $(2 \times 0.4) = \textbf{0.8}$	SCORE = 8 FINAL SCORE $(8 \times 0.4) = \textbf{3.2}$	**OVERALL SCORE = 5.2**

CHALLENGE 6: SECURING THE APPROVAL OR ENACTMENT OF A PROPOSAL

Policy advocates have to develop effective strategy if they wish to secure policy reforms. They have to establish policy goals, hone their proposal, establish a style, and select and use influence resources.

Developing Policy Goals

Policy advocates have to decide whether they want incremental change or basic change. They often have to downsize a proposal in the give-and-take of the political process. Policy advocates sometimes decide they want basic (or major) policy changes even if they encounter substantial opposition. They often develop fall-back strategies if they cannot obtain fundamental changes.

Honing the Proposal

Policy advocates often develop an initial proposal but fine-tune it as they proceed. When asked to identify his most difficult challenge, a top aide to President Bill Clinton said that he and the president constantly had to decide when to hold fast to specific policy proposals and when to accept compromises in the push-and-pull of the political process.

Developing a Style

Policy advocates sometimes use a high-conflict strategy that may include emotion-laden language and use of the mass media, particularly if they wish to appeal to relatively liberal or conservative constituents with strong ideological views. They often use a low-conflict strategy that emphasizes the technical details of their proposals and shared goals of different legislators. They select a style that they believe will be most effective in a specific situation. They may change their style as deliberations proceed. Stylistic options include:

- Focusing on technical details versus underlying principles
- Inviting substantive changes in the proposal versus resisting changes
- Expanding the number of people who participate versus limiting participation
- Seeking rapid resolution versus encouraging an extended process

Implementing and Assessing the Strategy

Even wise strategy choices come to naught, however, if advocates do not implement them skillfully. They need to be flexible; for example, they need to revise their strategies as events change. These revisions may include expanding the number of people that they consult, developing or expanding a coalition, or making concessions to others as they shape their policy proposal. Advocates sometimes soften their initial positions if they believe they cannot attract others to their cause or if they fear negative responses from members of their own party or their constituencies.

CHALLENGE 7: SECURING IMPLEMENTATION OF A POLICY REFORM

Enacted policies sometimes come to naught because they are not implemented at all, such as when they fail to receive needed budgetary resources or are poorly implemented, such as when executives and staff are not committed to them. Advocates may decide that perhaps government agencies need to monitor implemented programs more stringently in certain cases, such as when they think their resources are being used unwisely. Perhaps the implementing staff need more training to be able to achieve positive results or to be true to the provisions of a statute.

CHALLENGE 8: ASSESSING IMPLEMENTED POLICIES

Policy innovations have to be evaluated to ascertain if they improve consumers' well-being (effectiveness) and if they achieve these gains at acceptable costs (cost-effectiveness). Rigorous evaluations are often not conducted, however. They take considerable expertise to conduct, as well as considerable resources— and their findings may not emerge for several years.

Evidence-based policies emerge only as implemented policies are evaluated. Gold-standard evaluations require an experimental design to ascertain if persons who receive services or benefits from a specific program benefit from them when compared to a control group that does not receive these services and benefits. In many cases, evaluators have to rely on evaluations with less rigor due to lack of necessary resources or expertise—or because agency directors block evaluations of specific programs. An array of evidence-based policies can be identified by going online to various sites, including the site of the Campbell Collaboration that provides a searchable list of reviews of social research in the United States and Europe (www.campbellcollaboration.org).

Many policy assertions are made by public figures *as if* they have been subjected to evaluations when this is not true. For example, Mitt Romney, the Republican candidate for the presidency, asserted in 2012 that most spending by the federal government on public programs, like SNAP, housing vouchers, and Medicaid, has "massive overhead (so that) very little of the money that's needed by those that really need help . . . actually reaches them." In fact, administration costs of these programs range from 1% to 8% of total federal spending (Greenstein, 2012).

POLICY ADVOCACY LEARNING CHALLENGE 6.3

Getting to the Truth

Go online to see if the following assertions, which are often made in the public arena, are true:

1. Few users of safety-net programs work, including those who use SNAP and Medicaid
2. Increases in Medicaid or welfare programs in one state will attract low-income people from another state to emigrate to it
3. Tax increases for millionaires will cut the nation's economic growth

Select any other assertion made by a public figure and inquire whether research has shown it to be true.

Improvising When Engaging in the Eight Challenges

Policy advocates rarely engage in the eight policy advocacy challenges in a sequential process. They may bypass a challenge. They may engage in a challenge only to return to it at a later point. They improvise as events change.

IDENTIFYING MACRO POLICY ADVOCACY SKILLS

We now discuss specific skills that are needed by macro policy advocates.

Developing an Overarching Strategy

Macro policy advocates have to develop *political strategy*, that is, a sequence of actions and verbal exchanges that will increase the likelihood that a proposal will be enacted. Development of a political strategy contains seven steps:

1. *Organizing a team or coalition* that will spearhead the project, with leadership provided by an existing advocacy group (such as Planned Parenthood in a specific state) or by a new group.

2. *Establishing policy goals*, such as deciding whether to advocate incremental change or basic change. Advocates may decide in some cases that they want to block someone else's proposal if they believe it to be contrary to their values and preferences.

3. *Specifying a proposal's content*—and moving quickly to find early sponsors. Advocates often write a "policy brief" that identifies a policy issue, summarizes why the existing policy is inadequate, discusses available options, and selects a preferred option.

4. *Establishing a style*, such as opting for a nonconflictual process versus a higher-conflict approach that may include considerable publicity.

5. *Deciding who does what*, including who meets with specific people, who makes certain presentations, who does the research, and who develops lists of supporters.

6. *Implement the strategy* using the various influence and power resources.

7. *Revising the strategy* in light of changing events as the process unfolds.

Diagnosing Who Stands Where—and Recruiting People to a Cause

Macro policy advocates seldom have the luxury of unanimous support for a specific policy proposal. They often have to determine who stands where by talking with legislators, members of key interest groups, public officials, and others. Some people are intractable opponents. Others are enthusiastic supports. Others are undecided, but potentially persuadable—and these people often "swing the balance."

Advocates have to be skilled in recruiting people to their cause. They have to decide what provisions of a policy can be altered or added to their proposed legislation in order to gain support. They have to identify legislative leaders who are willing to persuade other legislators to support it.

Framing Issues to Gain Support

Macro policy advocates have to use words and concepts that elicit support for a policy among those legislators who are critical to its enactment. They often appeal to cultural symbols that attract support, like "prevention," "improving health," "increasing opportunity," "increasing fairness," "saving public resources," "increasing upward mobility," "helping children," "increasing transparency," "decreasing overhead," and "decreasing fraudulent use of public funds."

POLICY ADVOCACY LEARNING CHALLENGE 6.4

Identifying and Using Cultural Symbols

Take a stab at identifying cultural symbols that might prove adverse to securing support for a legislative measure, particularly with relatively conservative legislators. Might President Barack Obama have considered a different title for the Affordable Care Act to enhance support for it among conservatives, and, if so, what might a better title have been?

Networking and Coalition Building

Successful macro policy advocates have remarkably inclusive networks that they cultivate over an extended period. They can sometimes decrease opposition from likely opponents by finding commonalities with them, such as shared experiences. They can sometimes establish personal relationships by sending them thank-you notes or get-well notes. As social work policy advocate Melissa Bird said, "Most legislators are used to getting negative comments from their constituents for *not* supporting a specific measure or *for* supporting another measure. They really like positive communications, such as thank-you notes or congratulatory notes or even birthday cards."

Managing Conflict

Conflict often occurs but often needs to be "managed," whether upward or downward. Conflict sometimes enhances a policy advocate's quest to enact a specific piece of legislation, such as when it draws attention to a specific measure from opponents of the persons who create conflict by attacking it. Liberal and moderate legislators may, for example, believe a measure *must* be meritorious if conservatives attack it!

Conflict can often be harmful, however, when it highlights perceived shortcomings or objections to a specific policy proposal. It is particularly harmful if it leads some legislators in the "undecided" group to shift to the opposing group. Policy advocates can use many tactics to decrease conflict. They can persuade specific legislators that their views of a policy proposal are based on incorrect assumptions about it or knowledge of it. They can stress specific facets of the proposal that spur opposition to it. They can seek support from influential legislators who are widely admired by other legislators. They can change the proposal itself to make it less controversial.

Macro policy advocates often diminish conflict even as they write legislative proposals. They touch base with likely opponents or swing voters so that they can decrease the level of their opposition to them. They can sometimes anticipate opposition by examining prior voting patterns of legislators on similar policy proposals.

Using Procedural Power

Macro policy advocates often use procedural power to increase the chances that a particular measure will be enacted. They convince prominent and influential legislators to sponsor their legislation. They try to route their measures to those legislative committees and subcommittees that will be favorable to them. They try to get hearings for their policy proposals before legislative committees, because few measures are enacted that do not receive hearings in a timely way.

Developing and Using Personal Power Resources

Consider power transactions to be transactional in nature. Person A interacts with Person B in a way that makes Person B adopt a position or take actions that she or he would not otherwise take. Assume, for example, that Person B is predisposed to opposing a specific policy, but changes her mind *after* Person A discusses it with her. If Person B would not otherwise have changed her mind, Person A has successfully used her personal power sources, such as her communication skills, to induce Person B to support legislation she would otherwise have opposed.

Each of us has a considerable number of personal power resources in specific situations, but only to the extent that other people *respond* to them. We possess *expertise* based on our professional and other knowledge. We possess *reward power* to the extent that others believe we have and will use inducements such as money, recognition, friendship, favors, or increased support from their constituents. We possess *coercive power* to the extent that other people believe we can withhold inducements or impose penalties, such as excluding them from deliberations, harming their reputations, decreasing support for them from their constituents, firing them, or otherwise harming them. We possess the power of *authority* to the extent that others believe we hold powerful or influential positions that might ultimately help or harm them. We possess *charisma* to the extent that other people respond positively to our requests because of our personal qualities. We develop *substantive power* as other people come to see us as able to improve policy proposals or to make changes in them that are viewed as correct or advisable.

We develop these and other power resources as others come to view us in positive terms as they interact with us or learn about us. Persons who come to be viewed as "straight shooters" often benefit from this reputation in legislative settings, because legislators want and need accurate information and truthful interactions. People come to be seen as "credible" as they develop a reputation, often over many years, for providing accurate information.

Developing Credible Proposals

Macro policy advocates have to develop credible proposals. They have to demonstrate that they will be effective in addressing specific problems or issues. They need the support of recognized experts or research. They have to show that they can be funded by existing resources.

Negotiating Skills

Macro policy advocates have to be effective negotiators. They need to make concessions that appear reasonable, yet they cannot be perceived as "pushovers" who will always back down. Negotiators often "test the waters" by floating relatively minor concessions—and then expanding them or withdrawing them as circumstances dictate.

Developing Power by Changing Legislators' Environment

Legislators do not live in cocoons, but in systems that expose them to multiple interactions with the external world. Macro policy advocates can often impact legislators' decisions by changing their external environment. They can place pressure on them by using social media to lead many people to send them messages on Facebook, Twitter, and other social media sites—messages that may urge them to take or refrain from specific actions. Working with advocacy groups, macro policy advocates can pressure legislators to take certain actions, not only through lobbying but by encouraging their constituents to take specific actions. Macro policy advocates can place pressure on legislators by obtaining stories in the mass media that give them positive or negative coverage for specific positions or actions that they have taken.

Macro policy advocates can place pressure on specific legislators by participating in electoral politics. They can elicit support for them by engaging in political campaigns or can work to defeat them. They can organize specific parts of legislators' constituencies, such as homeless people, low-income people, residents of public housing, and other constituencies. They can raise funds for specific candidates.

Developing Personal Connections

It is easy to forget that public officials are people with the same problems and issues as everyone else. Policy advocates need skills to forge personal relationships with public officials, even getting to know names of their family members, learning their hobbies, discovering mutual friendships, and seeing them at a number of occasions. Nor does it hurt to empathize with them about the significant challenges public life brings to them, such as loss of anonymity, hectic working schedules, and exposure to criticism in the mass media.

POLICY ADVOCACY LEARNING CHALLENGE 6.5

Key Skills and Personal Assets

Identify some of the skills needed by macro policy advocates in the preceding discussion—but also identify some additional skills *not* discussed in the preceding pages. Discuss which of these skills you think you possess—and which you would like to further enhance.

Read the vignette in Policy Advocacy Learning Challenge 6.2 to identify key skills needed by macro policy advocates like social worker Melissa Bird, who successfully persuaded members of the legislature of the State of Utah to enact a specific piece of legislation. What specific policy advocacy skills did Melissa Bird use? What attributes does she possess that contributed to her success in enacting legislative proposals?

Can you imagine becoming a macro policy advocate for an issue that interests you, whether as someone like Melissa Bird or in some other capacity, such as working on a political campaign or helping an advocacy group?

POLICY ADVOCACY LEARNING CHALLENGE 6.6

A Social Worker Persuades the Utah Legislature to Advance Women's Reproductive Rights

By Melissa Bird, MSW and PhD candidate
at the School of Social Work at the University of Southern California

In my second year of my MSW program at the University of Utah, I engaged in research on homeless youth. It was my intent to discover how many homeless youth

(Continued)

(Continued)

identified as lesbian, gay, bisexual, transgender, or questioning (LGBTQ). At the time, there was no homeless youth shelter, and I partnered with Volunteers of America's Homeless Youth Resource Center (HYRC), a nonprofit agency in Salt Lake City which provided drop-in services to homeless youth under the age of 25. Estimates by advocates indicated that over 1,000 young people were homeless, oftentimes forced to sleep in subzero temperatures. As my working relationship with HYRC evolved, I became aware that the law in Utah stated that youth could not be sheltered for longer than eight hours without parental consent or emancipation, and there was no emancipation statute in the state of Utah.

This policy situation was untenable to me as a social welfare advocate. Armed with the policy advocacy skills I had learned in my MSW program, the data I had collected, and the knowledge that hundreds of young people were sleeping in the streets, I decided to tackle the issue of emancipation. Using the principles of social work and the science of social change, I sat at my dining room table and wrote my first piece of legislation. Building on the emancipation statutes from 26 other states, I crafted my bill (six more policies would be drafted over the next eight years, five of which were passed into law). As I combed through the policies from other states, it became clear that if I were to be successful in my endeavor to pass legislation, I would have to tailor my words carefully so that they would be palatable in a conservative political environment. After my draft was written, I contacted former Utah representative Roz McGee and asked her if she would look at my bill. Within minutes of reading it, not only did Representative McGee say that it was an incredible document but that she would be honored to sponsor it. Thus HB 77 Emancipation of a Minor was born.

The number-one social work principle that has carried me throughout my macro practice career has been working with people where they are, not where I want them to be. Working with politicians, stakeholders, nonprofit advocates, state agencies, and lobbyists can be an incredibly complicated and daunting task. I honed my skills and learned the legislative process with patience and an open mind. I understood that emancipation of youth was a complicated subject, especially in a conservative state where family and the rights of parents are paramount above all else. There is a saying that laws are like sausages: You don't want to see how either one is made. Being a social welfare advocate and a professionally trained social worker meant that I was ready and able to deal with the messiness of the Utah Legislature.

Honing My Skills

Representative McGee worked with me closely as I honed my skills as a macro-level practitioner. Not only did I need to learn how a bill becomes a law, but I needed to understand the fundamental difference between the words *may* (permissive) and *shall* (mandate), why budgets are important (the fiscal note had to be minor in order to get it through the process), who the people in power were (in Utah, the conservatives held the keys to the kingdom), and how to deal with conflicts and setbacks in a professional (read *unemotional*) manner. Strategically, you must get to know your legislature. Members of the legislature can be broken into three categories: *saints* (the legislators who support you 100% of the time), *sinners* (the legislators who never support you 100% of the time), and *savables* (the legislators who are on the fence). When developing macro policy strategy, you want to target the savables. Those are the legislators who you can move to your side. They are the ones who help you win.

Building a Coalition

Since I was the person who brought the issue of emancipation to Representative McGee, coalition building became my main task after the final draft of the bill was introduced. I went to the usual sources (the Health and Human Services' Division of Child and Family Services and Juvenile Justice Services) but also got creative. The best example of this is my cold-calling the attorney general of Utah, Mark Shurtleff. From the local media, I was aware of his special interest in the "lost boys" of polygamous communities throughout Utah. Young men were being kicked out of their homes and forced into homelessness by their parents, and it was my hope that his passionate interest in this issue would give me the backing I needed from the attorney general's office. Not only did I gain the valuable support of the attorney general, but my willingness to be candid and honest with him in our initial meeting led to a professional relationship that lasted years, even though we were on very different spectrums politically and philosophically.

Learning to Deal With Conflict

When engaging in macro-level policy, you will encounter an unusual amount of conflict, not just from people you know are your enemies (the one who will vote or work against you 100% of the time), but also from people you would have thought would be inherent allies. Despite this conflict, your success as a macro policy practitioner is dependent on your being able to work with everyone, even people you don't think you can work with. I cannot begin to tell you how many times I was shocked when meeting with peers and fellow social workers to hear things like, "You will never pass this legislation," "We can't support you because it would be detrimental to our agency," and "This is too controversial and you won't be successful anyway." If I had listened to everyone who told me this was impossible, hundreds of youth in Utah would still be sleeping in the snow. The person who became my main source of conflict was a conservative lobbyist named Gayle Ruzicka. She is the head of the Eagle Forum and was dead set on killing my emancipation bill. Gayle could have been a "sinner," and she was successful in killing the bill the first year it was introduced.

(Continued)

(Continued)

In 2006, HB 30 Emancipation of a Minor was reintroduced. This time I worked with Gayle to insert one crucial line about parents' fundamental rights over their children. This ensured that the bill passed, and we both ended up feeling like it was a good piece of legislation that would help children and their families.

I remember asking my policy professor if there were macro-level jobs for me in Utah; she told me no. I proved her wrong when my experience as a citizen lobbyist, a macro-level social worker, and a professional that works with people in a nondivisive manner led to a job as the executive director of the Planned Parenthood Action Council and vice president of public policy for Planned Parenthood of Utah. Never did I believe that one piece of legislation would lead to six. I continue to attribute my success as a lobbyist to successfully making the connection with the missing half of advocacy: bringing case advocacy skills together with policy advocacy skills to improve the lives of women and children throughout Utah.

LEARNING OUTCOMES

You are now equipped to:

- Use macro policy advocacy skills
- Analyze the context of macro policy advocacy
- Discuss how macro policy advocates engage the eight challenges
- Use a macro policy advocacy vignette to review content in this chapter

REFERENCES

Arnold, R. D. (1990). *The logic of Congressional action.* New Haven, CT: Yale University Press.

Bell, W., & Bell, B. (1982). Monitoring the bureaucracy: An extension of legislative lobbying. In M. Mahaffey & J. Hanks, *Practical politics: Social work and political responsibility.* Silver Spring, MD: National Association of Social Workers.

Greenstein, R. (2012, April 17). *Testimony before the House Budget Committee hearing on strengthening the safety net.* Center on Budget and Policy Priorities. Retrieved January 10, 2013, from http://www.cbpp.org/cms/index.cfm?fa=view&id=3745

Holtzman, A. (1970). *Legislative liaison: Executive leadership in the Congress.* Chicago, IL: Rand McNally.

Lynn, L. (1987). *Managing public policy.* Boston, MA: Little, Brown.

McIver, J. W. (1981). *Tribes on the Hill.* New York, NY: Rawson Wade.

Richan, W. (1991). *Lobbying for social change.* New York, NY: Haworth Press.

Smith, H. (1988). *The power games: How Washington works.* New York, NY: Ballantine Books.

Chapter 7

Becoming Policy Advocates in the Healthcare Sector

LEARNING OBJECTIVES

In this chapter, you will learn how to:

1. Analyze the evolution of the healthcare system in the United States

2. Analyze how health disparities are powerfully linked to economic inequality in the United States

3. Describe the political economy of the health sector, including powerful players and interests, as well as underrepresented ones—and identify some key advocacy groups in the health sector

4. Analyze seven core problems in the American health system and identify examples of Red Flag Alerts with respect to each of them

5. Identify background information about the causes and scope of each of the seven core problems

6. Identify important regulations, statutes, and programs that are important resources for advocates

7. Drawing upon vignettes in this chapter, discuss how advocates can move from micro policy advocacy to mezzo and macro policy advocacy

8. Learn about "breaking news" in the healthcare system

9. Discuss a major proposal for reforming the American healthcare system

The health sector will likely consume as much as 20% of the gross domestic product of the United States soon—or nearly one in five dollars spent by Americans. Yet it has been plagued by many problems, including inequitable access to medical services by low-income Americans, health disparities, and poor health outcomes when compared to other industrial nations, even as many Americans benefit from its medical care.

ANALYZING THE EVOLUTION OF THE AMERICAN HEALTHCARE SYSTEM

The evolution of the American healthcare system from the colonial era to the present is depicted by the following timeline:

- In the 19th century, the United States develops a two-tiered health system consisting of private-fee-paying individuals and low-income people who use public institutions.
- In the early 20th century, a national network of private nonprofit hospitals emerges. They are typically started by Jewish, Protestant, and Catholic religious groups.
- In the early 20th century, states enact laws for the licensing of physicians and hospitals as the American Medical Association (AMA) emerges as the most powerful lobbying group in the various states.
- From 1915 to 1920, various states reject proposals to enact state health insurance plans funded by public resources.
- In the late 19th century and early 20th century, public systems of healthcare emerge in many big cities, primarily serving low-income individuals who cannot afford private care.
- In the 1930s, Franklin Roosevelt decides *not* to include national health insurance in the Social Security Act because he fears that opponents, led by the AMA, will block the Social Security Act itself.
- Private health insurance begins in the 1930s and early 1940s but rapidly expands during World War II and afterward—the 1950s and 1960s—so that a vast majority of Americans receive private health insurance from their employers.
- After World War II, the Veterans Administration is established—and soon establishes a national network of hospitals.
- After World War II, the National Institutes of Health (NIH) is established.
- In 1949, Congress fails to enact President Harry Truman's proposal for national healthcare.

- After World War II, a national system of health benefits for federal civilian employees and their dependents is established. (It covers about 9 million people by 2014.)
- Congress enacts Medicare in 1965 to help finance acute care among seniors. Medicare provides inpatient care to people over 65 for relatively short-term health conditions (Part A), which is financed by payroll deductions of employers and employees. It also provides hospital care (Part B), which is financed by monthly premiums from seniors and from general revenues. (Other groups were added to Medicare in subsequent years, such as people with kidney disease who need dialysis and kidney transplants.)
- Congress enacts Medicaid in 1965 to serve two populations: (1) low-income nonelderly individuals who do not have private health insurance, whose medical costs bankrupt them, or who are on welfare rolls, and (2) seniors who become medically bankrupted when their medical costs exceed Medicare's benefits and their private savings. Medicaid is financed by a combination of federal payments and state payments. It covers many people who were previous uninsured.
- During the 1970s through the 1990s, Congress fails to enact national health insurance proposals put forward by Presidents Richard Nixon, Jimmy Carter, and Bill Clinton.
- In 1997, the Children's Health Insurance Program (CHIP) is established to finance healthcare for children not eligible for Medicaid.
- In 2010, President Barack Obama enacts the Affordable Care Act (ACA), the most significant health enactment since the passage of Medicare and Medicaid. We discuss its provisions subsequently in this chapter as well as its implementation in succeeding years.

IDENTIFYING HEALTH PROBLEMS CAUSED BY ECONOMIC INEQUALITY

VIDEO LINK 7.1
Improving Healthcare for Foster Children

Low-income consumers and consumers with low levels of education have higher rates of morbidity and shorter lives than other people (Kawachi, Daniels, & Robinson, 2005). Health disparities are caused by a combination of economic and social factors, including lack of nutrition and adequate housing, lack of stable employment, lack of health knowledge, community violence, fatalism, mental disorders linked to poverty, inaccessible healthcare, inability to finance healthcare, substance abuse, and unstable support systems (Jacobs, Kohrman, Lemon, & Vickers, 2003).

The nation has made remarkable progress in lengthening life spans and improving public health during the last century, but health disparities remain unacceptably high in the United States when we compare white Americans with specific racial groups and when we compare people in the top fifth of the economic distribution with those in the bottom fifth (Kawachi et al., 2005; Satcher et al., 2005). If relatively affluent African Americans have better health than low-income members of their races, *even they* often have poorer health outcomes than relatively affluent Caucasians (Kawachi et al., 2005).

Low-income Americans are more marginalized economically and educationally than their counterparts in Canada, the UK, and Japan. They are less educated and lack strong supports from safety-net programs (California Newsreel, 2008). They have lower rates of civic participation, with voting rates of only 49.1% as compared to 56.1% in Canada and 83.2% in Sweden (Jackson, 2002).

Some researchers have contended that Latino/as appear to have escaped the nexus between race, poverty, and poor health in the so-called Mexican American paradox. Mexican Americans have a life expectancy of 77 years for men and 83 years for women, for example—and this longevity, they contend, extends even to low-income Mexican Americans (Lee & McConville, 2007). They conjecture that social factors, such as cohesive families and religiosity, as well as diet, may have caused these positive effects. Other researchers argue, however, that sampling errors may account for some of these results. They note that immigrants to the United States have better health than migrants who have resided in the United States for a considerable period, which would suggest that Latino/as' health will erode as more of them are residents for longer periods. They also note that Latino/as have been plagued by an epidemic of obesity and diabetes that already is eroding these positive health outcomes. If 6.4% of Caucasians are diabetic, 11.1% of Latino/as are now afflicted with this disease (Office of Minority Health, 2009). Latino/as also suffer from increasing rates of HIV/AIDS and heart disease (Lee & McConville, 2007).

Poverty is associated with shorter lives and greater illness for several reasons. Poor people are more likely than affluent people to lack insurance and to lack accessible health practitioners and services. Some theorists contend that poverty causes adverse biological changes (Barr, 2008). Poverty is associated with poorer diets and less exercise, as well as higher rates of smoking. Some theorists contend that inequality in American society marginalizes American poor people as compared to poor people in nations with lower levels of inequality, creating stressors that undermine physical health.

ANALYZING THE POLITICAL ECONOMY OF THE AMERICAN HEALTH SYSTEM

The American health system places extraordinary power in the hands of its large funders, including private health. insurance companies and large employers. It places great power in nonprofit hospitals, for-profit hospitals, and managed care plans, which maintain powerful lobbies in state and federal capitols. The American Medical Association wields considerable influence, but its power has eroded as increasing numbers of physicians have taken salaried positions in managed-care plans and in hospitals. Trial lawyers oppose policies that would disallow or place caps on awards from malpractice insurance. State governments lobby federal authorities and Congress not to decrease the federal share of Medicaid's costs. Pharmaceutical companies and companies that make medical devices contribute heavily to political campaigns and lobby government officials to block regulations that limit the development and marketing of their products. Many conservative Republicans have sought to repeal the ACA. The U.S. Supreme Court has already made key rulings that overturned key portions of the ACA while also supporting other portions.

Many advocacy groups seek an American health system that is in accord with ethical principles of social justice (see Table 7.1).

Table 7.1   Advocacy Groups Seeking a Just American Health System

American Medical Student Association
American Nurses Association
American Public Health Association
California Nurses Association/National Nurses Organizing Committee
Families USA
Kaiser Family Foundation
Medicare Rights Center
National Association of Social Workers
National Physicians Alliance
Robert Wood Johnson Foundation

The power of state and federal governments has grown with the size of Medicare and Medicaid, which are administered by the federal Centers for Medicare and Medicaid Services (CMS). Republicans have failed to cut these programs' size or change them in major ways despite repeated attempts to do so, such as by seeking to turn Medicaid over to the states or replace Medicare with individual savings accounts.

The politics of healthcare often centers on technical issues, like the size of specific reimbursements, eligibility standards, various legal issues, and jockeying between states and the federal government over funding issues. Ideological conflict powerfully shapes the development of American health policies. Conservatives thwarted the passage of national health insurance in the presidencies of Richard Nixon, Jimmy Carter, and Bill Clinton. They sought to block enactment of the ACA in 2010—and then sought to repeal it or to slow its implementation in years following 2010. The ACA survived an important legal challenge in 2012 when the Supreme Court ruled that it was constitutional, but the Court also ruled that individual states could decide whether or not to expand the Medicaid program to include many noninsured persons who did not quality for health insurance offered by so-called state exchanges. The ACA faced yet another challenge in the Supreme Court in 2015 when conservatives hoped it would rule that the federal government could not provide subsidies to low- and moderate-income persons that would enable them to afford health insurance offered by state exchanges run by the federal government. They have often attempted to diminish federal funding and policy roles with respect to Medicaid. Other hot-button issues include proposals to allow physicians to prescribe life-ending medications to terminally ill patients, to legalize marijuana for medical purposes, to limit or enhance women's reproductive rights, and to limit malpractice suits.

Powerful interests dominate debates about healthcare in the United States. Health consumers, people of color, immigrants, and members of vulnerable populations have relatively little power in policy debates. Advocates of preventive services command less than 3% of health resources. Yet innovations of the ACA, if properly funded and implemented, could bring many positive reforms into place in the coming years.

ANALYZING SEVEN CORE PROBLEMS

Core Problem 1: Engaging in Advocacy to Promote Patients' Ethical Rights, Human Rights, and Economic Justice—With Some Red Flag Alerts

Many ethical issues arise in the American health system. Patients have to make difficult choices, often involving life-and-death issues. Health systems collect extensive data from patients about sensitive issues. Patients and parents have to make difficult decisions about preserving and ending lives. Decisions must often be made in a brief time span. Medical errors frequently occur, including hospital errors that cause between 100,000 and 400,000 preventable deaths per year ("Survive Your Stay," 2014). A power imbalance often exists between physicians and their patients that can lead to poor communication.

- **Red Flag Alert 7.1.** Specific patients do not give informed consent to procedures because health professionals fail to discuss the possible benefits, dangers, or side effects of treatment options—or do not inform them about certain treatment options, including the option of not proceeding with invasive procedures or specific medications.
- **Red Flag Alert 7.2.** The confidentiality of specific patients' medical information is not preserved because it is divulged to others without their consent.
- **Red Flag Alert 7.3.** Medical professionals perform surgery or provide medications to patients who are not competent to give informed consent, such as patients with limited cognitive function.
- **Red Flag Alert 7.4.** A patient is not informed of her right to sign an advance directive that tells health professionals what kinds of treatments she does not want under specified circumstances—for example, if she is comatose or has a terminal health condition such as incurable cancer. Advance directives also allow patients to name others who will act on their behalf if they are unable to express their own wishes. Health professionals sometimes do not honor patients' advance directives even when they exist.
- **Red Flag Alert 7.5.** A patient is given misleading information or insufficient information so that he cannot give informed consent as required by specific regulations and court rulings.
- **Red Flag Alert 7.6.** Inequitable or inferior treatment of specific patients takes place against members of specific vulnerable populations, such as members of racial minorities, women, LGBTQQ individuals, homeless people, people with mental health or substance abuse conditions, and low-income people.
- **Red Flag Alert 7.7.** The health system is financed in ways that lead to inferior care for people who cannot afford its care.
- **Red Flag Alert 7.8.** Health professionals fail to disclose conflicts of interest to patients, such as by referring them to nursing or convalescent homes that they wholly or partly own.

Background

We do not have data about the frequency of violations of patients' ethical rights in the United States. In a recent survey of 300 frontline health professionals (social workers, nurses, and medical residents), many respondents reported that they had seen considerable numbers of patients with the seven kinds of unresolved problems during the prior two months (Jansson et al., in press).

Resources for Advocates

Health advocates can draw on many existing policies to promote patients' ethical rights at the micro level, including accreditation standards, statutes and constitutional rights, state and federal regulations, and court rulings, as well as the standards of state-level boards that license health professionals.

Accreditation Standards. A chapter of the Joint Commission *accreditation standards* for hospitals is devoted to "rights and responsibilities of the individual" (Joint Commission, 2009). It asks hospitals to develop written policies on patient rights, including their right to refuse care, treatment, and services in accordance with laws and regulations, and to disseminate those policies to consumers. It requires patients to give informed consent. It requires that patients be informed about advance directives, including their right to forgo or withdraw life-sustaining treatment and to withhold resuscitative services. It identifies patients' right to participate in care decisions and to be treated in a dignified and respectful manner. It discusses patients' right to privacy, including their right to decline being filmed or recorded. It requires that patients receive caring treatment, including knowing the names of physicians or other practitioners that care for them. It discusses patients' right to participate in end-of-life decisions. It says that consumers have the right to receive information in a manner that they understand (since "communication is a cornerstone of patient safety and quality care"), including the right to translation services and communication that addresses the needs of people with visual or hearing impairments, children, and people with cognitive impairments. It asks hospitals to respect consumers' cultural and personal beliefs and preferences—as well as their right to religious and other spiritual services. It asks hospitals to allow consumers access to their health information. It requires each hospital to "put its respect for the patient's rights into action by showing its support of these rights in the ways that staff and caregivers interact with the patient and involve him or her in care, treatment, and services" (Joint Commission, 2009). It asks hospitals to involve surrogate decision makers when consumers are unable to make their own decisions. It asks them to involve consumers' families in making health decisions to the extent permitted by specific patients or surrogates. It requires hospitals to inform consumers or their surrogates of unanticipated outcomes of care, treatment, and services.

It asks hospitals to respect consumers' rights during research, investigation, and clinical trials. It requires hospitals to give consumers copies of some of its policies, including those about informed consent and advance directives.

These accreditation standards ask hospitals to develop measures to determine the extent to which they implement many of these policies, whether through documentation (such as in medical records) or consumer surveys. The accrediting team grades the hospital as achieving insufficient compliance, partial compliance, or satisfactory compliance with these ethical standards. It can recommend loss of accreditation or probationary status for hospitals that violate ethical standards—a decision that could lead to loss of Medicare and Medicaid funding and make it difficult to attract qualified staff.

Statutes and Constitutions. Many court rulings, as well as the federal Patient Self-Determination Act of 1990, give consumers the right to make their own medical decisions as long as they are not minors and are competent. They can decline treatment even when informed that they will suffer harm, or even death, without it. The Patient Self-Determination Act requires medical personnel to educate consumers about so-called advance directives that allow them to state what medical procedures they want, or do not want, if they are unable to communicate their wishes. The Fourteenth Amendment to the Constitution gives people a right to privacy that protects their right to informed consent for medical procedures (Stein, 2004).

Congress enacted the Health Information Portability and Accountability Act of 1996 (HIPAA; Annas, 2003). It protects individually identifiable health information from disclosure to others without the patient's consent. HIPAA calls this information "protected health information or PHI," and it includes patient information identified by name, address, telephone, or email address; transmitted via "any form or medium"; and consisting of "any information, oral or recorded, relating to the health of an individual, the health care provided to an individual, or payment for health care provided to an individual" (California Hospital Association [CHA], 2008, p. 16.4).

Providers must obtain advance authorization, in "plain language," from consumers to release their PHI. Some exceptions to HIPAA requirements include the release of information to researchers that is not personally identifiable, the release of HIV test results to public health officials in many states, and psychotherapy notes used by students, trainees, or mental health practitioners to develop their treatment skills. HIPAA allows release of information with respect to victims of abuse, neglect, or domestic violence to specific authorities.

Health advocates can advance social justice by helping patients gain access to federal programs that have improved access to healthcare for tens of millions of patients including Medicare, Medicaid, CHIP, and programs established by the ACA.

Regulations. Many state and federal regulations protect consumers' ethical rights, covering such diverse topics as determining when medical interventions can be terminated for dying patients, advance directives, safeguards for consumers who participate in research on human subjects, privacy rights, and informed consent. People who do not heed regulations can be subject to fines and criminal sanctions.

Regulations sometimes allow release of patients' information to appropriate authorities, but only under specific circumstances. Physicians, hospitals, and other healthcare providers must report all AIDS cases, HIV infections, and viral hepatitis infections, including those caused by blood transfusions, to the local health officer or other designated agency within a specific time frame.

Consumers who have been subject to sexual and other assaults often visit emergency rooms, clinics, and other health providers. Health practitioners are required to make reports to local law enforcement when they treat patients with specified injuries from possible assaults. "Assaultive or abusive conduct" includes (in California) a wide range of offenses, including murder; manslaughter; mayhem; aggravative mayhem; torture; assault with intent to commit mayhem, rape, sodomy, or oral copulation; administering controlled substances or anesthetics to aid in commission of a felony; battery; sexual battery; incest; throwing corrosive materials with intent to injure or disfigure; assault with a deadly weapon; rape; spousal rape; procuring any female to have sex with another man; child abuse and endangerment; abuse of a spouse or cohabitant; sodomy; lewd and lascivious acts with a child; oral copulation; sexual penetration by a foreign object; elder abuse; and attempts to commit any of these offenses (CHA, 2008). Patients who are victims of abuse or domestic violence must be informed that a report has been or will be made, unless (in California) the providers fear a report could place the patient at risk of serious harm *or* fear that they would be informing a personal representative who was responsible for the abuse, neglect, or other injury, which could result in injury to the victim (CHA, 2008). Health practitioners often enter into the medical record comments by the injured person regarding past domestic violence or the names of those suspected of inflicting injuries or assaultive or abusive conduct, as well as a map of the injured person's body showing where wounds were inflicted and a copy of the law enforcement reporting form (CHA, 2008). Failure to report is a misdemeanor punishable by fines, imprisonment, or both. Those suspected or accused of inflicting injuries, and their attorneys, cannot be allowed access to the injured person (CHA, 2008).

It is important to realize that regulations in one state are often different from those in other states—so you need to find experts to help you navigate the regulations in your own state. Take the case of regulations about HIV tests. Many states, such as California, require patients to consent to HIV tests; thus, physicians must inform the patient that the test is planned, provide information about the test, inform the patient of treatment options if he or she tests positive, and advise the patient that he or she has the right to decline the test. In some states, the medical care provider has to make a note in the medical record if the patient declines the HIV test. Different procedures exist for minors 12 years and older and children under age 12, as well as criminal defendants and inmates. Some states declare results of HIV tests to be confidential, as do federal privacy regulations. However, disclosures can be made to specific organizations or individuals, including health personnel who may have had contact with someone who tests positive. Physicians who order HIV tests in California may, but are not required to, disclose confirmed positive test results to the consumer's spouse, people reasonably believed to have been a sexual partner of the consumer, people who shared hypodermic needles with the consumer, or local health officers—but they must first discuss the results with the consumer, counsel him or her, and attempt to obtain voluntary consent prior to notifying the consumer's contacts. (When contacts are notified, the physicians must refer them for appropriate care.) Improper disclosures can bring civil penalties, including fines (CHA, 2008). First responders and healthcare personnel who have experienced significant exposure to patients' blood or other potentially infectious materials can ask for HIV testing of those patients under certain conditions (CHA, 2008).

Parents face difficult choices when they have infants who have serious medical conditions that may terminate their lives. Using information from their physicians, parents make final decisions unless they are incompetent or can't agree with one another. Nonetheless, various court rulings state that physicians should always act in the best interests of the child and provide life-sustaining treatment unless and until a court resolves the dispute. In general, life-sustaining treatment for newborns should not be withdrawn or withheld merely because they have a disability such as Down's syndrome or because their medical care will be costly. When parents and members of the healthcare team can't agree, they should generally turn to a multidisciplinary hospital ethics committee before resorting to the courts. The committee does not make treatment decisions or decide whether to disqualify parents but facilitates communication and provides advisory guidance when ethical conflicts exist (CHA, 2008). Health staff often need legal advice when making these decisions, because the federal Child Abuse Amendments of 1984 allow withholding of life-sustaining treatment only if infants are comatose and if treatment merely prolongs dying and would be medically futile (CHA, 2008, pp. 5–15).

Court Rulings. The U.S. Supreme Court, as well as lower courts, have ruled on such diverse topics as the right of states to enact legislation allowing physicians to prescribe lethal drugs to terminally ill patients, the use of medical marijuana for patients in pain, women's right to abort a fetus, informed consent, and the right of physicians to discontinue medical care for comatose patients.

Consumers can sue physicians, hospitals, and clinics for violating their ethical rights as established in constitutions, statutes, regulations, and accreditation standards. Failure to obtain proper consent to treatment can result in battery, professional negligence (malpractice), and/or unprofessional conduct charges against the physician or other healthcare provider *for even the simplest of procedures* (CHA, 2008). (Battery is defined legally as "the intentional touching of a person in a harmful or offensive manner without his or her consent"—and battery charges can be filed against any healthcare provider who performs a medical procedure without a patient's consent or performs a procedure that exceeds the scope of the consent *even* when the physician has no wrongful intent [CHA, 2008].) Physicians who fail to disclose the risks and alternatives open to consumers can be sued for malpractice. They must inform consumers of potentially conflicting interests, such as research or financial interests (CHA, 2008). Courts have frequently ruled that patients have the right of self-determination—even the right to decline treatment against physicians' advice.

Regulating Professionals' Conduct

Physicians, nurses, and social workers are licensed and regulated by state boards or commissions. These boards have the right to place practitioners on probation or to prohibit them from practicing if they violate specific ethical standards, such as by engaging in fraudulent behavior, battery, or malpractice; using drugs; or sexually abusing their patients.

POLICY ADVOCACY LEARNING CHALLENGE 7.1

Connecting Micro, Mezzo, and Macro Policy Advocacy to Protect a Patient's Ethical Rights

Mary was in the hospital for weeks. The nurse reported that there were reports that Mary had specifically stated that she did not want dialysis or life-sustaining measures if her health worsened. Yet Mary was on dialysis. She had been transferred to institutions far from her home in San Diego. Her caseworker, Joanne, was still in San Diego and called me yesterday morning. She sounded flabbergasted: "She's on dialysis?!? I've been her worker for over five years. I haven't been able to get there, but I'm coming this week and we'll settle this." Mary's wishes had been blatantly disrespected despite the voices of advocates who had attempted to bring attention to Mary's wishes and how her current level of care contradicted those desires.

Joanne arrived. Furious, she had already put motions into action to obtain a court order to stop the heroic measures that were artificially keeping Mary alive against her will and her previously stated desires. Joanne received her court order and came directly to the hospital with it. Joanne and I stood in the room as the nurse stopped the dialysis and ventilator, which were supporting Mary's weak last moments of existence. Just then, the doctor who had been opposing Mary's wishes and who was adamant about keeping her alive walked in, equally angry and demanding that the heroic measures continue. We observed as Joanne, Mary's case advocate, showed the physician the court order and assured him that Mary's wishes and needs were being met by her being allowed to pass with dignity as she had wanted. The physician was angry, but finally left as Mary died.

LEARNING EXERCISE

1. What preventive strategies might have averted this outcome at the micro policy level?
2. Should this case be taken to the risk manager or bioethics committee to see if it represents systemic problems in this hospital with honoring advance directives at the mezzo policy level?
3. It is not obvious how a social worker might initiate a macro policy intervention, but see if you can identify an option.

Core Problem 2: Engaging in Advocacy to Promote Quality Health Services—With Some Red Flag Alerts

- **Red Flag Alert 7.9.** Specific patients do not receive evidence-based care—or do not even discuss evidence-based options with the health professionals who care for them.
- **Red Flag Alert 7.10.** Specific patients do not inquire about a health professional's track record with respect to treating specific kinds of medical problems.
- **Red Flag Alert 7.11.** Specific patients do not use online and other resources to find information about performance indicators of specific professionals or providers who wish to care for them.
- **Red Flag Alert 7.12.** Specific patients do not seek second opinions for non-routine medical procedures.
- **Red Flag Alert 7.13.** Specific patients do not use the Internet to gain information about nonroutine medical problems.

- **Red Flag Alert 7.14.** Specific patients do not know how to search for information about clinical trials for their medical condition.
- **Red Flag Alert 7.15.** Specific patients have been subjected to medical error, but do not know how to proceed.
- **Red Flag Alert 7.16.** Specific patients do not know how to contest premature discharge from hospitals.

Background

A study from the RAND Institute discovered that roughly half of physicians in a national sample failed to use EBM (evidence-based medicine) findings to treat patients with asthma and depression—and even more of them failed to use an array of preventive measures (Adams et al., 2003). Researchers reached similar conclusions about failure to use evidence-based medicine for common health conditions when surveying providers for Medicaid enrollees in a broad survey of hospitals and when examining ambulatory care for children (Mangione-Smith et al., 2007).

People of color are often less likely than Caucasians to receive gold-standard medical care. For example, African Americans who present themselves to emergency rooms with acute chest pain are often less likely to be admitted or triaged into the coronary care unit (Council on Ethical and Judicial Affairs, 1990; Institute of Medicine, 2003; McBean & Gornick, 1994). More African Americans receive the poorest quality of care for congestive heart failure, acute myocardial infarction, pneumonia, and stroke than Caucasians, and African Americans are less likely to undergo angioplasty and bypass surgery, even after accounting for patient refusals of treatment—and receive poorer care for coronary heart disease (Fincher et al., 2004; Institute of Medicine, 2003; Kahn et al., 1994; Paschos et al., 1994; Taylor, Cano, Sanderson, Rogers, & Hilbe, 1998). Physicians spend less office time with Hispanic patients than Caucasians (Hooper, Comstock, Goodwin, & Goodwin, 1982). Summarizing considerable research, Beach et al. (2006) contend that provider behaviors and practice patterns contribute to health disparities—and that African Americans and other minority patients often receive different care than Caucasians (Cooper-Patrick et al., 1999).

Women often don't respond to specific medications or medical procedures that are effective with males and younger patients (Wartik, 2002). They sometimes don't receive state-of-the-art care as compared to males, such as for diagnosing myocardial infarctions (Willingham & Kilpatrick, 2005). Medical care is often insensitive to many of the needs of older women (Mayo, Nasmith, & Tannenbaum, 2003). Older women often receive contradictory and uncoordinated care (Lawrence, 2003).

Many critics contend that Americans often receive suboptimal health care. *Consumer Reports* maintains that between 98,000 and 400,000 patients suffer preventable fatalities each year from medical errors and infections in American hospitals ("Survive Your Stay," 2014). Considerable evidence suggests, as well, that specific physicians and hospitals provide poorer health care than others, as revealed by federal data that compare rates of mortality and injury for the people who use them (Institute of Medicine, 2000; "Survive Your Stay," 2014).

Researchers have discovered that medical errors substantially decline in intensive care units and elsewhere when staff follow checklists as they provide specific medical treatments. In intensive care units (ICUs), for example, staff provide mechanical ventilators, insert tracheotomy tubes, conduct dialysis, use aortic balloon pumps, feed patients through tubes, provide direct infusions into the bloodstream, and care for open wounds—providing 178 individual actions per patient per day. If they use checklists for these procedures, death rates plummet by as much as 66% in ICUs (Gawande, 2010).

Considerable research suggests that people who have chronic diseases or obesity, are at the end of life, or have certain other health conditions benefit from care from multidisciplinary teams (Brumley et al., 2007; Lin et al., 2000). Many health providers who are used to solo practice need to be trained in new practitioner roles that facilitate partnerships, such as the mental health integration (MHI) model developed for helping people with depression (Reiss-Brennan, 2006). Team-based chronic disease management (CDM) models have widely evolved in health settings, even if many health providers still rely on solo-based care (Bower & Gask, 2002).

Resources for Advocates

Federal Agencies That Disseminate EBM. The Agency for Healthcare Research and Quality (AHRQ) was established in 1997 to promote EBM as a tool for using scientific standards of evidence to discover what clinical practices were most effective in preventing and treating specific medical problems, using such outcome measures as mortality and morbidity rates, numbers of infections, numbers of readmissions, adverse drug events, and costs (Lefton, 2008). The National Guideline Clearinghouse, which is supported by the AHRQ, now supports over 2,200 guidelines. The volume of medical research has greatly increased, with more than 500,000 articles having been indexed by MEDLINE annually in recent years (Institute of Medicine, 2008). Many other organizations establish clinical guidelines and recommendations, including the American Heart Association, the American College of Physicians, the American Diabetic Association, the American Society of Clinical Oncology, and the National Heart, Lung, and Blood Institute. Many other organizations synthesize evidence collected by medical scientists, including the AHRQ, the Blue Cross and Blue Shield Association Technology

Evaluation Center, the Cochrane Collaboration, the ECRI Institute, and Hayes Inc. (Institute of Medicine, 2008).

The ACA created an Innovation Center in the Centers for Medicare and Medicaid Services (CMS) in 2011 as well as a national quality improvement strategy to improve the delivery of healthcare services and advance patient health outcomes.

Evaluations of specific physicians, clinics, and hospitals have increasingly been released to the public by state departments of public health, Medicare, state Medicaid programs, and state departments of health. These have included results of patient satisfaction surveys, overall mortality rates, mortality rates for specific kinds of cancer and heart disease, and rates of complications after specific kinds of surgery. They have evaluated the extent specific managed care plans provide preventive services. They have evaluated the extent to which specific providers use outdated equipment or equipment that isn't properly maintained.

The federal government, as well as many states, places data about the health outcomes of specific hospitals and physicians on the Internet (see www.medicare.gov/hospitalcompare/search.html), including the extent of "adverse events" that cause consumers to develop serious disabilities, such as surgeries performed on the wrong body parts or on the wrong patient; surgical procedures to which the consumer has not given informed consent; death of a healthy patient up to 24 hours after surgery; and disability from contaminated drugs, devices, or biological agents. Some states place data online about the extent to which specific physicians have caused adverse events as well as data about the extent to which specific physicians have been disciplined by state boards that regulate medical practitioners.

Consumers' Litigation. Consumers sometimes take matters into their own hands when they believe that they have been provided medical care that diverges from accepted norms, particularly if they believe they have suffered injuries because of subpar care. Millions of consumers have engaged private attorneys in past decades to litigate such issues as alleged malpractice or violation of their ethical rights. They have often sued hospitals, as well, when they have believed a certain hospital has lacked sufficient quality controls in its procedures, hiring of staff, in-service training, or monitoring of the quality of care provided within it. Consumers often litigate against pharmaceutical companies when they believe the company has failed to disclose potential side effects of medications or adverse drug interactions—or when they believe the company overstated the likely benefits from them. Consumers have also sued manufacturers of medical devices that they believe have malfunctioned.

The extent of consumers' litigation is considerable, but should not be exaggerated. Its elimination would only modestly cut American health costs. Consumers have directed their litigation against a relatively small number of physicians. Some states have placed limits on the size of allowable malpractice awards, such as

$250,000 in California. Many managed-care plans require enrollees to sign agreements when they enter their plans, where they agree to forgo litigation through the courts and to rely instead on the findings of internal administrative boards and the awards they suggest, which are often limited to a specific ceiling.

POLICY ADVOCACY LEARNING CHALLENGE 7.2

Connecting Micro, Mezzo, and Macro Policy Advocacy to Advance Quality of Care

Assume that you work in a neonatal intensive care unit (NICU) that currently lacks a protocol for deciding how to treat infants born before 23 weeks of gestation. Upon examining evidence-based research, you discover that babies born before 23 weeks rarely survive, but their survival rate increases from 29% to 65% between 23 and 25 weeks. You further discover that two thirds of infants born at 23 weeks have some form of functional disabilities when they reach two to three years of age—and one third of these assessed survivors have a severe disability. Infants born at 25 weeks have much better outcomes, with only one third possessing functional disabilities and 13% having a severe disability at two to three years of age (Singer, 2007). (No babies born before 26 weeks have survived without entering a neonatal intensive care unit). You want to be a micro policy advocate for traumatized parents with babies who were born before 23 weeks.

- At the micro advocacy level, would you refer these traumatized parents to evidence-based literature or to Internet sites that give them these probabilities, as well as information on economic, marital, and mental health issues related to premature births?
- At the mezzo advocacy level, might you want to consult the hospital's legal counsel to determine whether and when it is legal to allow some infants to perish by not giving them medications and other advanced medical treatment when their parents favor this policy?
- Can you think of possible macro policy advocacy interventions at the regulatory or government level?

Core Problem 3: Engaging in Advocacy to Promote Culturally Competent Health Services—With Some Red Flag Alerts

- **Red Flag Alert 7.17.** A specific patient's culture is not honored in interactions with health professionals.
- **Red Flag Alert 7.18.** A specific patient with limited English proficiency (LEP) is not given appropriate translation services.

- **Red Flag Alert 7.19.** A patient with limited health knowledge or literacy fails to receive health information that she can understand.
- **Red Flag Alert 7.20.** Health professionals do not communicate effectively with a patient with cultural perceptions of health and disease that are different from theirs.
- **Red Flag Alert 7.21.** Health professionals fail to honor a patient's specific religious and spiritual practices.
- **Red Flag Alert 7.22.** Health professionals fail to honor a patient's desire to use complementary and alternative medicine (CAM).
- **Red Flag Alert 7.23.** Members of specific vulnerable populations are not treated with respect.
- **Red Flag Alert 7.24.** Individuals from a specific cultural group are provided poorer services than other people.

Background

It is not surprising that many patients receive culturally incompetent care in a nation formed by successive migrations of people from other cultures. Physicians are disproportionately white and male compared to the patients they see, despite recent progress in diversifying health professionals. Many health professionals, too, fail to make sufficient accommodations to people with limited health literacy.

People with low levels of health literacy also face health-related challenges. Evidence strongly shows that health literacy is significantly related to both health and healthcare (DeWalt, Berkman, Sheridan, Lohr, & Pignone, 2004). People with low health literacy are more likely than those with higher health literacy to self-report fair or poor health (Kutner, Greenburg, Jin, & Paulsen, 2006). This health disparity may be linked to their lower level of knowledge about diseases and risk factors, such as smoking, contraception, HIV/AIDS, diabetes, and asthma. It may also be linked to under-use of preventive services such as mammography. Parents with low literacy may be less able to diagnose health problems in their children. Consumers with low literacy may be less likely to adhere to physicians' recommended treatments (DeWalt et al., 2004).

Racial discrimination and intolerance remain widespread but now assume more subtle forms. Minorities who face racial discrimination may be less likely or less willing to access the healthcare system and tend to exhibit worse health outcomes, such as self-reported health or chronic conditions (Williams & Mohammed, 2009). In its 2003 report on racial health disparities, *Unequal Treatment*, the Institute of Medicine argued that real or perceived racial discrimination can shape the expectations, attitudes, and behaviors of minority patients toward the healthcare system and health providers. African Americans tend to have less trust in their healthcare providers than Caucasians (Halbert, Armstrong, Gandy, & Shaker, 2006). Minority patients who are treated by a doctor of the same race or ethnicity (as in a racially concordant patient–physician relationship) tend to be more satisfied with the services they receive, possibly due to perceived personal or ethnic similarities (Street, O'Malley, Cooper, & Haidet, 2008). Relatively few minority physicians practice in many settings in the United States (Reede, 2003).

Compared to the U.S.-born population, immigrants and their children are less likely to have access to health services (Brown, Wyn, Yu, Valenzuela, & Doug, 1999; Huang, Stella, & Ledsky, 2006; Ku & Matani, 2001; Leclere, Jensen, & Biddlecom, 1994). Some qualitative studies suggest that culture may powerfully shape interactions between many immigrant and refugee families and the U.S. health system. Ngo-Metzger et al. (2003) found, for example, that Chinese and Vietnamese immigrants often encountered negative reactions regarding their use of traditional practices and commonly felt disrespected and devalued by their physicians.

The inability to speak or understand English can also lead to less access to health services and worse health outcomes. LEP individuals are less likely to have a usual source of care, utilize fewer preventive services, and tend to be less satisfied with their health services (Carrasquillo, Orav, Brennan, & Burstin, 1999; Ponce, Ku, Cunningham, & Brown, 2006). Consumers' lack of linguistic and cultural competency can also lead to medical errors. In a study of six randomly selected accredited hospitals, for example, Divi, Koss, Schmaltz, and Loeb (2007) found that almost 50% of adverse events with LEP patients resulted in some physical harm (and in some cases, death), compared to only 30% of those with English-speaking patients. The majority of these adverse events involved communication errors, such as questionable documentation, inaccurate or incomplete information, questionable assessment of patient needs, and questionable advice or interpretation.

Resources for Advocates

The right to communicate in one's own language is protected under the nation's anti-discrimination laws. Title VI of the 1964 Civil Rights Act provides the foundation for these protections:

> No person in the United States shall, on the ground of race, color, or *national origin*, be excluded from participation in, be denied the benefits of, or be subjected to discrimination under any program or activity receiving Federal financial assistance (42 U.S.C. §§ 2000d; emphasis added).

"National origin" has been interpreted in the courts to also include an individual's primary language so that no one should be excluded from federally funded programs because of his or her inability to speak, read, or understand English (Perkins, Youdelman, & Wong, 2003). President Bill Clinton issued Executive Order 13166 (EO 13166), which reinforced the protections afforded to LEP individuals under Title VI and instructed all federal agencies and federally funded programs to provide "meaningful access" to LEP people. Because most health providers receive some federal funding (e.g., in the form of Medicare or Medicaid), hospitals, clinics, and health providers have a legal obligation to provide linguistically appropriate services to LEP individuals. However, the implementation of Title VI regarding LEP people varies greatly across health providers. The actual enforcement of Title VI is largely driven by lawsuits or complaints, so the burden often falls on those who are facing discrimination.

The DHHS Office for Civil Rights' LEP Policy Guidance—first published in 2000 under the Clinton administration but later finalized in 2003 under the Bush administration—requires that provision of interpreter services be offered at no cost, that they be offered in the languages spoken most frequently in the given area, and that interpreters be qualified by having demonstrated proficiency (Perkins et al., 2003). Many state-level policies also govern the linguistic accessibility of healthcare services in specific states.

Most statutes, regulations, and litigation focuses on provision of translation and interpretation services rather than provision of culturally competent health services. The DHHS Office of Minority Health's (2001) CLAS standards are an exception (see Table 7.2).

Table 7.2   National Standards on Culturally and Linguistically Appropriate Services (CLAS).

Standard 1:	Healthcare organizations should ensure that patients/consumers receive from all staff members effective, understandable, and respectful care that is provided in a manner compatible with their cultural health beliefs and practices and preferred language.
Standard 2:	Healthcare organizations should implement strategies to recruit, retain, and promote at all levels of the organization a diverse staff and leadership that are representative of the demographic characteristics of the service area.
Standard 3:	Healthcare organizations should ensure that staff at all levels and across all disciplines receive ongoing education and training in culturally and linguistically appropriate service delivery.

Source: U.S. Department of Health and Human Services, Office of Minority Health.

Accreditation standards may have the greatest influence on how hospitals, clinics, and other healthcare provider organizations actually deliver their services. The Joint Commission has released requirements dealing with cultural competency that can be obtained from the Joint Commission's website. The National Committee for Quality Assurance (NCQA), a nonprofit organization that assesses and accredits health organizations and plans, has multicultural health care standards that apply to health plans. The ACA mandated enhanced collection and reporting of data on race, ethnicity, gender, primary language, disability status, and underserved rural populations in 2012.

POLICY ADVOCACY LEARNING CHALLENGE 7.3

Connecting Micro, Mezzo, and Macro Policy Advocacy for Patients' Unresolved Problems Regarding Culturally Competent Care

As I sat with my mother in the tiny, crowded clinic waiting room, I wondered why she had made me drive her for 45 minutes to receive medical services at a clinic that appeared dirty and required a lengthy wait. I finally asked my mother why she had dragged me down to the middle of Los Angeles for her to see a doctor when there were perfectly good clinics and hospitals in the region where we lived. She quickly reminded me that there were few Spanish-speaking doctors and nurses in the hospitals near our home and that the costs were much too high for someone with no health coverage. Although my brother and I had frequently played the role of translator when it came to my mother's communication between her and doctors, she felt the need to speak directly to the doctor to truly convey what she was feeling. She expressed that she was tired of having to communicate her ailments through someone else and believed it was a major reason why she had not received the medical treatment that she needed.

As our wait continued on, we suddenly heard my mother's name being called by the nurse who was admitting clients. We quickly gathered our belongings and made our way toward the nurse. While we maneuvered through the crowd toward her, she began to verify the symptoms that had brought my mother into the clinic—out loud, in front of the other patients in the waiting room.

Upon hearing the information being disclosed, I could see my mother nodding her head, with a look of embarrassment, to confirm the reasons that had brought her to the clinic. She looked around to scan the crowd to see if the other patients had heard. It was clear that everyone had heard what was ailing my mother. Upon approaching the nurse, I asked her if she was aware of her responsibility to maintain client confidentially, and I openly verbalized my anger at the manner in which she

(Continued)

(Continued)

had just violated my mother's privacy. My mother pulled me aside and asked that I stop challenging the nurse's authority, as she did not want to upset her. I explained to my mother that I had every intention of filing a formal complaint against the woman so that this would never happen to any other individual again. My mother asked that I do no such thing, as she felt it would make it impossible for her to return to this clinic again, which allowed her to pay a fee that was affordable while having access to Spanish-speaking doctors. I respected my mother's wishes and never filed a formal complaint. Upon leaving the clinic that afternoon, I left with a sense of helplessness and frustration at my inability to protect my mother's right to adequate, affordable, and culturally competent health services.

LEARNING EXERCISE

1. How does this vignette demonstrate that case advocates have to begin with the wishes of the consumer rather than proceeding without heeding their wishes?
2. How might the social worker consider mezzo policy advocacy at the organizational level? *Hint:* Recall that actual policies, such as HIPAA, are not actualized until they are implemented, so policy advocates can focus on strategies for bringing about this result.
3. Can you think of a macro policy advocacy intervention you could initiate?

Core Problem 4: Engaging in Advocacy to Promote Preventive Health Services—With Some Red Flag Alerts

- **Red Flag Alert 7.25.** Someone has not been helped to identify personal risk factors through family history and diagnostic tests.
- **Red Flag Alert 7.26.** Someone has not been tested for a possible chronic disease or diseases at a possible early stage.
- **Red Flag Alert 7.27.** People fail to receive assistance in addressing medical conditions such as obesity, lack of physical activity, poor nutrition, and smoking.
- **Red Flag Alert 7.28.** Adults and children are not given help in receiving vaccines.
- **Red Flag Alert 7.29.** A person who lives in an inner-city area is not given assistance in obtaining better nutrition and more exercise.
- **Red Flag Alert 7.30.** Specific members of vulnerable populations are not given access to prevention.

Background

Corporations have often blocked enactment of important prevention measures by lobbying politicians. Tobacco companies, fast-food companies, food manufacturers, automobile companies, and manufacturers and purveyors of alcoholic beverages have often resisted regulations, such as warning or information labels, safety devices, and restrictions on sale of their products. Corporations have often opposed regulations to combat pollution by toxic chemicals, whether in the air, water, or soil. In places like Fresno County, California, air pollution has led nearly one in three of its children to contract asthma (Anderson, 2007).

Considerable resistance to preventive care exists among health practitioners. Only 19% of primary care physicians discuss exercise with consumers, 22% discuss diet, and 10% discuss weight reduction. Only 4% encourage consumers to stop smoking, only 14% refer overweight persons to dieticians, and only 1% recommend exercise to overweight individuals (Centers for Disease Control, 1998; Knight, 2004). Only 11% of the contact time of primary care physicians is devoted to disease prevention—or seven minutes per patient per year on average (Knight, 2004; Rafferty, 1998). Only 50% of physicians follow the National Cholesterol Education Program guidelines, even with patients with high-risk coronary heart disease (Frolkis, Zyzanski, Schwartz, & Suhan, 1998; Knight, 2004). A survey of medical practice discovered that physicians give consumers only 54.9% of recommended preventive care (Knight, 2004; McGlynn et al., 2003).

Many experts hoped that managed-care plans would provide more preventive services than traditional medical arrangements for two reasons: They require consumers to access their plans through gatekeeper primary care physicians, and they cut their overall costs by emphasizing prevention rather than treatment. Physicians in managed care plans are no more likely, however, to provide many preventive services than other physicians (Pham, Schrag, Hargraves, & Bach, 2005).

American culture sometimes adversely affects health. Americans work harder than residents of many other nations, taking only 10 days' vacation per year as compared to 17 days for Canadians and 24 days for those in the UK (but only 8 days for those in Japan; Expedia.com, 2009). Whereas Americans consume 97 pounds of beef per year, Canadians consume 69 pounds, UK residents consume 38 pounds, and the Japanese consume 21.3 pounds (Red Meat Industry Forum, 2007). Forty-one percent of Americans eat at least once a week in fast-food restaurants, including 59% of 18- to 29-year-olds (Pew Research Center, 2006). Many Americans have become addicted to television, with adults watching it 8 hours per week, compared to only 3 hours in Canada, 3 hours in the UK, and 3.5 hours in Japan (Ramsay, 2008). Whereas 5.2 Americans per 100,000 die from homicides each year, only 1.7 Canadians, 1.4 people from the UK, and

0.5 Japanese die from them (United Nations Office on Drugs and Crime, 2010). Whereas 626 Americans per 100,000 are injured in automobile accidents each year, only 312 people in England per 100,000 are injured per year (Economist, 2009). Roughly 30% of young people 18 to 24 years old still smoke, and the percentage of female smokers has increased significantly since 1950. About 87% of the 159,000 lung cancer deaths in 2008 were linked to smoking (American Cancer Society, 2009).

More people in the United States than in Canada, the UK, or Japan have chronic diseases such as diabetes that are closely linked to lifestyle factors. Whereas 10.3% of people in the United States have diabetes, 9.2% of people in Canada, 3.6% of people in the UK, and 5% of people in Japan have this disease (International Diabetes Federation, 2010).

The United States ranks only 45th in the world in infant mortality (6.2 deaths per 1,000 live births), while Japan ranks fourth (2.8 per 1,000 live births), Canada ranks 35th (5 deaths per 1,000), and the UK ranks 31st (4.85 deaths per 1,000 births; Central Intelligence Agency, 2009). One in eight babies is born prematurely in the United States, partly because many women do not receive sufficient prenatal care (March of Dimes, 2009).

The high poverty rate in the United States also contributes to relatively high rates of sickness and mortality in the United States, as we discussed earlier in this chapter.

Many uninsured Americans receive less preventive care than insured Americans. They often use emergency rooms for healthcare rather than possessing ongoing relationships with primary care physicians. They receive less healthcare per year than insured consumers—or $583 per year as compared to $3,915—and self-fund 35% of it as compared to 17% for insured people (Hadley, Holahan, Coughlin, & Miller, 2008). Between 35,000 and 45,000 uninsured people die unnecessarily each year (Wilper et al., 2009).

Resources for Advocates

Resources and Data. The Centers for Disease Control and Prevention (CDC) has many programs within it, such as the National Center for Chronic Disease Prevention and Promotion, the Division for Heart Disease and Stroke, the Division of Cancer Prevention and Control, the Diabetes Prevention Program, the National Breast and Cervical Cancer Early Detection Program (B&C), the Office of Public Health Genomics, the Division of Reproductive Health, and the Division of Adolescent and School Health. (Each of these programs has a website that can be accessed through www.cdc.gov.) These programs not only conduct research about the incidence of specific diseases, but they mobilize coalitions in different states and tribes to promote and fund screening programs that are funded and implemented by states (Collins, Koplan, & Marks, 2009). All states have screening and wellness programs in such areas as tobacco use, diabetes, breast and cervical screening, and comprehensive cancer control, as well as the Behavioral Risk Factor Surveillance System, which surveys consumers and collects information on health risk behaviors, preventive health practices, and healthcare access, primarily related to chronic disease and injury.

The CDC often issues reports geared to mobilizing action, such as *A Public Health Action Plan to Prevent Heart Disease and Stroke* as well as *Healthy People 2000, Healthy People 2010*, and *Healthy People 2020*, which each established health and prevention goals for a specific decade. It helps fund a network of 33 Prevention Research Centers that fund collaborative research of community, academic, and public health partners with the use of participatory research that seeks implementation of public health programs, such as the Enhance Fitness program to increase physician exercise by senior citizens at 300 sites in 26 states. It develops evidence-based prevention strategies, such as a study that found that type 2 diabetes can be prevented or delayed with moderate weight loss, improved nutrition, and greater exercise (Collins et al., 2009). It promotes programs, such as the Health Communities Program that mobilizes action in local communities, including schools, work sites, and healthcare settings, to increase physical activity, improve nutrition, and curtail smoking to prevent chronic diseases. It targets women between ages 50 and 64 who are uninsured or underinsured in its Well-Integrated Screening and Evaluation for Women Across the Nation (WISEWOMAN) to enhance lifestyle changes as well as monitor blood pressure and cholesterol. The CDC promotes early detection of public health issues in different states by helping them implement surveys of citizens that probe the extent to which they have such problems as obesity and specific mental health problems.

The Department of Health and Human Services (DHHS) has developed many prevention programs, not just in its Medicare and Medicaid programs but in many specific divisions and programs. The Center on Medicare and Medicare Services (CMS) currently administers the Medicare and Medicaid Programs. Medicare promotes prevention by covering immunizations; screening for cancer, cardiovascular disease, glaucoma, and diabetes; bone density measurement; and smoking cessation programs. It will cover additional prevention programs under the ACA. Medicaid promotes prevention by covering smoking cessation, preventive health and dental care, prescription drugs, laboratory tests and x-rays, family planning, and prenatal care. Coverage and services vary by state. Public health staff are out-stationed in STD (sexually transmitted disease), TB (tuberculosis),

HIV/AIDS, WIC (the Special Supplemental Nutrition Program for Women, Infants, and Children), and prenatal clinics that are scattered throughout urban and some rural areas, but that often aren't closely linked with primary care clinics or hospitals.

The federal Agency for Health Care Quality (AHCQ) oversees and funds considerable research on prevention. It contains the U.S. Prevention Services Task Force that grades specific preventive interventions from A to D depending on their cost-effectiveness in preventing specific health conditions. This task force will have expanded roles under the ACA.

Regulations. Many local jurisdictions ban smoking in public places. Federal regulations require food labeling on many products—and require fast-food establishments to post the level of these ingredients in their food. Some local jurisdictions have banned the use of partially hydrogenated oils in cooking French fries, as well as ending the use of trans fats in fast-food and other food establishments. The ACA requires chain restaurants and vending machine companies to post the nutritional content and calories of their food.

Congress enacted legislation that defined tobacco as a drug in 2009, giving the Food and Drug Administration the power to regulate it by establishing, expanding, and monitoring local and state regulations that prohibit the placement of smoking advertisements and vending machines near schools, sales to minors, the giving of free samples, and smoking in public places. Forty-three states currently allow employers *not* to hire people who smoke. Many jurisdictions prohibit smoking in public places or in places at work where others will breathe their secondhand smoke.

Some local jurisdictions have regulated the number of fast-food outlets in specific neighborhoods where they are disproportionately located, such as low-income neighborhoods. Some have placed restrictions on food provided in local schools, requiring lunches with lower fat content and more vegetables. Some have prohibited vending machines in schools that sell soda and candy. Some jurisdictions place limits on the number of bars in specific communities, as well as locations near schools. Many jurisdictions take away the driver's licenses of people who drive while intoxicated (DWI)—and may give them prison sentences.

The Occupational Safety and Health Administration (OSHA) establishes specific regulations to protect workers' safety; state chapters administer them and establish some of their own regulations. OSHA regulates emissions of toxic chemicals within plants, requires the use of safety practices and equipment, and requires employers to monitor hazards and maintain records of workplace injuries and illnesses.

Statutes. The ACA has created a Prevention and Public Health Fund to modernize disease prevention and improve access to clinical preventive services in schools, as well as Medicare annual wellness programs getting it started by funding $11 billion to community health centers beginning in 2011. It will fund health prevention programs in occupational settings. It will subsidize many not-for-profit community-based clinics.

Prevention in Places of Work. Many corporations, such as the rail company CSX Transportation, Johnson & Johnson, and Coors Brewing, have instituted wellness programs in their work sites (Brink, 2008; CSX, 2005). Many technology companies, such as Google and Microsoft, have wellness programs, as well as exercise facilities at their work sites. As of 2014, the Affordable Care Act of 2010, as amended by Congress, permits employers to offer employees rewards of up to 30%, increasing to 50% if appropriate, of the cost of coverage for participating in a wellness program and meeting certain health-related standards. It will establish state pilot programs in 10 states to offer similar rewards to consumers in wellness programs who purchase individual policies.

POLICY ADVOCACY LEARNING CHALLENGE 7.4

Connecting Micro, Mezzo, and Macro Policy Advocacy With Respect to Prevention

This case is drawn from: Gawande, A. (2010, April 5). Now what? *New Yorker*, p. 22.

Clinicians at Children's Hospital, Boston, were concerned about the sheer number of asthma attacks among low-income youth in Boston's inner city. They developed an innovative prevention strategy that included:

- Having nurses visit parents after their children's discharge to educate them about adherence to medications and follow-up visits to their pediatricians
- Home inspections for mold and pests
- Provision of free vacuum cleaners to parents who lacked them
- Funding of these interventions from the hospital's budget, since insurance covered only the cost of a prescribed inhaler

This strategy was so successful that hospital readmissions of these children dropped by more than 80%—and costs of treatment dropped precipitously. This intervention threatened to bankrupt the hospital, however, because it had depended on revenues from public and private insurances and programs for the many beds that had been occupied by these children.

LEARNING EXERCISE

1. If you worked in this hospital and wanted to be an advocate for this creative program, what conflict of interest would you confront—and what ethical issues might you face?
2. How might you have to shift from micro policy advocacy to mezzo policy advocacy?
3. What macro policy advocacy might you consider launching?

Core Problem 5: Engaging in Advocacy to Promote Affordable and Accessible Health Services—With Some Red Flag Alerts

- **Red Flag Alert 7.31.** A person does not receive help in selecting an insurance plan; gaining eligibility to Medicaid, CHIP, or portions of the Medicare program, or in obtaining Medicare Supplemental Insurance; or becoming dually eligible for Medicare and Medicaid.
- **Red Flag Alert 7.32.** A person is not given assistance in accessing charitable health funds in those clinics and hospitals that have them.
- **Red Flag Alert 7.33.** A person is not given assistance in contesting specific decisions made by Medicare, Medicaid, CHIP, Supplemental Security Income (SSI), Social Security, or specific private health insurance plans.
- **Red Flag Alert 7.34.** An uninsured person is not helped to find free clinics, public clinics or hospitals, or private hospitals that serve uninsured individuals through the Medicaid DSH (Disproportionate Share Hospital) program.
- **Red Flag Alert 7.35.** A person does not receive help in obtaining disability health benefits.
- **Red Flag Alert 7.36.** A person does not receive assistance in obtaining in-home supportive care from Medicare, Medicaid, or private insurance.
- **Red Flag Alert 7.37.** An undocumented immigrant is not given help in finding healthcare.
- **Red Flag Alert 7.38.** A senior citizen who has exhausted her Medicare benefits is not helped to understand her options.
- **Red Flag Alert 7.39.** Patients are not given help in financing their out-of-pocket costs.

Background

The United States finances healthcare through a combination of private insurance, government programs, corporations, and out-of-pocket payments—a chaotic system that has left many consumers without insurance or access to public programs. The ACA seeks to decrease medically uninsured people from 45 million to 16 million by 2020—an ambitious goal—by employing a series of strategies. Its proponents want to decrease the number of uninsured individuals by using the following strategies in tandem:

- Requiring private insurance to cover people with preexisting conditions— and allowing parents to keep children on their policies until age 26
- Making uninsured people pay penalties if they do not obtain insurance
- Providing tax credits to small businesses to encourage them to fund health insurance for their employees
- Providing subsidies to individuals who fall beneath relatively high income levels to induce them to purchase private health insurance
- Establishing "insurance exchanges" in the states—whether under the aegis of specific states or of the federal government
- Raising the eligibility level of Medicaid and expanding its coverage to single individuals as well as families—and requiring Medicaid to raise its reimbursements of providers to the same levels as Medicare
- Greatly expanding federal funding of Medicaid

If the ACA is successful in reaching this goal, lack of coverage will be greatly diminished—and healthcare should improve because lack of coverage adversely affects health outcomes in several ways:

- It delays care when consumers don't initiate recommended care because they fear it will bankrupt them or make them destitute.
- It interrupts care when consumers discontinue care because they fear it will bankrupt them or make them destitute.
- It makes specialists unavailable to low-income patients because Medicaid has paid them at such low levels.
- It causes inadequate primary care because consumers use emergency rooms excessively due to lack of insurance.
- It leads to hostile or shunning actions by health providers because they don't want to serve uninsured or underinsured people.
- It increases angst arising from uncertain or inadequate health coverage.
- It encourages patients not to take their prescriptions or to split their pills because they can't afford expensive drugs.

It is estimated that roughly 30,000 uninsured people were losing their lives each year due to lack of coverage prior to the enactment of the ACA in 2010.

Core Problem 6: Engaging in Advocacy to Promote Care of Health Consumers' Mental Distress

We will discuss mental health services in the two succeeding chapters. We will note how most mental health services are delivered by primary care physicians in the United States as well as by prisons.

Core Problem 7: Engaging in Advocacy to Promote Healthcare Linked to Households and Communities—With Some Red Flag Alerts

- **Red Flag Alert 7.40.** A clinic or hospital fails to promote referrals of patients to community-based agencies.
- **Red Flag Alert 7.41.** A hospital fails to commit sufficient staff to helping with patients' transitions to assisted-living and nursing homes.
- **Red Flag Alert 7.42.** A clinic or hospital fails to monitor community nursing homes and convalescent homes so that it does not refer patients to those of poor quality.
- **Red Flag Alert 7.43.** A clinic or hospital fails to link its patients to community-based preventive services.
- **Red Flag Alert 7.44.** A clinic or hospital lacks community workers.

Background

Many physicians view health as mostly confined to the physiological realm, failing to factor culture, social class, community realities, fiscal constraints, family dynamics, emotions, and consumers' mental conditions into their diagnoses and treatments (Glasgow et al., 1999). Many physicians also assume that most consumers will adhere to treatment regimens, rather than exploring financial, family, mental, cultural, and community factors that might contravene them (Glasgow et al., 1999). In fact, health consumers live in ecosystems that profoundly shape their health, as well as their use of health systems (DuBois & Miley, 2002). They may live in housing that causes or exacerbates asthma (Bell & Standish, 2005). They may live in neighborhoods with relatively Spartan health services so that they are less likely to use them. They may lack transportation services to health programs. They may reside in housing that is not designed for people with disabilities or be unable to access health services because of physical limitations. The medical problems of consumers who come to emergency rooms are often linked to mental trauma, family violence, malnutrition, exposure, drug overdoses, gang violence, homelessness, and other social and economic problems that cause or exacerbate their medical problems.

Effective healthcare systems need to have information about their patients' ecosystems—and have the ability to provide outreach services. The term *hard to reach* is used in the disability literature to define disabled consumers who won't typically be reached unless a dedicated effort is made to engage with them, such as women whose visual, auditory, or mobility limitations make it difficult for them to leave their homes (Smeltzer, Sharts-Hopko, Ott, Zimmerman, & Duffin, 2007). They need to have resources and personnel to locate people who don't return for appointments when they have serious health conditions.

Many ER physicians, nurses, and social workers engage in referral, brokerage, and liaison services, including with law enforcement, mental health, child welfare, substance abuse, assisted living, and nursing home agencies, as well as shelters. They often help consumers gain eligibility to specific safety-net programs such as Medicaid, CHIP, the Supplemental Nutrition Assistance Program (SNAP), and Section 8 programs.

Resources for Advocates

Social workers are uniquely equipped to link health services to communities, since they have been in the network of community-based nongovernmental organizations. Several developments should speed these linkages. The ACA is requiring hospitals to establish "medical homes" for patients where they receive a broad array of outpatient and inpatient services and where hospitals provide them with those services needed to prevent illness and to slow the development of chronic diseases. The ACA would like to move reimbursement of health providers from the current fee-for-service approach to so-called capitated care, where they receive flat fees. Such fees will give hospitals incentives to cut their costs by helping patients prevent health problems by working with an array of community agencies.

The ACA will establish a national Medicare pilot program to develop and evaluate a bundled payment for acute inpatient hospital services, primary care services, outpatient hospital services, and post-acute care services for an episode of care. It will evaluate whether this approach will decrease medical silos and improve outcomes.

Medicare and Medicaid are giving hospitals additional reasons to link themselves with community agencies by penalizing them financially if patients who are given surgery return to hospitals sooner than 30 days after their inpatient care. These penalties will prompt hospitals to identify factors in patients' households and communities that *cause* them *not* to recover rapidly, such as their diet, their inability to obtain needed medications, poor life habits like substance abuse, poor housing, mental illness, and failure to adhere to suggested treatments.

Health professionals can promote community-oriented care for consumers—including care for mental health, family, substance abuse, shelter, income assistance, health insurance, public health, housing, employment, physical therapy, speech and language, and other health-related problems—by establishing links between community agencies. These links can take place between autonomous agencies (linkage), can include more systematic relationships (coordination), or can involve "joint goals, very close and highly connected networks . . . and high degrees of mutual trust and respect" (integration), as discussed by Glendinning (2002).

Emerging technology—including video conferencing, electronic monitoring, and video cameras—allows providers to link providers with consumers in their homes and communities.

Several policies give hospitals incentives to relate to their communities. The federal Emergency Medical Treatment and Active Labor Act (EMTALA) established procedures that apply not only to consumers who are transferred from ERs to other locations, but to all transfer cases (CHA, 2008). Hospitals are legally responsible "for the safety, appropriateness, and monitoring of the transfer process and protocol" (CHA, 2008). Medicare, Medicaid, and the Joint Commission add additional requirements. EMTALA prohibits transfers before consumers are medically stabilized. Some states prohibit transfers of consumers from specific vulnerable populations (e.g., those of a certain race, with disabilities, or with a certain sexual orientation) for financial reasons because they are *suspected* of lacking resources to fund their medical care without having been determined to actually be medically indigent. Some states and federal law also require emergency services to be given to consumers without first investigating to see if they can fund them (even though payment can be sought *after* they have been treated) and prohibit discrimination in providing emergency services on the basis of race, gender, and other characteristics (CHA, 2008).

Transition planning is often inadequate because hospitals and clinics don't hire sufficient social workers and discharge nurses to provide effective interventions. These professionals are often pressured to speed the release of consumers from hospitals to save them resources when they are reimbursed with capitation or with prospective payments such as Medicare's DRGs (diagnosis-related groups). Some populations may be most subject to poor discharge planning. Many states have specific regulations regarding the discharge of homeless people, for example, who in the past have been inappropriately transported to skid row areas in such cities as Los Angeles, sometimes in their hospital gowns, and without ensuring that they receive a place in shelters.

POLICY ADVOCACY LEARNING CHALLENGE 7.5

**Connecting Micro, Mezzo, and Macro Policy
Advocacy to Help Fugitive Patients Obtain Needed Services**

A Good Samaritan Nurse

A nurse in a health clinic used primarily by low-income consumers in the Bronx decided to follow up on consumers who had received biopsies that indicated they had cancer at relatively advanced stages, but who had failed to keep appointments to receive their biopsy results. She often assumed the role of a detective because many of them lacked telephones and frequently changed addresses. She was not asked to undertake this assignment by clinic staff, but felt ethically impelled to locate these fugitive consumers in after-work hours. She was able to locate many of them and to convince them to come to the clinic so that they could begin treatments.

LEARNING EXERCISE

1. How does this vignette illustrate a tendency to define medical practice as confined to the four walls of specific clinics and hospitals?
2. Why does this clinic rely on a Good Samaritan nurse to perform this life-preserving function—and what are some disadvantages of this informal practice?
3. Could a social worker in this clinic have engaged in mezzo policy advocacy to persuade clinic administrators to hire an outreach worker with this assignment?
4. Can you think of a possible macro policy intervention at the state or federal level?

"THINKING BIG" AS ADVOCATES IN THE HEALTHCARE SECTOR

Several major proposals for reforming social policy currently exist in healthcare. Discuss these proposals as you think they do or do not have merit.

1. Reform the ACA in major ways, such as moving toward a universal payer model or making Medicare cover most of the population.

2. Move the health system toward a wellness model by requiring insurance companies, Medicare, and Medicaid to place greater emphasis on wellness programs and services. If the nation fully endorses a "wellness" model, what policies might it consider regarding fast-food outlets, lack of places to exercise for many Americans, and new approaches for balancing work and recreation? How might particular assistance be given to low-income and other vulnerable populations to engage in wellness programs?

LEARNING OUTCOMES

You are now equipped to:

- Identify stages in the evolution of the American health system in seven eras
- Identify key interest groups in the political economy of the American health system, as well as groups that are not well represented
- Analyze why income inequality in the United States exacerbates health disparities
- Identify seven major problems encountered by consumers of American healthcare in their policy and regulatory context
- Develop Red Flag Alerts at the micro level
- Develop micro, mezzo, and macro policy advocacy initiatives
- Discuss and analyze a major proposal for reforming the healthcare system

REFERENCES

Adams, J., Asch, S. M., DeCristofaro, A., Hicks, J., Keesey, J., Kerr, E. A., & McGlynn, E. A. (2003). The quality of healthcare delivered to adults in the United States. *New England Journal of Medicine, 348*(26).

American Cancer Society. (2009, December). *Tobacco-related cancers fact sheet.* Retrieved February 25, 2010, from http://www.cancer.org/docroot/PED/content/PED_10_2x_Tobacco -Related_Cancers_Fact_Sheet-asp?sitearea=PED

Anderson, B. (2007, December 12). Fresno is state's asthma capital. *Fresno Bee.* Retrieved from http://www.fresnobee.com/2007/12/12/263218/fresno-is-states-asthma-capital.html

Annas, G. (2003). HIPAA regulations: A new era of medical-record privacy? *New England Journal of Medicine, 348,* 1486–1490.

Barr, D. (2008). *Health disparities in the United States: Social class, race, ethnicity, and health.* Baltimore, MD: Johns Hopkins University Press.

Beach, M. C., Gary, T. L., Price, E. G., Robinson, K., Gozu, A., Palacio, A., & Cooper, L. A. (2006). Improving healthcare quality for racial/ethnic minorities: A systemic review. *BioMed Central Public Health, 6,* 104. Retrieved April 10, 2010, from http://www.biomedcentral .com/1471-2458/6/104

Bell, J., & Standish, M. (2005). Communities and health policy: A pathway for change. *Health Affairs, 24*(2), 339–342.

Bower, P., & Gask, L. (2002). The changing nature of consultation-liaison in primary care: Bridging the gap between research and practice. *General Hospital Psychiatry, 24*(2), 63.

Brink, K. (2008, April 29). *Wellness programs at work.* Retrieved from http://www.asociated content.com/article/724387/wellness_programs_at_work_pg3.html?cat=5

Brown, E. R., Wyn, R., Yu, H., Valenzuela, A., & Dong, L. (1999). Access to health insurance and healthcare for children in immigrant families. In D. J. Hernandez (Ed.), *Children of immigrants: Health, adjustment, and public assistance* (pp. 126–186). Washington, DC: National Academy Press.

Brumley, R., Enguidanos, S., Jamison, P., Seitz, R., Morgenstern, N., Saito, S., . . . Gonzalez, J. (2007). Increased satisfaction with care and lower costs: Results of a randomized trial of in-home palliative care. *Journal of the American Geriatrics Society, 55*(7), 993–1000.

California Hospital Association. (2008). *Consent manual: A reference for consent and related healthcare law.* Sacramento, CA: Author.

California Newreel (Producer). (2008). *Unnatural causes: Is inequality making us sick?* [Television series]. Washington, DC: Public Broadcasting Service.

Carrasquillo, O., Orav, E. J., Brennan, T. A., & Burstin, H. R. (1999). Impact of language barriers on patient satisfaction in an emergency department. *Journal of General Internal Medicine, 14*(2), 82–87.

Centers for Disease Control and Prevention. (1998). Missed opportunities in preventive counseling for cardiovascular disease—United States, 1995. *Journal of the American Medical Association, 279,* 741–742.

Central Intelligence Agency. (2009). *The world factbook.* Retrieved from https://www.cia .gov/library/publications/download/download-2009/index.html

Collins, J. L., Koplan, J. P., & Marks, J. S. (2009). Chronic disease prevention and control: Coming of age at the Centers for Disease Control and Prevention. *Preventing Chronic Disease, 6*(3).

Cooper-Patrick, L., Gallo, J. J., Gonzales, J. J., Vu, H. T., Powe, N. R., Nelson, C., & Ford, D. E. (1999). Race, gender, and partnership in the patient–physician relationship. *Journal of the American Medical Association, 282*(6), 583–589. doi: 10.1001/Journal of the American Medical Association.282.6.58

Council on Ethical and Judicial Affairs. (1990). Black–white disparities in healthcare. *Journal of the American Medical Association, 263,* 2344–2346.

CSX. (2005). *Safety is a way of life.* Retrieved April 26, 2010, from http://www.csx .com/?fuseaction=about.safety

DeWalt, D. A., Berkman, N. D., Sheridan, S., Lohr, K. N., & Pignone, M. P. (2004). Literacy and health outcomes. *Journal of General Internal Medicine, 19*(12), 1228–1239.

Divi, C., Koss, R. G., Schmaltz, S. P., & Loeb, J. M. (2007). Language proficiency and adverse events in US hospitals: A pilot study. *International Journal for Quality in Health Care, 19*(2), 60–67.

DuBois, B., & Miley, K. K. (2002). *Social work: An empowering profession* (4th ed.). Boston, MA: Allyn & Bacon.

Economist. (2009). *The Economist pocket world in figures, 2010 edition.* London, UK: Profile Books.

Expedia.com. (2009). *2009 international vacation deprivation survey results.* Retrieved from http:/media.expedia.com/media/content/expus/graphics/promos/vacations/Expedia_International_Vacation_Deprivation_Survey_2009.pdf

Fincher, C., Williams, J. E., MacLean, V., Allison, J. J., Kiefe, C. I., & Canto, J. (2004). Racial disparities in coronary heart disease: A sociological view of the medical literature on physician bias. *Ethnicity and Disease, 14,* 360–371.

Frolkis, J. P., Zyzanski, S. J., Schwartz, J. M., & Suhan, P. S. (1998). Physician noncompliance with the 1993 national cholesterol education program (NCEP-ATPII) guidelines. *Circulation, 98*(9), 851–855.

Gawande, A. (2010). *The checklist manifesto: How to get things right.* New York, NY: Henry Holt.

Glasgow, R. E., Wagner, E. H., Kaplan, R. M., Vinicor, F., Smith, L., & Norman, J. (1999). If diabetes is a public health problem, why not treat it as one? A population-based approach to chronic illness. *Annals of Behavioral Medicine, 21*(2), 159–170.

Glendinning, C. (2002). Breaking down barriers: Integrating health and care services for older people in England. *Health Policy, 65,* 139–151.

Hadley, J., Holahan, J., Coughlin, T., & Miller, D. (2008). Covering the uninsured in 2008: Current costs, sources of payment, and incremental costs. *Health Affairs, 27*(5), w399–w415.

Halbert, C. H., Armstrong, K., Gandy, O. H., Jr., & Shaker, L. (2006). Racial differences in trust in health care providers. *Archives of Internal Medicine, 166*(8), 896.

Hooper, E. M., Comstock, L. M., Goodwin, J. M., & Goodwin, J. S. (1982). Patient characteristics that influence physician behavior. *Medical Care, 20,* 630–638.

Huang, Z. J., Stella, M. Y., & Ledsky, R. (2006). Health status and health service access and use among children in US immigrant families. *Journal Information, 96*(4).

Institute of Medicine. (2000). *To err is human: Building a safer health system.* Washington, DC: National Academy Press.

Institute of Medicine. (2003). *Unequal treatment: Confronting racial and ethnic disparities in healthcare.* Washington, DC: National Academy Press.

Institute of Medicine. (2008). *Knowing what works in healthcare.* Washington, DC: National Academy Press.

International Diabetes Federation. (2010). *IDF diabetes atlas.* Retrieved April 22, 2010, from http://www.diabetesatlas.org/content/regional-data

Jackson, A. (2002). Canada beats USA—but loses gold to Sweden. *Women, 81*(79.2), 81–83.

Jacobs, E. A., Kohrman, C., Lemon, M., & Vickers, D. L. (2003). Teaching physicians-in-training to address racial disparities in health: A hospital–community partnership. *Public Health Reports, 118,* 349–355.

Jansson, B., Nyamathi, A., Duran, L., Kaplan, C., Heidemann, G., & Ananias, D. (in press). Validation of the Patient Advocacy Scale for health professionals. *Research in Nursing and Health.*

Joint Commission. (2009). *Comprehensive accreditation manual for hospitals: The official handbook: Refreshed core.* Oakbrook Terrace, IL: Joint Commission Resources.

Kahn, K. L, Pearson, M. L., Harrison, E. R., Desmond, M. S., Rogers, W. H., Rubenstein, L. V., & Brook, R. H. (1994). Healthcare for black and poor hospitalized Medicare patients. *Journal of the American Medication Association, 271,* 1169–1174.

Kawachi, I., Daniels, N., & Robinson, D. E. (2005). Health disparities by race and class: Why both matter. *Health Affairs, 24*(2), 343–352.

Knight, J. A. (2004). *A crisis call for new preventive medicine: Emerging effects of lifestyle on morbidity and mortality.* Hackensack, NJ: World Scientific.

Ku, L., & Matani, S. (2001). Left out: Immigrants' access to health care and insurance. *Health Affairs, 20*(1), 247–256.

Kutner, M., Greenburg, E., Jin, Y., & Paulsen, C. (2006). The health literacy of America's adults: Results from the 2003 National Assessment of Adult Literacy (NCES 2006-483). *National Center for Education Statistics.*

Lawrence, D. (2003). My mother and the medical care ad-hoc-racy. *Health Affairs, 22*(2), 238–242.

Leclere, F. B., Jensen, L., & Biddlecom, A. E. (1994). Health care utilization, family context, and adaptation among immigrants to the United States. *Journal of Health and Social Behavior,* 370–384.

Lee, H., & McConville, S. (2007). Death in the Golden State: Why do some Californians live longer? *California Counts: Population Trends and Profiles, 9*(1). Retrieved from http://www.ppic.org/content/pubs/cacounts/CC_807HLCC.pdf

Lefton, R. (2008). Reducing variation in healthcare delivery. *Healthcare Financial Management: Journal of the Healthcare Financial Management Association, 62*(7), 42.

Lin, E. H., VonKorff, M., Russo, J., Katon, W., Simon, G. E., Unützer, J., . . . Ludman, E. (2000). Can depression treatment in primary care reduce disability? A stepped care approach. *Archives of Family Medicine, 9*(10), 1052.

Mangione-Smith, R., DeCristofaro, A., Setodji, C., Keesen, J., Klein, D., Adams, J., . . . Glynn, F. (2007). Quality of ambulatory care delivered to children in the U.S. *New England Journal of Medicine, 357*(15), 1515–1523.

March of Dimes. (2009, October). *PeriStats: Born too soon and too small in the United States.* Retrieved from http://www.marchofdimes.com/peristats/pdflib/195/99.pdf

Mayo, N., Nasmith, L., & Tannenbaum, C. B. (2003). Understanding older women's healthcare concerns: A qualitative study. *Journal of Aging and Women, 15*(4).

McBean, A. M., & Gornick, M. (1994). Differences by race in the rates of procedures performed in hospitals for Medicare beneficiaries. *Healthcare Financial Review, 15,* 77–90.

McGlynn, E. A., Asch, S. M., Adams, J., Keesey, J., Hicks, J., DeCristofaro, A., & Kerr, E. A. (2003). The quality of health care delivered to adults in the United States. *New England Journal of Medicine, 348*(26), 2635–2645.

Ngo-Metzger, Q., Massagli, M. P., Clarridge, B. R., Manocchia, M., Davis, R. B., Iezzoni, L. I., & Phillips, R. S. (2003). Linguistic and cultural barriers to care. *Journal of General Internal Medicine, 18*(1), 44–52.

Office of Minority Health. (2009, December). *Diabetes and Hispanic Americans.* Retrieved from http://minorityhealth.hhs.gov/templates/content.aspx?ID= 3324

Paschos, C. L., Normand, S. L., Garfinkle, J. B., Newhouse, J. P., Epstein, A. M., & McNeil, B. J. (1994). Trends in the use of drug therapies in patients with acute myocardial infarction: 1988 to 1992. *Journal of the American College of Cardiology, 23,* 1023–1030.

Perkins, J., Youdelman, M., & Wong, D. (2003). *Ensuring linguistic access in health care settings: Legal rights and responsibilities.* National Health Law Program.

Pew Research Center. (2006, April). *Eating more, enjoying less.* Retrieved from http://pewresearch.org/pubs/309/eating-more-enjoying-less

Pham, H. H., Schrag, D., Hargraves, J. L., & Bach, P. B. (2005). Delivery of preventive services to older adults by primary care physicians. *Journal of the American Medical Association, 294*(4), 473–481.

Ponce, N. A., Ku, L., Cunningham, W. E., & Brown, E. R. (2006). Language barriers to health care access among Medicare beneficiaries. *Journal Information, 43*(1).

Rafferty, M. (1998). Prevention services in primary care: Taking time, setting priorities. *Western Journal of Medicine, 169*(5), 269.

Ramsay, N. (2008, May 24). *TV viewing figures vs. IQ ranking by country* [Web blog post]. Retrieved from http://www.longcountdown.com/2008/05/24/tv-viewing-figures-vs-iq-ranking-by-country/

Red Meat Industry Forum. (2007, May). *Beef and veal consumption and choosing the right cut.* Retrieved from http://www.redmeatforum.org.uk/supplychain/BVConsumption.html

Reede, J. Y. (2003). A recurring theme: The need for minority physicians. *Health Affairs, 22*(4), 91–93.

Reiss-Brennan, B. (2006). Can mental health integration in a primary care setting improve quality and lower costs? A case study. *Journal of Managed Care Pharmacy, 12*(2), 14.

Satcher, D., Fryer, G. E., McCann, J., Troutman, H., Woolf, S. H., & Rust, G. (2005). What if we were equal? A comparison of the black–white mortality gap in 1960 and 2000. *Health Affairs, 24*(3), 459–464.

Singer, P. (2007, January 3). Early births fade to grey. *The Australian*, p. 10.

Smeltzer, S. C., Sharts-Hopko, N. C., Ott, B. B., Zimmerman, V., & Duffin, J. (2007). Perspectives of women with disabilities on reaching those who are hard to reach. *Journal of Neuroscience Nursing, 39*(3), 163–171.

Stein, T. (2004). *Role of law in social work practice and administration.* New York, NY: Columbia University Press.

Street, R. L., O'Malley, K. J., Cooper, L. A., & Haidet, P. (2008). Understanding concordance in patient–physician relationships: Personal and ethnic dimensions of shared identity. *Annals of Family Medicine, 6*(3), 198–205.

Survive your stay at the hospital. (2014, May). *Consumer Reports,* pp. 44–46.

Taylor, H. A., Jr., Cano, J. G., Sanderson, B., Rogers, Q. J., & Hilbe, J. (1998). Management and outcomes for black patients with acute myocardial infarction in the reperfusion era. National Registry of Myocardial Infarction 2 Investigators. *American Journal of Cardiology, 82,* 1019–1023.

United Nations Office on Drugs and Crime. (2010). *Homicide statistics, criminal justice, and public health sources: Trends 2003–2008.* Retrieved from http://www.unodc.org/unodc/en/data-and-analysis/homicide.html

Wartik, N. (2002, June 23). Hurting more, helped less? *New York Times,* pp. 1, 6.

Williams, D. R., & Mohammed, S. A. (2009). Discrimination and racial disparities in health: Evidence and needed research. *Journal of Behavioral Medicine, 32*(1), 20–47.

Willingham, S., & Kilpatrick, E. (2005). Evidence of gender bias when applying the new diagnostic criteria for myocardial infarction. *Heart, 91,* 237–238.

Wilper, A. P., Woolhandler, S., Lasser, K. E., McCormick, D., Bor, D. H., & Himmelstein, D. U. (2009). Health insurance and mortality in US adults. *Journal Information, 99*(12).

Chapter 8

BECOMING POLICY ADVOCATES IN THE GERONTOLOGY SECTOR

Bruce Jansson and Dawn Joosten

LEARNING OBJECTIVES

In this chapter, you will learn how to:

1. Recognize how Americans created a gerontology sector in which older adults have historically been perceived as weak and dependent

2. Recognize political aspects of the gerontology sector, including powerful players and interests as well as underrepresented ones

3. Understand some social injustices in the gerontology sector

4. Analyze seven core problems in the gerontology sector

   - Identify barriers in remedying each of them
   - Recognize important policies, regulations, and organizational factors that provide the context for each of them
   - Understand some Red Flag Alerts for each problem
   - Understand some connected micro, mezzo, and macro policy interventions by social workers seeking to ameliorate the seven problems
   - Understand gerontology-related initiatives

5. Drawing upon vignettes in this chapter, discuss how advocates can move from micro policy advocacy to mezzo and macro policy advocacy

ANALYZING THE EVOLUTION OF THE AMERICAN GERONTOLOGY SECTOR

The following timeline depicts how policies for the aging and perceptions of older adults historically in the United States have created the seven problems we discuss throughout this book:

Christian Morality and Civil War, 1800–1860

- Elders occupied a high position in society in the colonial period. Veneration of them, which was based on Puritan beliefs that elders should be revered because spirituality and wisdom peaked in old age and because they provided moral leadership to younger generations, began to decline in the early to mid nineteenth century (Quadagno, 2008).
- By 1820, elders no longer held the best seats in churches and legislatures established requirements for public officials to retire between the age of 60 and 70 (Quadagno, 2008).
- The cultural value of a youthful society began to emerge as elders' manner of dress became designed to make them appear younger.
- The attitude of seeing older adults as unproductive emerged, and retirement became a practice that further reinforced negative stereotypes of older adults as poverty rates among older adults rose (Quadagno, 2008).

Post–Civil War Degradation, 1860–1920

- As manufacturing employers focused on mass production with the assembly line to increase profits, ageist stereotypes well embedded in American culture by this period often led employers to perceive older adults as less productive than younger workers, further degrading the value of the older adult in the new industrial workforce.
- The demographic profile of the population in the United States in 1905 resembled a pyramid shape, consisting of a small proportion of adults ages 65 and older, reflecting mortality rates that were high, and a larger proportion of infants and children, reflecting fertility rates that were high (Aldwin & Gilmer, 2004).

Addressing Destitution in the New Deal and Its Aftermath

- Stereotypes of older adults as frail, abandoned by their children, and impoverished became deeply embedded in the attitudes of Americans toward older adults (Quadagno, 2008).
- President Franklin Roosevelt sought to alleviate widespread poverty among the elderly by enacting the Social Security Act in 1935, as well as Old Age Assistance.

- In 1959, poverty rates of older adults 65+ were slightly more than double those in the 18–64 age group: 35.2% and 17%, respectively (U.S. Census Bureau, 2011).
- The nursing home industry began to grow during the 1950s and 1960s, taking the place of traditional "almshouses."

Growth of Public Social Services, Personal Rights, and Social Programs, 1960–1980

- The proportion of older adults 65+ below the poverty rate continued to decline during this time period, from the high of 35.2% in 1959 to a low of 15.7% in 1980 (U.S. Census Bureau, 2011).
- A new stereotype of older adults emerged in society as the economic condition of older adults improved: They were now viewed, according to Binstock, as "a prosperous, selfish, and politically powerful group that is gobbling up scarce societal resources" (as cited in Quadagno, 2008, p. 103).
- The Kerr-Mills Act of 1960 was a small means-tested program to enhance the income of seniors (Quadagno, 2008).
- Medicare and Medicaid (as Titles XVIII and XIX, respectively, of the Social Security Act) soon replaced it in 1965 (Midgley, Tracy, & Livermore, 2000).
- The means-tested Supplementary Security Income (SSI) program was created in 1972 to provide income to low-income seniors as well as low-income nonelderly individuals with disabilities and blind individuals (Torres-Gil & Villa, 2000).
- The National Aging Network was established to meet the needs of noninstitutionalized older adults through the enactment of the Older Americans Act (OAA) on July 14, 1965.
- The OAA established the Administration on Aging (AoA) (Angel & Angel, 1997) which accomplished its mission through local and state Area Agencies on Aging (AAAs) (Angel & Hogan, 2004).

Devolution of Federal Programs to States and Individuals in the Presidencies of Ronald Reagan and George W. Bush

- President Ronald Reagan enacted Social Security amendments in 1983 intended to keep Social Security solvent. These reforms included "advancing the age of eligibility for benefits, increasing the federal withholding tax, including federal and nonprofit employees in the program, and a 6 month delay in benefit increases" (Midgley et al., p. 145).
- The American's with Disabilities Act (ADA; P.L. 101-336) was enacted during George H. W. Bush's presidency, creating a national mandate of anti-discrimination for disabled individuals in the workplace, the community, public places, and public and transportation services (Hayden, 2000).

Social Reform in a Polarized Context During
the Presidencies of Bill Clinton and Barack Obama

- President Bill Clinton enacted the Balanced Budget Act of 1997 seeking to end the budget deficit in five years and promised to "divert any federal budget surplus resulting from the budget balancing to the Social Security trust fund so that baby boomers would be assured of benefits on their retirement" (Stosz, 2000, p. 149).

- Medicare provided health insurance to 38 million older and/or disabled adults and Medicaid to 36 million low-income individuals (Pear, 1998, as cited in Midgley et al., 2000).

- Political and public debates took place during the Clinton administration surrounding concerns about the future of the three entitlement programs (Medicare, Medicaid, and Social Security) amid the "graying of the federal budget."

- President Obama released his plan for reducing the federal deficit in September, 2011—a plan that included spending caps and other cuts in Medicare and Medicaid for programs used by seniors (Office of Management and Budget, 2011, p. 1).

- These cuts came on top of the $424 billion in cuts in Medicare over a 10-year period when the Patient Protection and Affordable Care Act was enacted in 2010 (Kaiser Family Foundation, 2011).

- The Affordable Care Act (ACA) allowed early retirees between the ages of 55 and 65 as well as their dependents an option to maintain employer-provided insurance until the State Insurance Exchanges established by the Act became available in 2014 (U.S. Department of Health and Human Services, 2011). Framers of the ACA chose, however, to eliminate a program that would have financed long-term care for people not on Medicaid.

ANALYZING PROBLEMS OF SENIORS CAUSED BY ECONOMIC INEQUALITY

Inegalitarian nations are characterized by social and economic inequalities. The baby boom and increased life expectancies have contributed to a dramatic demographic shift among older adults in the United States. The number of adults 65 and older will increase from 12.4% of the total population in 2004 to 20% in 2030 (Administration on Aging, 2005b). The percentage of adults 85 and over, as a proportion of adults 65 and over, will increase from 12% in 2000 to 24% in 2050 (Administration on Aging, 2004), and the number will increase from 4.6 million in 2002 to 9.6 million in 2030 (Administration on Aging, 2005b). Mortality rates from 1950 to 2002 dropped for the following age groups: (1) 27% for 85 and over, (2) 40% for 75 to 84, and (3) approximately 20% for ages 65 to 74 (National Center for Health Statistics, 2004, as cited in Joosten, 2008).

Many of these seniors will face severe financial straits. Roughly half of retirees have no assets when they retire—and many of them have credit card debt and other forms of debt. They will have to rely only on Social Security benefits. Many of them—particularly women—have no pensions or pensions that pay low amounts. Many of them will exhaust their Medicare benefits when they develop chronic health conditions. Many will be hard-pressed to meet their survival needs of rent, food, and transportation. Many will have to live in unsafe areas to find rental costs they can afford (Angel & Hogan, 2004, as cited in Joosten, 2008).

ANALYZING THE POLITICAL ECONOMY OF THE GERONTOLOGY SECTOR

Our discussion reveals a complex political economy of aging. Older people have had many advocates over the past century, including the sheer clout of older individuals in elections and groups defending Social Security and Medicare. Social Security, Medicare, Medicaid, and SSI, once enacted, created huge constituencies favorable to seniors. Indeed, the Democratic Party made many electoral gains in the 1980s and beyond when they attacked efforts by leading Republicans to cut or privatize these programs. Interest groups catering to hospitals, nursing homes, and convalescent homes, as well as retirement homes, often fought cuts in Medicare and Medicaid that funded their operations. Growing numbers of younger people defended seniors' programs as well, as they realized that their aging parents and grandparents relied on government programs for seniors. (See Table 8.1 for advocacy groups that seek greater social justice in the gerontology sector.)

No longer a national organization, the Gray Panthers now exists in many cities, such as Sacramento and Detroit. Formed in 1970 by Maggie Kuhn, who was angry that she was forced to retire at age 65, the Gray Panthers militantly sought greater rights for seniors. Kuhn established a collection of local networks that used advertising and guerrilla theater and sought universal healthcare, lower-cost medications, greater patient rights, affordable housing for all, and a patient bill of rights. Kuhn believed that ageism was a potent ideology that restricted elderly individuals' participation in society. She favored house sharing for seniors as well as intergenerational living as compared to nursing homes.

Table 8.1   Some Advocacy Groups Seeking Greater Social Justice in the Gerontology
Sector

AFL-CIO

Alliance for Retired Persons

American Association of Retired Persons

Center for Economic and Policy Research

Century Foundation: Social Security Network

Institute of America's Future

National Committee to Preserve Social Security and Medicare

New York Network for Action on Medicare and Social Security

These forces defending seniors' programs have increasingly faced opposition to seniors' publicly funded programs. These include growing numbers
of conservatives who seek deep cuts in government programs. They include
Republicans' efforts to convert Medicare into a voucher program during the
past two decades, as well as their efforts to cut funding of Medicaid and devolve
it to the states. They include members of both parties who want to cut huge government deficits by downsizing seniors' programs. They include some members
of the baby boomer generation born between 1946 and 1962 who believe that
they can avert chronic health conditions by dieting and exercising. They include
many public officials who oppose a federally financed program for long-term
care or insurance.

We suspect that the sheer growth of the number of older people in the next
three decades will lead to a resurgence of senior power. Older adults are a strong
political force. In comparison to adults ages 30 to 49, older adults along with baby
boomers are more likely to vote, convey more enthusiasm toward voting, and
have demonstrated an increase in election engagement since 1994 (Kuhn, 2010).
In fact, a Gallop Poll of registered voters for the 2012 presidential election suggested that "age is a predictor of voter turnout," as 87% of registered voters ages
60 to 69 reported that they definitely would vote compared to 59% of registered
voters ages 19 to 29 (Newport, 2012, para. 8). They will constitute a massive part
of the American electorate—as much as 25% in some jurisdictions. A majority of
seniors have voted for Republican candidates in the last several national elections,
but this may change as more elderly people lack adequate living standards, health,
and long-term care.

ANALYZING THE SEVEN CORE PROBLEMS IN THE GERONTOLOGY SECTOR

VIDEO LINK 8.1
Improving
Healthcare
for Seniors

Core Problem 1: Engaging in Advocacy to Promote Ethical Rights, Human Rights, and Economic Justice for Older Adults—With Some Red Flag Alerts

- **Red Flag Alert 8.1.** Older individuals do not receive adequate information to make an informed decision about the options for end-of-life care, such as palliative care, hospice, and legal options like advance directives or living wills.
- **Red Flag Alert 8.2.** Patients' right to self-determination is violated when competent older adults are not included in decision making about their care or preferences for care.
- **Red Flag Alert 8.3.** The wishes of elderly individuals with advance directives are not honored.

Background

Older adults 65+ account for 55.8% of all intensive care unit stays in the United States, and the rates are expected to increase (Balas, Casey, & Happ, 2007) with the graying of America over the next three decades. The oldest-old (ages 85+) have the highest rates of functional limitations and hospitalizations. The prevalence of chronic diseases is greatest among older adults; 80% of older adults 65+ have at least one chronic disease (Centers for Disease Control and Prevention [CDC], 2011). Each year in the United States, 70% of deaths are due to chronic diseases, with prevalence rates for heart disease, cancer, and diabetes among adults 65 and older in 2008–2009 being 31.7%, 26.9%, and 17.1%, respectively (CDC, 2011).

Many of these ethical issues arise during end-of-life situations where seniors must make difficult decisions about many issues, including whether to sustain support or treatments such as mechanical ventilation, dialysis, nasal or gastric feeding tubes, and cardiopulmonary resuscitation. They often must make these decisions when they have diminished decision-making capacity. When they are declared to be mentally incompetent by courts, surrogates such as spouses or adult children must make these decisions.

Social workers, bioethicists, and bioethics committees at healthcare institutions are crucial advocates in resolving and addressing violations of older adults' ethical rights. They often act on behalf of those with diminished capacity or empower proxy decision makers or other healthcare providers to request bioethics consultations and review of cases by bioethics committees at healthcare institutions where ethical dilemmas occur.

End-of-life care is an area where conflicts between medical ethics and individual rights can create barriers in access to medical treatments and services that enable older adults to remain in the community and out of institutions. The major moral principles used in bioethics when considering ethical dilemmas include:

- Autonomy (or self-determination), that is, the right to accept or refuse medical treatment by competent individuals based on informed consent where they are told about the benefits and risks of specific treatments
- The principle of not harming people unnecessarily through injury or the taking of life—and the corresponding principle of helping people (often called beneficence)
- The principle of honesty, where people are given accurate and timely information
- The principle of confidentiality
- The principle of equity so that some people do not receive better treatment than others based on their social class, ethnicity, gender, sexual orientation, or any other personal characteristic (Csikai & Chaitin, 2006).

Many factors can impede ethical treatment of patients. Family members may want medical options at variance with an elderly person. Time pressures may lead physicians to not fully consult with patients and their families. The availability of medical technology may skew decisions toward their use even when patients do not want them. Some physicians impose their judgments on patients or are unable to communicate effectively with them. Some medical choices are made to avert medical costs. Some family members may seek to influence medical choices because they want to inherit money and other goods from a parent or relative.

Social work advocates are in a unique position to intervene on behalf of vulnerable older adults and their family members to ensure that their ethical rights are not being violated. Advocates trained in advance care planning, bioethics, and end-of-life care ensure that terminal older adults and those facing life-threatening illnesses are informed about the range of options available to them and have access to them.

Older adults' ethical rights can be violated if they fail to document their preferences for end-of-life care. It is estimated that between 2% to 15% of adults in the general population and 55.7% of patients with terminal cancer have advance directives in the United States (Ott, 1999). In contrast, 57% of patients in primary care have an estate will (Ott, 1999), indicating that there are more Americans who are prepared to handle their estate at the time of their death than those who have made decisions about care leading up to their death.

There is a need for increasing the workforce of physicians who specialize in end-of-life care. In 2007, the specialty became recognized, and currently 86 new palliative care physicians acquire accredited training for the subspecialty annually. It is estimated that there is currently one palliative care physician for every 1,200 individuals with chronic diseases in comparison to "one cardiologist for every 71 people experiencing a heart attack and one oncologist for every 141 people with cancer" (Cantlupe, 2012).

Resources for Advocates

End-of-life care involves services such as hospice and palliative care. According to Field and Cassel (1997), hospice care is defined by the Institute of Medicine as a program that provides dying individuals and their families with supportive and medical services at a specific cite of care, emphasizing a philosophy that incorporates spiritual, clinical, social, and metaphysical principles (as cited in Reese & Raymer, 2004). The Dana Farber Cancer Institute (2015) describes palliative care as a type of care that focuses on the whole person (mind, body, and spirit) to allow individuals to be more comfortable during medical treatments and to reduce pain and suffering in later stages of disease. Unlike most hospice programs, palliative care is not defined by a patient's life expectancy, since it can be provided at the time of diagnosis and for years for individuals managing chronic diseases (Morrison & Meier, 2011). Both programs, however, provide a team of professionals that include physicians, nurses, social workers, and chaplains to work with patients and their families. A study sponsored by the Robert Wood Johnson Foundation that sought to understand the prognosis and preferences for outcomes and risks of treatment (SUPPORT) by looking at 5,000 dying patients in American hospitals concluded that most Americans "die alone in institutions, in pain, and attached to machines against their wishes" (Berzoff & Silverman, 2004, p. 7).

Hospice seeks to reduce some of these problems by giving patients the choice to receive nonheroic treatment for terminal conditions. It allows them to die in their homes if they wish. It provides them with social work and nursing services geared toward helping them avoid pain.

Hospices are accredited by the Community Health Accreditation Program (CHAP) that also conducts surveys of community-based and other public health programs (National League for Nursing, 1999). The Joint Commission accredits hospitals, including their palliative care and ICU programs. Both CHAP and the Joint Commission may sanction programs and hospitals that violate ethical standards.

Medicare covers inpatient care at skilled nursing facilities, hospice services, and home health services for Medicare beneficiaries in need of long-term, end-of-life, and intermittent care. The Medicare benefit for hospice services was established in 1982 as part of the Tax Equity Fiscal Responsibility Act—and became a national guaranteed benefit under the administration of President Bill Clinton (National Hospice and Palliative Care Organization, 2011). Patients must have a physician's order that confirms they have a terminal illness with six months or less to live to qualify for hospice coverage. They can receive the benefit at home, at a hospital, or at a skilled nursing facility at no charge with a copayment of up to $5 for medication that manages patients' pain and symptoms (Centers for Medicare and Medicaid Services [CMS], 2011).

Palliative care is a board-certified specialty that is similar to hospice care. Patients are often contacted in hospitals where they have come for treatment of chronic and terminal conditions. They confer with palliative care physicians and other health professionals, including social workers, as they make choices about how to have dignified deaths under terms and conditions that they select.

The Patient Self-Determination Act of 1991 requires hospitals to provide patients with advance directives in which they indicate whether they want specific medical procedures if they become terminally ill and are not able to request them due to their medical condition. They might decide, for example, not to have a feeding tube inserted into their stomach if they are unable to swallow. They can also decide they want to designate a person, such as a spouse or an adult child, to make medical choices for them if they are unable to make their own choices—often called "durable power of attorney."

Federal courts have generally supported patients' right to make end-of-life choices—and the right of relatives to make them for them when they are unable to make these choices due to their medical condition. In the landmark case of *Cruzan vs. Director, Missouri Department of Health*, for example, the court upheld a request by Nancy Cruzan's parents to have her feeding tube removed due to her expressed preference not to have life supportive measures prior to the automobile accident that left her in a vegetative state.

Some states, such as Oregon and Washington, have enacted ballot measures that allow people declared by two physicians to have less than six months of life to request the medical infusion of lethal substances to hasten death—often called "euthanasia." These ballot measures state many procedural safeguards to ensure ethical decisions, including:

- It must be medically determined that the patient is not depressed and does not have another mental condition that might make him or her suicidal.
- The patient must state his or her preference to physicians on multiple successive occasions.
- Physicians must administer the lethal substances.

Researchers have discovered that relatively few people choose euthanasia in these states.

Physicians are allowed in all states to issue "Do Not Resuscitate" orders (DNRs) for patients with end-of-life conditions because physicians can choose not to provide "medically futile" treatments. The Physician Order for Life Sustaining Treatment, or POLST, replaced the Do Not Resuscitate order in California. It is a physician order for providing or withholding cardiopulmonary resuscitation (CPR) and other end-of-life and life-sustaining measures. The document informs responding medical professionals what measures to take or not take—and this order follows patients across the continuum of care from their home to the ambulance, the emergency room and hospital, and a skilled nursing facility if transfer is arranged.

POLICY ADVOCACY LEARNING CHALLENGE 8.1

Connecting Micro, Mezzo, and Macro Policy Advocacy to Protect Patients' Ethical Rights

Social workers are often the healthcare professionals that family and patients reach out to when making end-of-life decisions. Social workers have an ethical obligation to advocate for the right to self-determination among competent patients with clearly executed advance directives and living wills indicating their preferences and instructions for withholding and withdrawal of care, as well as among the surrogate decision makers they appoint, that is, individuals with power of attorney.

Mr. K was an 80-year-old Caucasian male who resided at his home with his spouse. He had advanced Parkinson's disease and was dependent on a ventilator/tracheotomy and artificial hydration/nutrition through a feeding tube.

Mr. K was bedbound and required total care. He was alert and oriented times four (person, time, place, situation) but was nonverbal. His only way of communicating was by writing on a whiteboard. Mr. K had a very active spouse and two adult children who were professionals. Mr. K received long-term home health care and had a visiting nurse. Mr. K had the financial resources to pay for around-the-clock 24-hour care. Mr. K identified his religious view of an afterlife as one source of hope and ability to cope. To Mr. K, the ability to communicate with loved ones and visitors via the whiteboard helped define his quality of life. He stated that once he could no longer write, he wanted life support discontinued. Mr. K had an advance directive which designated his spouse as his healthcare proxy/decision maker. In Mr. K's advance directive, he requested that his life not be prolonged if he had "an incurable and irreversible condition that would result in his death within a relatively short time." About two weeks after the social worker met with Mr. K and his spouse, the spouse contacted the social worker, indicating that the time had come that Mr. K could no longer write on the whiteboard, that he wanted to be taken off life support according to his instructions in his advance directive, and that he wanted to die at home surrounded by his family.

LEARNING EXERCISE

1. How should the social worker proceed with a micro policy intervention?
2. Does Mr. K have a right to die at home?
3. What are the legal requirements or programs available?
4. What are the goals and timeline for executing the actions?
5. Should an interdisciplinary team meeting, bioethics consult, and/or psychiatric evaluation be requested to establish a plan of care and determine whether the patient still has the mental capacity to make such a decision?
6. How can the end-of-life options be best explored with the patient and family?
7. Assume that a physician insisted that all medical means be used to prolong this patient's life. How might a social worker initiate a macro policy intervention at the organizational level to decrease the likelihood of incidents like this?

Core Problem 2: Engaging in Advocacy to Promote Quality Services and Programs for Seniors—With Some Red Flag Alerts

- **Red Flag Alert 8.4.** Conflicting values between an older adult and her family members and healthcare providers result in violations of her right to autonomy, which in turn creates a barrier to her receiving quality care in a setting she prefers.
- **Red Flag Alert 8.5.** People with disabilities are sometimes placed in institutions in violation of the Olmstead decision made by the U.S. Supreme Court in July 1999 that prohibits unnecessary institutionalization of individuals with disabilities.
- **Red Flag Alert 8.6.** Elderly individuals receive other kinds of medical care that fall short of gold-standard care, including excessive numbers of medications, fragmented care where physicians fail to communicate with one another, and excessive use of surgical remedies before less invasive strategies are attempted.
- **Red Flag Alert 8.7.** A patient does not receive adequate information to make an informed decision about the options for long-term care available across the continuum of health care and residential care.
- **Red Flag Alert 8.8.** A competent older patient's right to self-determination is violated when he is not included in the decision making about his care.
- **Red Flag Alert 8.9.** A resident of a nursing home, board-and-care, or assisted living facility experiences a violation in the Residents' Bill of Rights.

- **Red Flag Alert 8.10.** Seniors lack a range of choices in specific communities other than nursing homes, including the community-based Village program or small group homes.

Background

The Geriatric Social Work Initiative was funded through the Hartford Foundation to provide training and establish competencies for geriatric social workers in 1999 to meet the biopsychosocial needs of the growing older adult population. The need for geriatric social workers will continue to grow as the population of older people expands. In 2009, there were only 7,162 geriatricians in the United States with a Certificate of Added Qualifications in Geriatric Medicine (AGS Foundation for Health in Aging, 2015) to address the needs of 39.6 million adults 65 and older— or a ratio of only one physician per 4,400 older adults 65+ (U.S. Census Bureau, 2011). This ratio will decline to a ratio of one geriatrician for every 9,833 older adults by 2050 if training rates remain the same.

Resources for Advocates

The Joint Commission's Long Term Care Accreditation program was created in 1966 and is responsible for the accreditation of over 15,000 skilled nursing facilities and 1,000 eligible long-term care organizations in the United States. It requires these facilities to undergo an on-site survey every three years to maintain accreditation (Joint Commission, 2011). The Joint Commission has developed long-term care standards in the following performance areas: environment of care; emergency management; human resources; infection prevention and control; information management; leadership; life safety; medication management; national patient safety goals; record of care, treatment, and services; rights and responsibilities of the individual; and waived testing (Joint Commission, 2011).

Inpatient care at skilled nursing facilities, hospice services, and home health services are covered benefits for Medicare beneficiaries in need of long-term, end-of-life, and intermittent care. Medicare Part A covers medically necessary intermittent care for community dwelling beneficiaries with a stay-at-home disability, including home nursing; physical, occupational, and speech therapies; personal assistance from certified home health aides; and psychosocial services from social workers at no charge (CMS, 2011). Once patients have spent three days in an acute care hospital, Medicare covers skilled needs such as IV antibiotics or physical therapy with no copays for the first 20 days and co-insurance for days 21 to 100 when Medicare coverage ends (CMS, 2011).

The Long-Term Care Ombudsman Program, begun under the Older Americans Act in 1972, provides advocacy for the vulnerable older adult residents in skilled nursing, board-and-care, and assisted living facilities (Administration on Aging, 2011b). Each state has a Long-Term Care Ombudsman Program that investigates and resolves complaints to ensure that residents' ethical rights are not being violated. The top five resident complaints in skilled nursing facilities in 2010 were:

> unanswered requests for assistance such as when residents with functional dependence require toileting or assistance with transferring out of the bed to a chair or the toilet; inadequate or no discharge/eviction notice or planning; lack of respect for residents, poor staff attitudes; and resident conflict, including roommate to roommate when residents were not transferred to a separate room or not provided conflict medication. (Administration on Aging, 2011b, para. 2)

Ombudsmen nationwide resolved 74% of all complaints at nursing homes and 39% of all complaints at assisted living and board-and-care facilities in 2010 (Administration on Aging, 2011b).

Congress passed the Nursing Home Reform Act in 1987 that required nursing homes to "ensure that the resident has the right to choose activities, schedules, and health care" and to "promote each resident's quality of life and maintain dignity and respect of each resident" (Nursing Home Abuse and Neglect Resource Center, 2011). The Nursing Home Reform Act established rights for residents under the Residents' Bill of Rights, such as the rights to exercise self-determination; communicate feely; privacy; participate in care; and be free from abuse, neglect, and physical restraints (Klauber & Wright, 2001). States have also enacted a variety of bills to ensure the protection of residents' rights in residential care facilities, such as (in California) the Nursing Home Resident's Rights in 2006 (California Advocates for Nursing Home Reform, 2011).

POLICY ADVOCACY LEARNING CHALLENGE 8.2

Connecting Micro, Mezzo, and Macro Policy Advocacy

Mrs. C is an 89-year-old resident in a skilled nursing facility, where she has resided for three years. Prior to entering the nursing home, she lived in her home with a private 24-hour caregiver. Once she required the assistance of a Hoyer lift, she decided she could not afford the extra caregiver to assist with transfers, and she made the decision to relocate to a nursing home. She is alert and oriented, suffers from no psychological disorders, has capacity to engage in all decision making, and signs all her own consents. She is obese, and had her left leg amputated four years ago due to complications with diabetes. She suffers from severe diabetic neuropathy and cannot ambulate without an assistive device and cannot transfer without assistance. Since entering the nursing home, she has required three attendants to assist with the use of a Hoyer lift to transfer her from her hospital bed to her wheelchair. You are the new social worker at this facility and are meeting with each resident to update psychosocial assessments and treatment plans. In your assessment interview, Mrs. C states that she would like to eat her meals in the dining room but is often brought her meals to eat alone in her room. She also reports that she would like to participate in the social activities such as bingo and music, but reports that when she asks the attendants, they say, "I'm too busy; I'll come back," but they "never come back, so I sit in my room watching television by myself."

LEARNING EXERCISE

1. How should the social worker proceed with a micro policy intervention?
2. Does the long-term care ombudsman need to be notified?
3. What are the legal requirements for the nursing home?
4. What resident rights have been violated?
5. How can the resident's rights be best addressed?
6. What policies may need to be updated at the organizational level to reflect state and/or national policies ensuring protection of residents' rights?
7. Could state regulations governing nursing homes be modified to limit seniors' isolation?

Core Problem 3: Engaging in Advocacy to Promote Culturally Competent Services for Seniors—With Some Red Flag Alerts

- **Red Flag Alert 8.11.** An older adult's culture is not honored in interactions with health and/or other professionals.
- **Red Flag Alert 8.12.** An older adult with limited English proficiency (LEP) is not given appropriate translation services.
- **Red Flag Alert 8.13.** An older adult with low literacy fails to receive health information that she can understand.
- **Red Flag Alert 8.14.** Older adults from a specific cultural group are provided poorer services than other persons.

Background

Myriad factors contribute to inequities in minority health: socioeconomic status, gender, environment, access, racial bias, and genetics. The National Institute on Aging identifies race, ethnicity, gender, socioeconomic status, age, education, occupation, and as-yet unknown lifetime and lifestyle differences, as well as less access to and use of healthcare and poorer health care (National Institute on Aging, 2010).

We have an increasingly diverse population of seniors, yet many of them fail to receive culturally competent care—an omission that could endanger their safety and health. The racial composition of the aging population is changing. As a proportion of adults 65 and older, minorities will increase from 15% in 2000 to 36% in 2050 (Quadagno, 2008). African Americans represented the largest minority subgroup as a proportion of older adults 65 and over in 2000—or 8% of elderly Americans, or 2.8 million people (Administration on Aging, 2005a). Hispanic adults 65 and over will increase from 5% of American elderly individuals in 2000 to 16% in 2050 (Quadagno, 2008). The percentage of Asian and Pacific Islanders will increase by 350%, from 2% to 7% of American seniors, between 2000 and 2050 (Quadagno, 2008). More African American and Hispanic elderly individuals live in poverty than Caucasian elderly individuals—or roughly 20% to 25% as compared to 5% to 10% in 2001 (Angel & Hogan, 2004). Their poverty puts them at greater risk for health disparities. It makes it more difficult for them to access services and healthcare.

Membership in a minority group is a risk factor for poor health. African American males are 30% more likely to die from heart disease than Caucasian elderly individuals (Centers for Disease Control and Prevention, n.d.). For all cancers combined, African American females are more likely to die from cancer than non-Hispanic whites, Hispanics, or Asian and Pacific Islanders. American Indian/Alaskan Native females are less likely than non-Hispanic whites to have cervical and breast cancers detected early (Centers for Disease Control and Prevention, 2014).

According to the American Society on Aging (2015), there are approximately 2 million lesbian, gay, bisexual, and transgender (LGBT) individuals in the United States. Risk factors for LGBT older adults include limited caregiver assistance and/or families that have excluded them because of their sexual orientation (9 out of 10 do not have a child who can help); fears of mistreatment by caregivers due to their sexual orientation, which exacerbates isolation in times of need (7 out of 10 live alone); and a lifetime of workplace discrimination and limited partner benefit access, which are factors that contribute to poverty. In comparison to heterosexuals, older LGBT persons are three times more likely to live in poverty (LGBT Older Adult Coalition, 2012, p. 1). Policy advocates must be aware of the myriad social, economic, and societal factors that create barriers to accessing healthcare, housing, and social services for this population. In an LGBT Older Adult Summit, 75 LGBT advocate participants identified the following areas as the greatest issues for LGBT older adults: isolation (38%), healthcare affordability (34%), and LGBT culturally incompetent care (13%; LGBT Older Adult Coalition, 2011). Advocates recommend improving access to culturally competent care for LGBT older adults through competency training for all providers in residential, community, and healthcare settings working with older adults as well as through education to individual care providers and families.

Resources for Advocates

The first investigation on health disparities comparing minorities to non-Hispanic whites began in 1984 when the secretary of health and human services established the Task Force on Black and Minority Health, which examined mortality rates for six leading causes of death at that time: stroke and cardiovascular disease, cancer, diabetes, infant mortality, chemical dependence, and accidents and homicides (National Institute of Minority Health and Health Disparities, 2013). The task force discovered that 80% of deaths among minorities were due to these six causes of death. A multitude of initiatives sponsored by both the National Institutes of Health and National Institute on Aging followed, beginning in the 1990s. In 1999, at the 25th anniversary of the National Institute on Aging, the director requested an evaluation of its past and current research efforts on minority aging and developed new initiatives to study minority aging research, training, and outreach activities (National Institute on Aging, 2010).

The U.S. Department of Health and Human Services has created a special link (www.hrsa.gov/culturalcompetence/index.html) under the Health Resources Services Administration website that provides resources and training materials for culture, language, and health literacy for organizations.

The ACA promotes cultural competence training for health care providers and improves collection and analysis of data on health disparities—and on disability status, primary language, race, sex, and ethnicity of persons who use healthcare (U.S. Department of Health & Human Services, 2011). Many states have passed their own laws and regulations to require and promote culturally competent healthcare and other services.

POLICY ADVOCACY LEARNING CHALLENGE 8.3

Connecting Micro, Mezzo, and Macro Policy Advocacy

Mr. A is a 66-year-old male referred to home health services by social work for crisis intervention and discharge planning; physical therapy for new DME (walker), strengthening and endurance, and gait training due to a fracture sustained to his hip when he fell; and nursing to monitor vitals and medication management/compliance. Mr. A was admitted via ambulance to the ER upon being found unconscious in a park. He flat-lined in the ambulance on the way to the ER but was brought back with CPR and chest compressions. He was admitted and transferred to the ICU, where he was on life support for three days. He was successfully weaned from the ventilator and transferred to the medical floor until he stabilized. The hospital social worker discovered that Mr. A had just been released from prison the day before he was brought to the ER. A Medicaid application was not completed at the hospital. Mr. A could not go to a shelter due to the change in his functional health. The hospital discharged Mr. A to a board-and-care facility, where his basic needs were met for 30 days, fully paid through a charity program by the hospital. He had no income, housing, insurance, transportation, ID, clothing, or adequate social support. He had been a janitor for 15 years on and off in between times he was in prison.

Mr. A reveals to the home health social worker that he missed his parole officer meeting and has a diagnosis of schizophrenia. He asks the social worker for help in changing his life circumstances. He tells his life story, leading to his present state, of getting caught in a cycle of committing crimes, using drugs, going to prison, and returning back to the same environment to repeat the cycle. One of the home health providers labels Mr. A as a "drug dealer" unlikely to change, and the hospitalist refuses to provide pain medication beyond the discharge prescription, requesting that the patient find a primary care physician.

LEARNING EXERCISE

1. How might the social worker intervene as a case advocate?
2. What might the social worker's plan of care look like?
3. What programs, services, and benefits is the client eligible for and in need of advocacy for in terms of coordination and implementation?
4. What state and national policies relate to this case?
5. How might the social worker advocate changes in policy at the organizational level?

Core Problem 4: Engaging in Advocacy to Promote Preventive Services and Programs for Seniors—With Some Red Flag Alerts

- **Red Flag Alert 8.15.** An older adult has not been helped to identify personal risk factors through family history and diagnostic tests.
- **Red Flag Alert 8.16.** An older adult has not been tested for a possible chronic disease or diseases at a possible early stage.
- **Red Flag Alert 8.17.** An older adult with a relatively sedentary lifestyle has not been given help in increasing her exercise or is not given modifications in her exercise program based on her functional health and chronic diseases.
- **Red Flag Alert 8.18.** An older adult has not been given help in improving her nutrition.
- **Red Flag Alert 8.19.** An older adult has not been given help in not smoking.
- **Red Flag Alert 8.20.** An older adult has not been given help in receiving vaccines.
- **Red Flag Alert 8.21.** A person who lives in an inner city area is not given assistance in obtaining better nutrition and more exercise.
- **Red Flag Alert 8.22.** An older adult is not given access to prevention.

Background

Health promotion is particularly important to older adults, as health behaviors, both negative (obesity, alcohol abuse, smoking) and positive (avoiding tobacco, exercise, drinking alcohol in moderation), impact their functional health and quality of life (Aldwin & Gilmer, 2004). Prevention activities to reduce functional limitations such as immunizations, well check-ups, screenings, and good nutrition are extremely important (Aldwin & Gilmer, 2004).

A myriad of barriers contribute to the overlooked need for health prevention among older adults, including the prevalence of chronic disease and functional limitations of older adults, the inappropriate provision of interventions designed for middle or younger adults to older adults by medical professionals, the lack of recognition and financing by Medicare for prevention (Richardson, 2006), and the tendency to prescribe medications over education on proper nutrition and exercise. Many professionals wrongly believe that prevention programs primarily help younger individuals rather than older individuals (Aldwin & Gilmer, 2004).

Development of preventive programs for seniors was a "young field" up to 2000 (Albert, 2004, p. 16). Prevention activities for older adults now include primary prevention, such as vaccinations for the flu and shingles, medication therapies, counseling and prosthetic devices; secondary prevention (for early disease detection and treatment), such as screenings for cognitive deficits, diabetes, hypertension, and osteoporosis; and tertiary prevention (for disease management and disability reduction). Primary care or geriatrician physicians can coordinate care, telemedicine, emergency response pendants, and education (Albert, 2004).

Many residents are still not provided opportunities for exercise and improved nutrition (Kayser-Jones, 2009). Prevention among geriatric persons is slowed because "many geriatric disorders have multifactorial risk factors, interventions, and expected outcomes; older adults are often not represented in clinical trials; and important outcomes may not be measured and reported in ways that are conducive to evidence synthesis and interpretation" (Leipzig et al., 2010).

Self-rated health is a greater predictor of health and mortality among older adults, even those with chronic illnesses, than physician ratings. Most seniors rate their health as excellent, very good, or good (Aldwin & Gilmer, 2004). Functional health is also impacted by mental health, as low self-esteem and depression can lead older adults to neglect their health through poor diet, lack of exercise, and isolation from a support network (Aldwin & Gilmer, 2004). A model of health behavior change appropriate for use with older adults is the self-regulation model proposed by Leventhal, Rabin, Leventhal, and Burns (2001) that focuses on motivational characteristics of an older adult in participating in disease prevention and health promotion activities through goal setting, progress monitoring, and rewards for behaviors or steps. The model also emphasizes sociocultural aspects of change, including the older adult's community, age, and culture as well as social and historical factors (Aldwin & Gilmer, 2004). For example, a health behavior change plan for an older adult who has never exercised before would connect the older adult's history of not engaging in exercise to his or her current social/community context of needing exercise to prevent further disability after an injury (Aldwin & Gilmer, 2004).

Resources for Advocates

The Evidence-Based Prevention Program was initiated by the Administration on Aging (AoA) in 2003 to ensure that older adults have access to evidence-based interventions to reduce their risk for disability, disease, and injury (Administration on Aging, 2010). As part of the Aging Network, the Department of Health and Human Services collaborates with the AoA to ensure that effective programs are implemented in older adults' community settings. The Aging Network also includes collaboration with 30+ private foundations, the Agency for Healthcare Research and Quality, the Centers for Disease Control and Prevention, the Centers for Medicare and Medicaid Services, the Substance Abuse and Mental Health Services Administration, and the Health Resources and Services Administration (Administration on Aging, 2010). Evidence-based health programs include physical activity, fall prevention, smoking cessation, medication management, diabetes, chronic disease management, and nutrition programs (Administration on Aging, 2010). AoA has funded evidence-based programs in many states, including Enhance Fitness, Matter of Balance, Healthy IDEAS, and the Stanford University Chronic Disease Management Program. These and other programs are provided to older adults in settings such as senior housing, faith-based organizations, senior centers, and nutrition programs (Administration on Aging, 2010).

The ACA has several initiatives that will benefit older adults and make prevention services more available. It funds improved access to primary care, making prevention activities such as well checks and screenings more available to at-risk and underserved populations (U.S. Department of Health and Human Services, 2011). It funds programs for preventive care for people with disabilities, including programs aiming to prevent chronic disease (U.S. Department of Health and Human Services, 2011). Yet other programs funded by the ACA give seniors greater access to primary prevention health services through physical exams and free preventive care, as do Medicare B deductibles or copayments for screenings such as those for colorectal cancer, cervical cancer, cholesterol, and cardiovascular disease; mammograms; and prostate screenings.

The National Prevention Strategy released in June 2011 by the National Prevention, Health Promotion, and Public Health Council establishes 10-year targets to improve screening of adults ages 50 to 75 for colorectal cancer from 54.2% to 70.5% and to increase the percentage of adults 65+ vaccinated annually against influenza from 67.0% to 90.0% (Office of the Surgeon General, 2011). The National Prevention Strategy seeks to promote injury- and violence-free living through home modifications such as improved lighting, grab bars, and railings; strength and balance exercise programs geared specifically to older adults; monitoring of polypharmacy to reduce side effects that contribute to falls; and improving access to and linkage between prevention programs in health- and community-based settings (Office of the Surgeon General, 2011). The National Prevention Strategy also prioritizes increased support for those older adults who prefer to "age in place" and remain in their community as a means of promoting their emotional and mental health (Office of the Surgeon General, 2011).

POLICY ADVOCACY LEARNING CHALLENGE 8.4

Connecting Micro, Mezzo, and Macro Policy Advocacy

Mrs. G is a 61-year-old LEP female patient hospitalized after fainting. She has high blood pressure, a family history of type 2 diabetes, and a history of high cholesterol; is overweight; and does not exercise. Her educational level is sixth grade. You are asked by the hospitalist (a physician who speaks only English) to identify a clinic that will accept Mrs. G's new PPO insurance that she received after September 23, 1010 (the date when the Affordable Care Act required new insurance plans to provide free preventive services for all new plans), for primary care follow-up of her hypertension. Mrs. G is instructed by the hospitalist to start exercising and modify her diet to a low-sodium diet (1,200 mg or less). You are brought in right at the time she is being discharged. You ask whether she was screened for diabetes, and she replies that she was not. She cannot recall her cholesterol levels from a test when she was 40. She indicates she does not know what type of exercise or diet to follow.

LEARNING EXERCISE

1. If you worked in this hospital and wanted to be an advocate for diabetes screening for this patient before discharge, what conflicts might arise, and how might you best mitigate them?
2. What procedures or protocols at the organization level should be in place to prevent a patient with risk factors for diabetes from not receiving screening tests before discharge?
3. How might you as the social worker best coordinate the patient's linkage to an outpatient physician and/or other services necessary to ensure that the patient has access to a physician in her community?
4. What policies or programs exist in the community you work in for older adults with diabetes or hypertension? How might you link an older LEP patient to such services?
5. How would you advocate policy change at the organizational level?

Core Problem 5: Engaging in Advocacy to Promote Affordable and Accessible Services for Seniors—With Some Red Flag Alerts

- **Red Flag Alert 8.23.** An older adult is not informed of financing options for home- and community-based services and programs to allow her to remain in her community and out of an institution.

- **Red Flag Alert 8.24.** An older adult is incorrectly informed about his eligibility for long-term Medicaid and receives services through In-Home Supportive Services, not knowing about the estate recovery aspect.
- **Red Flag Alert 8.25.** A person is not linked to programs and services in his community that can help subsidize services he cannot afford, such as housekeeping and errands.
- **Red Flag Alert 8.26.** An older adult is unaware of the costs associated with programs and services as her functional health changes and she requires more assistance in the future.
- **Red Flag Alert 8.27.** An older adult needs insurance counseling about how to finance out-of-pocket costs related to services he may use.

Background

Advocates must be aware of the multiple options available for funding for services to allow older adults to remain in their communities and out of institutional facilities. Low-income older adults are at a higher risk for premature institutionalization when they have utilized all public programs available to finance their care and still require additional personal assistance with ADLs (activities of daily living) and IADLs (instrumental activities of daily living) to remain safely in their homes. Middle-class older adults who own a home but have limited income and savings are at risk for having unmet needs when their income covers only their monthly expenses and they are overqualified for public means-tested programs and services. To be effective advocates, social workers should be aware of the variety of funding options, services subsidized through programs in communities, and experts who can assist older adults with financial planning.

Resources for Advocates

Medicare does not finance services for older adults to help them to stay safely in their homes when changes in their functional health undermine their ability to perform tasks of daily living. Medicare will finance home health services for Medicare beneficiaries with a stay-at-home disability that prevents them from leaving their homes without the assistance of others, provided that they have a need for skilled nursing or rehabilitative services such as physical or occupational therapy. Under these circumstances, a certified home health aide can be provided for personal care assistance for an intermittent period. However, for those who do not regain their prior level of functioning and still require assistance, few options exist to help them finance services for assistance with tasks of daily living. Some older people are eligible for means-tested personal assistance services through

Medicaid. Such individuals may also qualify for In-Home Supportive Services offered by Medicaid in some areas, as well as Multipurpose Senior Services and integrated care management programs and adult day care, but these programs have been severely cut in many areas and may not exist in other areas, so social worker advocates have to ascertain what programs exist in their areas and states for low-income seniors who need personal services. Many other middle-income older adults, such as many individuals with Social Security whose income is too high to qualify for Medicaid, must finance these personal assistance services themselves or with the help of family members. Unfortunately, many of these individuals cannot afford the expenses associated with privately financed services, such as caregiver agencies who charge between $12 and $20 per hour (or more) in major urban areas, not to mention the cost of transportation services and home-delivered meals.

The Older Americans Act funds many services for older adults (age 60+) through the Administration on Aging. They include:

- Title III provides allocations to states for community programs for the aging, including supportive services, congregate meals, home meals, preventive services, and the National Family Caregiver Support Program (NFCSP). The budget allocated to these services increased from $1.1 billion in 2006 to $1.2 billion in 2011 (Administration on Aging, 2011a).
- Title III-NSIP funds the Nutrition Services Incentive Program. The budget allocated to these services increased from $143.5 million in 2006 to $154.2 million in 2011 (Administration on Aging, 2011a).
- Title VII funds the Vulnerable Elder Rights Protection Activities. The budget allocated to these services increased from $19.9 million in 2006 to $ 21.8 million in 2011 (Administration on Aging, 2011a).
- Title VI provides the Tribal Organization Allocation for Native Americans, including the Nutrition Services Incentive Program. The budget allocated to these services increased from $33.7 million in 2006 to $ 37.1 million in 2011 (Administration on Aging, 2011a).
- Higher proportions of the budget are allocated to states with large populations of older adults, such as Florida, California, Massachusetts, Pennsylvania, and New York (Figure 8.1). In accordance with the mission statement of the AoA to target services to those in need, the states of California and Texas have the highest proportions of older adults in poverty receiving AoA services in comparison to other states (Figure 8.2).

Medicare provides funding for 100 skilled nursing days per year, covers intermittent home health services, and covers hospice services for those with

Figure 8.1 Total expenditures for all states for all AoA programs and services

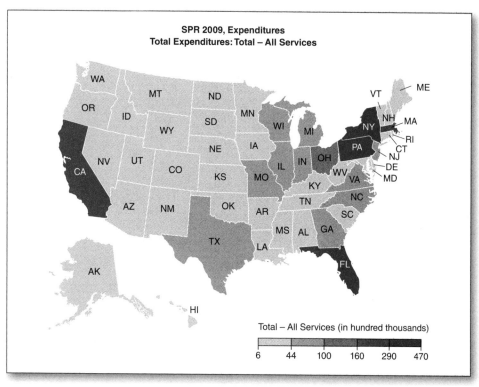

SPR 2009, Expenditures
Total Expenditures: Total – All Services

Total – All Services (in hundred thousands)

6   44   100   160   290   470

Source: Total Expenditures for All States for all AoA Programs and Services. Administration on Aging (2011). Aging Integrated Database.

a diagnosis of six months or less to live. With trends among several presidential administrations to control costs of aging programs over the past several decades, long-term care benefits provided under Medicare have faced cuts. In particular, the Medicare home health benefit implemented in 1975 under Title XX of the Social Security Act has been dramatically cut over the last 20 years to reduce costs, as at "one point home care was the fastest growing segment of the Medicare budget, reaching almost 10 percent of the Medicare budget and increasing four-fold in 10 years" (Ferrinni & Ferrinni, 2008, p. 457). Title XX under the Social Security Act ensured federal matching with states for some social services (Ferrinni & Ferrinni, 2008). Medicaid provides a long-term care benefit that subsidizes custodial care at a skilled nursing facility for older and disabled adults. In an attempt to recover money states spend on long-term Medicaid programs, in 1993 the Federal Budget Reconciliation Act permitted states to begin claiming assets of long-term Medicaid beneficiaries through estate recovery programs, provided

Figure 8.2   Older adults in poverty receiving AoA services

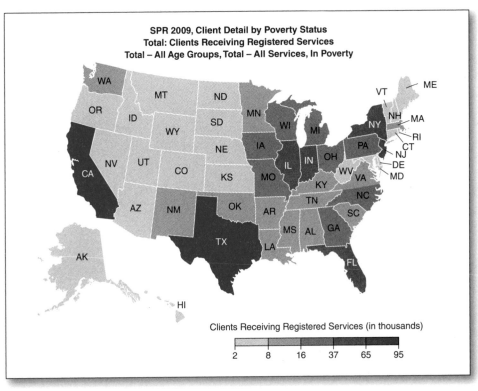

Source: Older Adults in Poverty Receiving AoA Services. Administration on Aging (2011). Aging Integrated Database.

that the recipient and the recipient's spouse are both deceased and/or there is not a surviving child or spouse that is either 18 or under, blind, or disabled (Ferrinni & Ferrinni, 2008).

Long-term care insurance has also been an option *to those who have the resources to purchase it.* These plans cover all or part of the cost of personal care services and skilled nursing home costs, as well as some other costs. Seniors must, however, begin paying premiums years before they use resources to make monthly premiums affordable, such as in their 60s. Moreover, many of these plans raise the level of premiums in the intervening years so that their cost becomes exorbitant—and some of the companies go out of existence before seniors can claim benefits. Considerable care should be given to researching specific plans before committing to one of them.

The ACA would have allowed individuals to contribute to a long-term care insurance benefit, but this feature was deleted due to its likely high costs.

POLICY ADVOCACY LEARNING CHALLENGE 8.5

Connecting Micro, Mezzo, and Macro Policy Advocacy

An affluent couple, who resided in a rural area, ran into financial difficulties when they encountered health problems that meant they could not perform many daily activities. The female member of this couple (Mary) became, in effect, the head of household because her husband (John) had been severely handicapped by a stroke. They found a woman (Joan) who had cared for others who had become, in effect, the head of their home health team. While a caring person, Joan had only a high school diploma and was often remiss in keeping the house clean or helping Mary and John to clean themselves because they could not ascend steps to the second floor to a bathroom with a shower. Joan recruited other younger women who also had not progressed beyond high school. She frequently had to recruit new people, as the women tended to leave this job due to the treatment they received from Mary, who viewed them as intruders in her house. Joan screened applicants by placing a $10 bill on the floor near John's bed. If they picked it up and did not give it to Joan, she did not hire them. Little did they know it was a fake $10 bill inscribed with "Take Jesus Into Your Everyday Life" on the side facing the floor. Almost bankrupted by the cost of this home health team, Mary had to endure the visit of a realtor to her home, organized by her children, to appraise its value in the event that she exhausted her savings and could not obtain Medicaid-financed home health services.

LEARNING EXERCISE

1. Millions of additional seniors will need home health teams in coming years. What does this situation tell us about the relative preparedness of the U.S. for this situation?
2. If a relatively affluent couple encountered this situation, what additional hardships would many less affluent couples encounter?
3. What macro policy initiatives might social workers consider in the state's capitol to shape programs offered by the state's Medicaid program?

Many seniors need financial planning so that they can preserve their estates in the event that they run into situations like Mary and John's. Advocates should be aware of where such services are in the communities of consumers they work with to ensure they have access to this specialized financial planning in advance. They need to be aware that in some states, Medicaid authorities will "go after" the resources and estates of older people who try to transfer their resources to their children shortly before they need help from Medicaid for home health costs.

Advocates who seek increases in funding of programs for seniors sometimes encounter opposition from people who fear that seniors' programs divert funds from children and youth, as well as other programs. Social Security expenditures currently represent one fifth of the federal budget at a cost of $733 billion, with 82% allocated specifically to Old Age and Survivor's Insurance (OASI) and 18% to Disability Insurance (DI; Congressional Budget Office, 2011). However, many of these costs are offset by payroll taxes of employers and employees.

Core Problem 6: Engaging in Advocacy for Services to Help Seniors With Mental Distress—With Some Red Flag Alerts

- **Red Flag Alert 8.28.** An older adult fails to receive needed clinical interventions to address diagnosed mental health disorders (counseling and medication; medication; counseling).
- **Red Flag Alert 8.29.** An older adult's physician discounts her depression, calling it normal, due to contextual changes associated with aging.
- **Red Flag Alert 8.30.** An older adult with chronic diseases who presents with depression, anxiety, or another mental disorder is not referred to a geriatric specialist for a differential diagnosis.

Background

According to the National Institute of Mental Health, more than 7.5 million older adults 55+, or one in five of them, have a diagnosable mental health illness each year—a number projected to increase to 15 million older adults by 2030 (Ferrinni & Ferrinni, 2008). Depression, anxiety, sleep disorders, substance use, dementia, and delirium are the most common mental disorders among older adults (Ferrinni & Ferrinni, 2008). For community-dwelling older adults, rates of depression or symptoms of depression range between 8% to 20% of the population (Ferrinni & Ferrinni, 2008). Research indicates that older adults whose depression is treated have improvements in their medical conditions and respond well to traditional best treatment practices that use either medication, medication, and psychotherapy, or psychotherapy alone (National Institute of Mental Health, 2011).

Estimates of the prevalence of anxiety disorders among older adults in the United States range between 3.2% and 14.2%. Diabetes, hyperthyroidism, and gastrointestinal medical conditions are often associated with anxiety among older adults (Wolitzky-Taylor et al., 2010). Anxiety disorders among some older adults present serious risks for their health and well-being. Anxiety increases the risk for mortality among older adults following heart surgery, and cardiovascular morbidity and associated mortality have been linked to panic attacks among older adults (Wolitzky-Taylor et al., 2010). Comorbidity prevalence estimates of chronic obstructive pulmonary disease (COPD) and anxiety among older adults range between 18% and 50%; those numbers are between 40% and 43% for Parkinson's disease and anxiety (Wolitzky-Taylor et al., 2010). Five percent to 21% of older adults with dementia have an anxiety disorder—and cognitive decline and anxiety disorders occur frequently (Wolitzky-Taylor et al., 2010). Anxiety has been identified as a likely risk factor for developing dementia for older adults with mild cognitive impairment (MCI); in one study, 83% of older people with anxiety went on to develop Alzheimer's disease (AD) three years later in comparison to only 40.9% of individuals with MCI only and 6.1% of cognitively intact individuals. Among individuals with both MCI and anxiety, the relative risk of developing AD almost doubled with each anxiety symptom, from 1.8% to 2.7 per symptom (Wolitzky-Taylor et al., 2010, p. 202).

Undetected mental disorders among older adults can have life-threatening consequences. Older adults have higher rates of suicide than any other age group, and older adult males have the highest suicide rates. In 2004, older adults 65+ accounted for 16% of deaths by suicide and non-Hispanic white males had the highest suicide rates of all age and ethnic groups, with 49.8 deaths per 100,000 for those ages 85 and older (National Institute of Mental Health, 2010). Even more startling is the fact that up to 75% of older adults who commit suicide visit their primary care physician shortly before their suicide (National Institute of Mental Health, 2010). Mental health professionals and social workers are needed to detect mental disorders among older adults in primary care settings.

Older adults who require home health care have depression rates estimated at 13.5% (National Institute of Mental Health, 2010). For older adults who cannot leave their homes without assistance, they may actively grieve the loss of their previous independence, engagement in work and community, lifestyle, youth, and leisure activities. Depression risk increases with functional dependence and poor health. Its prevalence in hospitalized older adults is 11.5% (National Institute of Mental Health, 2010). Typical definitions of normal mental health may not provide the best fit for older adults with functional dependence, since the general definition of mental health is "the ability to engage in productive activities and fulfilling relationships and to cope successfully with change and adversity" (Ferrinni & Ferrinni, 2008). Among the difficult tasks for older individuals are accepting the multiple changes they experience and readjustment of what it means to engage in productive activities and fulfilling relationships, recognizing how it may be different or similar from prior periods. Models of successful aging may not provide the best fit for older adults with unmet mental health needs and chronic diseases causing functional dependence. For example, three conditions characterize successful aging under Rowe and Kahn's (1998) definition: "(1) positive self-attitude, (2) high cognitive and physical functional capability, and (3) active engagement in life, including maintaining personal relationships and sustaining productive activity" (Ferrinni & Ferrinni, 2008, p. 193). Depression can be a normal reaction to the multiple losses older people encounter, making it difficult to detect mental disorders among older adults (National Institute of Mental Health, 2010).

Older adults must adjust to myriad changes, including changes in their functional health due to chronic diseases and subsequent needs for assistance (physical losses), changes in their cognition or facing their mortality (psychological losses), shrinking social support networks, surviving a spouse or child (interpersonal losses), relocating to a residential care facility or home of a family member, loss of ability to drive (social losses), and retirement and living on a fixed income (economic losses).

Barriers exist within the medical profession for differential diagnosis of mental disorders among the older adult population. Differential diagnosis and detection of mental health disorders is complicated by the comorbidity of medical conditions among older adults. Primary care physicians most frequently treat older adults for mental disorders, and differentiating between medical conditions and mental disorders can be difficult (Ferrinni & Ferrinni, 2008). Social workers should advocate geriatric assessment and/or geropsychiatric assessment to ensure proper diagnosis of underlying mental health disorders among older adults. The scarcity of medical and mental health professionals specializing in geriatric care, assessment, and psychiatry impedes detection of mental disorders among older adults.

Resources for Advocates

Lack of parity in coverage among insurance companies for treatment of mental disorders in comparison to physical conditions has historically existed and has created barriers to mental health services for older adults. The Mental Health Parity Act of 2007 has eased this problem.

Changes to mental health services coverage under Medicare have been made with the implementation of the ACA. Medicare Part A covers inpatient hospital care for a mental health disorder; Part B covers outpatient mental health services, such as visits with a psychiatrist or physician, clinical psychologist, social worker, nurse specialist, nurse practitioner, or physician assistant and laboratory tests ordered by a physician; and Part D covers medications prescribed to treat mental disorders (Centers for Medicare and Medicaid Services, 2009). Although certain deductibles and coinsurance may apply, Part B covers the following outpatient mental health services: group and individual psychotherapy, family counseling, testing, evaluation by a psychiatrist, management of medications, occupational therapy, education and training, partial hospitalization if a physician certifies that the patient would otherwise require inpatient treatment, diagnostic tests, and depression screening during the one-time physical exam under the "Welcome to Medicare" benefit (for beneficiaries within the first 12 months of Part B enrollment; Centers for Medicare and Medicaid Services, 2009). Parity was further addressed under the ACA, ensuring that Medicare beneficiaries' coinsurances for mental health services are similar to coinsurances for medical care services, with the coinsurance rates for outpatient treatment falling to 20% in 2014 (Centers for Medicare and Medicaid Services, 2009). Medicare beneficiaries pay 20% of the accepted Medicare rate for diagnosis of their mental health condition (Centers for Medicare and Medicaid Services, 2009). Medicare Part A covers 190 lifetime days of inpatient psychiatric care at a psychiatric hospital rather than a general acute care hospital (Centers for Medicare and Medicaid Services, 2009). At a general hospital, a deductible of $1,100 applies for benefit periods of 1 to 60 days, $275 coinsurance for days 61 to 90 of the benefit period, and $550 coinsurance per day after the 90th day of the benefit period (Centers for Medicare and Medicaid Services, 2009).

Medicaid is the largest funder of mental health services in the United States, paying $26 billion (representing 26% of all expenditures in the U.S.) for mental health in 2003 (Substance Abuse and Mental Health Services Administration, 2007). Medicare made up 7% of all mental health expenditures in the Unites States in 2003 (Substance Abuse and Mental Health Services Administration, 2007).

Under the ACA, access to mental health services will be implemented through two key provisions: integration of mental health services across the continuum of care within the healthcare system, and the provision of annual well visits that provide risk assessments for cognition and health along with a plan for health promotion tailored to the individual (American Association for Geriatric Psychiatry, 2011).

POLICY ADVOCACY LEARNING CHALLENGE 8.6

Connecting Micro, Mezzo, and Macro Policy Advocacy

Anna Gorman contended in a *Los Angeles Times* article on September 5, 2011, that "ERs are becoming costly destinations for mentally disturbed patients: Budget cuts are creating added safety risks at hospitals and placing a burden on already crowded emergency rooms." She noted that many hospitals discharge patients with unaddressed

(Continued)

(Continued)

mental health disorders into local communities. (By contrast, hospitals in affluent areas often have psychiatric services available.) The outcome is that many mentally ill people are released homeless into communities without their mental health needs being addressed, posing a danger to themselves and the local community.

Imagine you are a social worker who works in the emergency room of the local hospital and there is no staff psychiatrist. Mr. S is a 70-year-old homeless male who is brought to the emergency room by a police officer after he threatened to harm a street vendor in the local community. The police officer reports that Mr. S displayed "bizarre behavior" and threatened to harm the officer as well. The patient presents in the emergency room with auditory hallucinations, is disheveled in appearance, and has poor hygiene. He is able to report his name, the date, and the city he is in (oriented times three). The attending physician requests a social work consultation. You identify a county hospital that can take this patient, because he cannot be admitted to this hospital. The patient has an identification card and no insurance. You find out that he has been homeless for over 15 years. The patient states he does not want to go to a shelter and denies that he needs help with his psychiatric symptoms.

LEARNING EXERCISE

1. How might this social worker intervene to provide case advocacy to address the mental health needs of this patient?
2. What policies and/or procedures/protocols exist in the agency you were in for intervening with homeless older adults with unaddressed mental health needs?
3. What programs and services (inpatient vs. outpatient) are available in the community you work in that can take uninsured older adults?
4. What local, federal, or state policies can help inform policy changes at the organization to improve services to older adults with unaddressed mental health needs?

Core Problem 7: Engaging in Advocacy for Home- and Community-Based Services (HCBS) for Seniors—With Some Red Flag Alerts

- **Red Flag Alert 8.31.** An older adult with changes in functional health or a new chronic disease is not provided with referrals to home- and community-based services at the time of discharge from an acute care setting.

- **Red Flag Alert 8.32.** An older adult who inquires about home- and community-based services at a primary care setting is unable to obtain information about relevant services due to a lack of social services at the primary care setting.
- **Red Flag Alert 8.33.** An older adult is unaware of the range of home- and community-based services that may be relevant to her over the remaining period of her life as her functional and residential status may change.
- **Red Flag Alert 8.34.** An older adult searches the yellow pages and cannot find relevant home- and community-based services, such as home-delivered meals or transportation with wheelchair access.
- **Red Flag Alert 8.35.** Hospitals or healthcare settings that serve older adults do not refer social workers for a consult for home- and community-based service options in advance of discharge to allow time for patients to make an informed decision and allow time to link them to the specific service or program of their preference.

Background

Most older adults live in traditional communities. In 2005, 93% of Medicare beneficiaries lived in traditional community settings, 5% in long-term care facilities, and 2% in community housing with assistance such as assisted living (Centers for Medicare and Medicaid Services, 2000). The functional needs of older adults vary across residential settings; in 2005, 37% of those living in traditional community settings required assistance with IADLs, ADLs, or a combination of both ADLs and IADLs (Centers for Medicare and Medicaid Services, 2000). Older adults with ADL and IADL limitations may need a variety of home- and community-based services to compensate for functional losses so that they can remain safely in their homes.

Eligibility criteria for home- and community-based services create barriers for older adults attempting to access services. Advocates must be informed of the various eligibility criteria for programs and services in older adult communities. Age and functional dependence are traditional criteria used to determine eligibility for long-term care assistance. For example, Meals on Wheels programs typically target adults aged 60 and over with physical limitations that affect their ability to shop or prepare meals on a daily basis. Specialty transportation services base eligibility on age and functional dependence. However, criteria related to functional dependence are much more stringent. For example, an older adult who uses a motorized scooter or wheelchair is ineligible for door-to-door wheelchair-accessible transportation. Such a client is considered capable of accessing public transportation services with wheelchair-accessible ramps (Joosten, 2008).

Eligibility criteria for services should be modified to reflect the diverse needs of the aging population. The addition of more eligibility criteria is a simplistic solution intended to facilitate targeting of services but can inadvertently create barriers to service access. For example, Meals on Wheels programs frequently do not serve disabled adults under age 60, even though they meet functional dependence criteria. An additional barrier pertains to living arrangements. Meals on Wheels programs with long waiting lists often exclude older adults who live with a family member, regardless of whether the family member works full time or may need respite care (Joosten, 2008).

The ability to identify programs and services in a community can also present challenges. Services for older adults are fragmented at the community level. Caregiver agencies, home-delivered meals, and transportation services are not combined at one location where an older adult can access all three services simultaneously. Each service requires a separate phone call and a separate application—and each has its own criteria for eligibility. Locating services to meet geographical needs of an older adult can create barriers to service access as well. For example, some transportation programs have service areas that do not go outside the city where they operate, so seniors in these areas cannot access their programs.

Community-dwelling older adults who receive long-term care from a home health agency have access to a clinical social worker who refers them to services that they need. Individuals without access to a social worker often do not know how to identify services in their community—or even realize that they need them, as in the case of people with chronic health conditions. Older adults often do not know what types of services they will need until they return to their home environment from an acute care center. Older adults accounted for 37% of all hospital discharges and more than 50% of the 1 million discharges related to fractures in 2007 (Hall, DeFrances, Williams, Golosinsky, & Schwartzman, 2010). More research is needed to see if the increasing use of nurses rather than clinical social workers as discharge planners impedes needed referrals for complex crisis intervention cases (Joosten, 2008).

Resources for Advocates

A relatively complex hierarchy of agencies exists to oversee, fund, and administer community programs for older people:

- Funding for AoA programs is allocated to each State Unit on Aging (SUA) based on each state's number of older adults 60+ and to the National Family Caregiver Support Program (NFCSP) based on the number of older adults age 70+ (Administration on Aging, 2011a).

- The funding of programs is administered by each SUA to Area Agencies on Aging (AAAs), which in turn designate funds within states to planning and service areas (PSAs) (Administration on Aging, 2011a).
- The AAAs determine the specific service needs of older adults in the PSA and work to address those needs through the funding of local services and through advocacy (Administration on Aging, 2011a)
- The PSAs customize program services to the specific needs of the older adults in the communities they serve (Administration on Aging, 2011a).

Yet another layer of complexity exists. Each state can request a "waiver" from the federal Center on Medical Services (CMS) for their Medicaid program that allows them to obtain funding for a program innovation. They have to demonstrate that providing waiver services to a target population is no more costly than the cost of services these individuals would receive in institutions such as hospitals or long-term care institutions. Currently, roughly 287 waiver programs exist in the U.S. that provide a wide array of community-based programs to decrease the extent to which older adults are institutionalized (Center for Medicare and Medicaid Services, 2011, para. 7).

A 1999 ruling of the U.S. Supreme Court in *Olmstead v. L. C.* increased emphasis on community-based programs when it ruled that segregation of disabled adults in institutions violates Title II of the Americans with Disabilities Act (Centers for Medicare and Medicaid Services, 2011). It led to development of waiver programs funded by CMS to serve disabled individuals in the "least restrictive environment" possible. Roughly 1 million disabled people, including many seniors, now receive community-based programs funded by the federal government.

The ACA also promotes community-based services. It made $45 million available in 2011 for the Money Follows the Person (MFP) demonstration program, and up to $3.7 billion was available to states between 2011 and 2014 in new funds for the Community First Choice Option through matching funds for attendant services and additional supports to Medicaid recipients (U.S. Department of Health and Human Services, 2011). The MFP program allows institutionalized individuals to relocate into traditional community settings with services and support (U.S. Department of Health and Human Services, 2011). Under the Community First Choice Option, attendant services will include assistance with activities of daily living, supervision, and assistance with health-related activities (U.S. Department of Health and Human Services, 2011). The ACA will fund improvements for older adults' care after they leave acute care hospitalizations under the "Community Care Transitions Program" to help high-risk Medicare beneficiaries avoid unnecessary readmissions "by coordinating care and connecting patients to services in their communities" (U.S. Department of Health and Human Services, 2011).

Intergenerational programs provide social, economic, and personal benefits to both older adults and youth (Generations United, 2006). Intergenerational environmental health programs provide a common goal of improving the environment and health through collaboration across generations in programs within communities in settings such as parks, environmental centers, community centers, farms, schools, and universities (Generations United, 2006). These programs provide opportunities for both civic engagement and lifelong learning across generations, and they enable important relationships to be built across generations as people come together to address environmental health issues that mutually affect them (Generations United, 2006). School-based intergenerational programs promote positive perceptions of older adults among youth and enhance positive relationships between the generations (Bales, Ekland, & Siffin, 2000). The benefits of intergeneration programs are mutual. Older adults who mentor at-risk youth report both greater meaning in their lives and opportunities to enhance positive emotions (Larkin, Sadler, & Mahler, 2005).

POLICY ADVOCACY LEARNING CHALLENGE 8.7

Connecting Micro and Macro Policy Advocacy

You are a home health social worker who is referred by the primary care physician for information on community resources for your 62-year-old single female patient, who has just undergone a mastectomy and will be receiving chemotherapy for three months. She was working full time up until the time of her surgery, and her doctor has informed her that she will be unable to work while she is receiving the chemotherapy. She was working as an engineer at a large aerospace organization and has no children. She does not have affiliations with religious or social supports beyond her co-workers, as she reports she worked 60 hours per week. She was not seen by a social worker at the hospital and has no help coming into the home with the exception of the nurse, physical therapist, and you, the social worker. She is now ambulating with a walker due to postoperative weakness and having had a prolonged hospital stay of five weeks as she underwent testing, surgery, and postoperative complications. There was a delay in the home health referral, causing the social worker not to make the first home visit until two weeks after the patient was already discharged. She has been ordering cabs to get to her chemotherapy and reports she fell getting out of the cab coming into her home because the cab was too low. Now that she is home, she reports she can barely make it to the bathroom, she has difficulty preparing food and has a low appetite, and she cannot drive to run errands, go shopping, or make it to her chemotherapy and doctor's appointments. She ran out of food yesterday and has prescriptions that needed to be picked up from the pharmacy.

LEARNING EXERCISE

1. How might the social worker intervene?
2. What home and community-based services might this patient need?
3. What programs are relevant for this patient?
4. What state or federal benefits might this patient be eligible for?
5. How would you advocate policy change at the hospital organization that discharged her without having her see a social worker?

"THINKING BIG" AS POLICY ADVOCATES IN THE GERONTOLOGY SECTOR

The United States clearly needs a comprehensive plan to deal with the tens of millions of people—so-called baby boomers—who will reach age 65 in the next three decades. We currently have a disjointed set of programs and policies, as our discussion in this chapter clearly reveals. Take a stab at trying to identify some components of a multifaceted policy proposal called "Addressing the Social, Medical, Community, and Resource Needs of Baby Boomers." Part of this plan should include a strategy for preventing the inhumane policy of "spend-down" where millions of seniors have to deplete their assets and savings to a welfare level to be eligible for long-term care financed by Medicaid. Yet other parts should involve far more alternatives to traditional nursing homes, including small residency facilities. Yet other parts should involve rigorous enforcement of civil rights for aging workers to prevent employers from firing them to obtain lower-cost younger workers.

LEARNING OUTCOMES

You are now equipped to:

- Analyze the evolution of the gerontology sector in seven eras
- Discuss the political economy of the gerontology sector
- Identify some injustices in the gerontology sector
- Analyze seven core problems of the gerontology sector, including:
    - Barriers to resolving or mitigating them
    - The policy and regulatory context of each of them

o Red Flag Alerts for micro, mezzo, and macro policy

o Connections between micro policy and macro policy interventions

- Write your own policy alert, as well as connected micro policy and macro policy interventions

- Develop a multifaceted policy proposal

REFERENCES

Administration on Aging. (2004). *Statistics on the aging population.* Retrieved from http://www .aoa.dhhs.gov/prof/Statistics/online_stats_data?AgePop2050.asp

Administration on Aging. (2005a). *Census 2000 data on aging.* Retrieved from http://www.aoa .gov/prof/Statistics/Census2000/census2000.asp

Administration on Aging. (2005b). *Statistics on the aging population.* Retrieved from http://www .aoa.gov/prof/Statistics/statistics.asp

Administration on Aging. (2010). *Evidence-based disease and disability prevention program.* Retrieved from http://www.aoa.gov/AoA_programs/HPW/Evidence_Based/index.aspx

Administration on Aging. (2011a). Aging integrated database. Retrieved October 21, 2011, from http://www.agidnet.org/DataGlance/SPR

Administration on Aging. (2011b). *Office of long-term care ombudsman programs.* Retrieved from http://www.aoa.gov/

AGS Foundation for Health in Aging. (2015). *How many board certified geriatricians and geropsychiatrists are there in the US?* Retrieved from http://www.americangeriatrics.org /advocacy_public_policy/gwps/gwps_faqs/id:3183

Albert, S. M. (2004). *Public health and aging: An introduction to maximizing function and well-being.* New York, NY: Springer.

Aldwin, C. M., & Gilmer, D. F. (2004). *Health, illness, and optimal aging: Biological and psychosocial perspectives.* Thousand Oaks, CA: SAGE.

American Association for General Psychiatry. (2011). *Legislative & regulatory agenda.* Retrieved from http://www.aagponline.org/index.php?submenu=pub_reports_submenu&sr c=gendocs&ref=LegislativeRegulatoryAgenda&category=pub_reports_submenu

American Society on Aging. (2015). *Diversity.* Retrieved from http://www.asaging.org/diversity

Angel, J., & Hogan, D. (2004). *Population and diversity in a new era* (pp. 1–12). In K. Whitfield (Ed.), *Closing the gap: Improving the health of minority elders in the new millennium.* Washington, DC: Gerontological Society of America.

Balas, M. C., Casey, C. M., & Happ, M. B. (2007). Geriatric nursing protocol: Comprehensive assessment and management of the critically ill. In Bolzt et al. (Ed.), Evidence-based geriatric nursing protocols for best practices (4th ed.). New York, NY: Springer. Retrieved from http://consultgerirn.org/topics/critical_care/want_to_know_more/

Bales, S., Ekland, S., & Siffin, C. (2000). Children's perceptions of elders before and after a school-based intergenerational program. *Educational Gerontology, 26*(7), 677–689.

California Advocates for Nursing Home Reform. (2011). *Twenty-eight years of advocacy.* Retrieved from www.canhr.org/legislation

Cantlupe, J. (2012). *Palliative care challenged by physician shortage.* Retrieved from http://www .healthleadersmedia.com/page-1/MAG-282158/Palliative-Care-Challenged-by-Physician-Shortage

Centers for Disease Control and Prevention. (n.d.). *Heart disease and race.* Retrieved from http://millionhearts.hhs.gov/abouthds/risk-factors.html#hdRace

Centers for Disease Control and Prevention. (2011). *Healthy aging: At a glance 2011.* Retrieved from http://www.cdc.gov/chronicdisease/resources/publications/AAG/aging.htm

Centers for Disease Control and Prevention. (2014). *Basic information about health.* Retrieved from http://www.cdc.gov/cancer/healthdisparities/basic_info/index.htm

Centers for Medicare and Medicaid Services. (2000). *Medicare current beneficiary study.* Retrieved from http://www.cms.gov/Research-Statistics-Data-and-Systems/Research/MCBS/Data-Tables-Items/CMS1253276.html

Centers for Medicare and Medicaid Services. (2009). *Medicare and your mental health benefits* (CMS Product No. 10184). U.S. Department of Health and Human Services.

Centers for Medicare and Medicaid Services. (2011). *Section 1915(c) home and community-based services waivers.* Retrieved from www.cms.gov/MedicaidStWaivProgDemoPGI/05_HCBS Waivers-SEction1915(c).asp

Congressional Budget Office. (2011). *CBO's 2011 long-term projections for Social Security: Additional Information.* Retrieved from http://www.cbo.gov/ftpdocs/123xx/doc12375/08-05-Long-TermSocialSEcurityProjections.pdf

Csikai, E., & Chaitin, E. (2006). *Ethics in end of life decisions in social work practice.* Chicago, IL: Lyceum Books.

Dana Farber Cancer Institute. (2015). *Adult palliative care.* Retrieved from http://www.dana-farber.org/Adult-Care/Treatment-and-Support/Treatment-Centers-and-Clinical-Services/Pain-Management-and-Palliative-Care.aspx

Ferrinni, A., & Ferrinni, R. (2008). *Health in the later years* (4th ed.). McGraw-Hill, NY: New York.

Field, M.J., & C. K. Cassel, (Eds.), *Approaching death at the end of life.* National Academies Press; Institute of Medicine.

Generations United. (2006). *Fact sheet: Environmental health for all generations.* Retrieved from http://www.gu.org/LinkClick.aspx?fileticket=itkytMumazE%3d&tabid=157&mid=606

Hall, J. H., DeFrances, C. J., Williams, S. N., Golosinsky, A., & Schwartzman, A. (2010). *National Hospital Discharge Survey: 2007 summary* (National Health Statistics Reports, No. 29). Hyattsville, MD: National Center for Health Statistics.

Hayden, M. F. (2000). Social policies for people with disabilities. In J. Midgley, B. Tracy, & M. Livermore (Eds.), *The handbook of social policy.* Thousand Oaks, CA: SAGE.

Joint Commission. (2011). *Facts about ambulatory care accreditation.* Retrieved from http://www.jointcommission.org/assets/1/18/Ambulatorycare_1_112.PDF

Joosten, D. (2008). *Aspects of clinical social workers' decision-making with older adult clients with unmet psychosocial and/or physical needs: Outcomes, patterns, and processes of referrals for services.* Doctoral dissertation, University of California, Los Angeles.

Kaiser Family Foundation. (2011). *Medicare spending and financing: A primer 2011.* Retrieved from http://kaiserfamilyfoundation.files.wordpress.com/2013/01/7731-03.pdf

Kayser-Jones, J. (2009). Nursing homes: A health-promoting or dependency-promoting environment? *Family and Community Health, 32*(1), S66–S74.

Klauber, M., & Wright, B. (2001, February). *The 1987 Nursing Home Reform Act.* Public Policy Institute. Retrieved from www.aarp.org

Kuhn, D. P. (2010). The senior wave: Older voters set for historic turnout. *RealClearPolitics.* Retrieved from http://www.realclearpolitics.com/articles/2010/10/18/the_senior_wave_older_voters_set_for_historic_turnout_107608.html

Larkin, E., Sadler, S., & Mahler, J. (2005). Benefits for older adults mentoring at-risk youth. *Journal of Gerontological Social Work, 44*(3–4), 23–37.

Leipzig, R. M., Whitlock, E. P., Wolff, T. A., Barton, M. B., Michael, Y. L., Harris, R., . . . Siu, A. (2010). Reconsidering the approach to prevention recommendations for older adults. *Annals of Internal Medicine, 153,* 809–814.

Leventhal, H., Rabin, C., Leventhal, E. A., & Burns, E. (2001). Health risk behaviors and aging. *Handbook of the Psychology of Aging, 5,* 186–214.

LGBT Older Adult Coalition. (2011). *Report: The needs of LGBT older adults in metro Detroit.* Retrieved from http://lgbtolderadults.files.wordpress.com/2012/02/report-needs-of-older-adults-6-12-11.pdf

Midgley, J., Tracy, B., & Livermore, M. (2000). *The handbook of social policy.* Thousand Oaks, CA: SAGE.

Morrison, S., & Meier, D. (2011). The National Palliative Care Research Center and the Center to Advance Palliative Care: A partnership to improve care for persons with serious illness and their families. *Journal of Pediatric Hematology/Oncology, 33,* S126–S131. doi: 10.1097/MPH.0b013e318230dfa0

National Hospice and Palliative Care Organization. (2011). *History of hospice care.* Retrieved from http://www.nhpco.org/history-hospice-care

National Institute of Mental Health. (2010). *Older adults: Depression and suicide facts* (Fact sheet). Retrieved from www.nimh.nih.gov/health/publications/older-adults-depression-and-suicide-facts-fact-sheet/index.shtml

National Institute of Mental Health. (2011). *NIH senior health: Depression.* Retrieved from www.nihseniorhealth.gov/depression/research/o1.html

National Institute of Minority Health and Health Disparities. (2013). *Health disparities.* Retrieved from http://report.nih.gov/nihfactsheets/viewfactsheet.aspx?csid=124

National Institute on Aging. (2010). *Research Goal E: Improve our ability to reduce health disparities and eliminate health inequities among older adults.* Retrieved from http://www.nia.nih.gov/about/living-long-well-21st-century-strategic-directions-research-aging/research-goal-e-improve-our

National League for Nursing. (1999). Hospice patients alliance. Retrieved from http://www.hospicepatients.org/chap-accredit.html

Newport, F. (2012). In presidential election, age is a factor only among whites. *Gallup.* Retrieved from http://www.gallup.com/poll/154712/Presidential-Election-Age-Factor-Among-Whites.aspx

Nursing Home Abuse and Neglect Resource Center. (2011). *Nursing Home and Abuse Neglect Resource Center.* Retrieved from http://www.nursinghomeabuseandneglectattorney.com/nursing-home-neglect-resources.aspx

Office of Management and Budget. (2011). *Living within our means and investing in the future: The President's plan for economic growth and deficit reduction.* Washington, DC.

Office of the Surgeon General. (2011). *National prevention strategy.* Retrieved from http://www.surgeongeneral.gov/initiatives/prevention/strategy/

Ott, B. B. (1999). Advance directives: The emerging body of evidence. *American Journal of Critical Care, 8*(1).

Quadagno, J. (2008). *Aging and the life course* (4th ed.). New York, NY: McGraw Hill.

Reese, D., & Raymer, M. (2004). Relationships between social work services and hospice outcomes: Results of the National Hospice Social Work Survey. *Social Work, 49*(3).

Richardson, J. P. (2006, May 17). Considerations for health promotion in disease prevention in older adults. *Medscape News Today.* Retrieved from www.medscape.com/viewarticle/531942

Rowe, J. R. & R. L. Kahn (2004). *Successful aging.* New York: Dell Publishing.

Stosz. D. (2000). Social policy: Reagan and beyond. In J. Midgley, B. Tracy, & M. Livermore (Eds.), *The handbook of social policy.* Thousand Oaks, CA: SAGE.

Substance Abuse and Mental Health Services Administration. (2007). *National expenditures for mental health services and substance abuse treatment 1993–2003* (Publication No. SMA 07-4227). U.S. Department of Health and Human Services.

Torres-Gil, F., & Villa, V. (2000). Social policy and the elderly. In J. Midgley, B. Tracy, & M. Livermore (Eds.), *The handbook of social policy.* Thousand Oaks, CA: SAGE.

U.S. Census Bureau, Social, Economic, and Housing Statistics Division. (2011). *Poverty.* Retrieved from www.census.gov/hhes/www/poverty/data/historical/people.html

U.S. Department of Health and Human Services. (2011). *The Affordable Care Act.* Retrieved from www.healthcare.gov

Wolitsky-Taylor, K. B., Castriotta, N., Lenze, E., Stanley, M. A., & Craske, M. G. (2010). Anxiety disorders in older adults: A comprehensive review. *Depression and Anxiety, 27,* 190–211.

Chapter 9

BECOMING POLICY ADVOCATES IN THE SAFETY-NET SECTOR

LEARNING OBJECTIVES

In this chapter, you will learn how to:

1. Analyze how the American safety-net sector evolved over time

2. Analyze how economic inequalities are powerfully linked to defects in American safety-net programs

3. Analyze the political economy of the safety-net sector, including powerful players and interests as well as underrepresented ones—and identify key advocacy groups

4. Use safety-net programs, as well as information you obtain from advocacy groups, as resources for your clients

5. Engage in policy advocacy to address seven core problems in the safety-net sector by recognizing Red Flag Alerts and connecting micro policy advocacy, mezzo policy advocacy, and macro policy advocacy

6. Discuss major proposals for reforming the safety-net sector

The United States has developed an array of safety-net programs that address the basic living needs of tens of millions of people. You need to know about these programs, because you will refer thousands of your clients or patients to these programs during your career. You will engage in micro policy advocacy for them—and this advocacy will allow some families to escape malnutrition, extreme poverty, and homelessness. You can engage in mezzo and macro policy advocacy to improve these programs. We cast a wide net when discussing safety-net programs, and you may be surprised to find how relevant many of them are to your specific clients.

We discuss both *universal programs* that are provided to most Americans, such as unemployment insurance, and *means-tested* programs that are provided to people who meet specific income, employment, and other criteria. We discuss government regulations over banks, other lenders, purveyors of credit cards, and landlords that prevent some practices that negatively impact low- and moderate-income individuals. We discuss *federal government programs* such as Social Security, Medicare, the Supplemental Nutrition Assistance Program (SNAP), and Supplemental Security Income (SSI); *federal and state government programs* such as Temporary Assistance for Needy Families (TANF) and Medicaid; *state programs* such as programs that give specific kinds of assistance or general assistance

Figure 9.1 Evolution of the American safety-net programs

The Great Depression and the "New Deal": 1929–1942
In response to massive unemployment and poverty following the stock market crash of 1929, President Franklin D. Roosevelt establishes numerous federal programs to put millions (mostly men) back to work, creates public housing, creates a progressive federal income tax, establishes a federal minimum wage, and provides huge subsidies to states to finance their welfare programe; federal government begins playing a major role in the social safety-net.

The Gilded Era: 1880–1900
Marked by growing economic inequality as the U.S. becomes world's largest economy; urban centers expand rapidly; a professional class emerges while workers' rights are stifled.

Colonial Era: Pre-1800
Marked by slavery, indentured servitude, and lack of property rights for women; "poorhouses" are erected for the destitute; the federal government plays no role in the social safety-net.

Modifications to Social Security in the 1950s
Social Security becomes a family-oriented program that provides benefits to widows and children of beneficiaries; Social Security Disability Insurance (SSDI) is added in 1956 for persons with "an impairment of mind or body" that precludes gainful occupation.

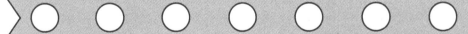

Westward Expansion, the Civil War, and Industrialization: 1800–1860
Marked in early years by subsistence living on farms; asylums and "wayward children's homes" are erected; the temperance movement grows.

The Progressive Era: 1900–1917
Policies and regulations are established mostly at state and local levels related to food, drugs, housing, and occupational safety; the federal government begins playing a major role in the social safety-net.

The Social Security Act of 1935
The backbone of the U.S. social safety net system is established; two means-tested programs — Aid to Dependent Children and Old Age Assistance — are established, along with two universal programs — Unemployment Insurance and Social Security.

to specific populations, like immigrants; *local government programs* such as specific shelters; and *private sector programs* such as food banks run by nonprofit or religious organizations. Regulations vary by state for some of these programs.

ANALYZING THE EVOLUTION OF THE AMERICAN SAFETY-NET SYSTEM

Figure 9.1 provides an overview of the evolution of the American safety-net system, from the colonial era to the present. It demonstrates that the federal government had little role in the safety-net system through the 19th century and up to the start of

VIDEO LINK 9.1
Plight of the
Working Poor

Safety Net Expansion: 1969–1980
Republican President Richard Nixon enacts the Employment and Training Act of 1973, expands the Food Stamps program, establishes the Supplemental Security Income Program (SSI), enacts the Earned Income Tax Credit, and establishes Section 8 housing; Democratic Presidents Ford and Carter subsequently do little to expand the safety-net.

Era of Devolution: 1981–1992
Presidents Ronald Reagan and George H.W. Bush enact "supply side" economic policies, such as tax cuts for the wealthy, cuts to Food Stamps and EITC programs, and restrictions on union organizing; many federal programs are devolved to the states through block grants.

Personal Responsibility and Work Opportunities Reconciliation Act of 1996
President Clinton "ends welfare as we knew it" by removing entitlement status, implementing lifetime limits and work requirements, allowing states to develop their own eligibility standards, and barring immigrants from a range of safety-net programs.

The Great Recession of 2007– 2009 and Beyond
President Barack Obama inherits the economic devastation wreaked by a banking crisis resulting from massive foreclosures in the housing market; millions are unemployed; "bailouts" for large institutions are enacted; despite the recession, the Democratic Congress successfully enacts the American Recovery and Investment Act of 2009, and the Affordable Care Act of 2010.

Lyndon B.Johnson's "Great Society": 1960–1969
Aimed at eliminating poverty and racial injustice; President Johnson initiates a "war on poverty," enacts the Civil Rights Act, the Economic Opportunity Act, the Food Stamp Act, and the Voting Rights Act, and establishes Medicare and Medicaid.

Era of Budget Surplus: 1992–2000
President Bill Clinton balances the national budget while keeping many safety-net programs intact; the Children's Health Insurance Program (CHIP) is enacted and the EITC program is expanded.

Era of Budget Deficits: 2000 – 2008
President George W. Bush vastly increases the national debt by slashing taxes and increasing military spending; funding for pharmaceutical benefits through Medicare is enacted.

the Great Depression in 1929. It shows how that role expanded in the New Deal, Great Society, and early part of the 1970s—only to contract substantially in the decades following 1980 with cuts in many programs and welfare reform, including passage of the Personal Responsibility and Work Opportunities Reconciliation Act (PRWORA) of 1996, otherwise known as "Welfare Reform," that transformed the largest income-supporting safety-net program, Aid to Families of Dependent Children (AFDC), from an entitlement program with no time limits to a time-limited means-tested program called Temporary Assistance for Needy Families (TANF). PRWORA also added work requirements, and instituted bars to many safety-net programs for immigrants. The American Recovery and Investment Act of 2009 (often called the Stimulus Program) greatly expanded funding of many safety-net programs during the presidency of Barack Obama, but only for a few years.

We discuss a wide array of safety-net programs that are needed and used by social workers' clients (see Table 9.1). You will learn about specific programs in other policy sectors that *also* allow people to escape deep poverty: Medicaid and Medicare as well as tax policies that allow some families to deduct medical expenses help people in the *health sector*; Medicaid, TANF, SNAP, subsidized rent and housing programs, and tax incentives for families that adopt foster children are vital to children and families in the *child and family sector*; the mental health services of Medicaid and Medicare and income supports for people with mental disabilities from SSI, TANF, and SNAP are widely used by individuals in the *mental health sector*; Medicare, Medicaid, Social Security, SSI, and senior citizen housing help people in the *gerontology sector*; General Relief, shelters, Medicaid, and SSI are beneficial in the *corrections sector*; and SNAP, TANF, and school lunch programs serve people in the *education sector*.

Table 9.1   Important Safety-Net Programs Discussed in This Chapter

Income-Enhancing Programs
1. Temporary Assistance for Needy Families (TANF)
2. General Assistance or General Relief (GA or GR)
3. Supplementary Security Income (SSI)
4. Social Security for permanently and totally disabled people (SSDI)
5. Social Security for survivors of deceased beneficiaries
6. Income-enhancing provisions of the federal tax code
7. The Earned Income Tax Credit (EITC)
8. Other provisions in the federal tax code relevant to low- and moderate-income families

9. Tax provisions in state and local jurisdictions relevant to low- and moderate-income individuals

10. Unemployment insurance

11. Workers' compensation

12. Minimum wage and living wage

Regulations Over Credit-Providing Agencies

1. Regulations of the lending practices of banks, payday lenders, and other providers of loans, mortgages, and credit cards

Job-Related Programs

1. Job-finding and placement programs

2. Job-training programs

3. Job creation programs

4. Transportation and childcare programs to help people work

Nutrition-Enhancing Programs

1. Supplemental Nutrition Assistance Program (SNAP; formerly the Food Stamp Program)

2. Special Supplemental Nutrition Program for Women, Infants, and Children (WIC)

3. Meals on Wheels

4. Food banks run by nonprofit and religious organizations

5. School breakfast and school lunch programs

Shelter-Enhancing Programs

1. Section 8 subsidized rental housing

2. Continuum of Care (COC) and other programs for homeless people funded by the McKinney-Vento Homeless Assistance Act

3. Public housing

4. Tax incentives to build affordable housing

Asset-Creating Programs

1. Private and public pensions

2. Home ownership programs

3. Individual development accounts (IDAs)

Safety-net programs cut across age groups. *Children* often benefit from SNAP, TANF, Medicaid, school breakfast and lunch programs, food banks, and subsidized housing. *Working individuals* benefit from Medicaid and SNAP. *Unemployed adults* benefit from General Assistance (GA) and unemployment insurance. *Elderly people* benefit from Medicare, Medicaid, SSI, Social Security, senior housing, Meals on Wheels, and deductions of mortgage interest from income. Each of these age groups benefits from subsidized rent programs, public housing, and temporary shelters.

ANALYZING HOW DEFECTS IN AMERICAN SAFETY-NET PROGRAMS OFTEN EXACERBATE INCOME INEQUALITY

Poverty is the most important social problem in the United States for multiple reasons. It affects roughly half the entire American population, who live near or beneath the poverty line. People near and in poverty experience far higher levels of physical and mental illnesses, as well as high levels of chronic disabilities and substance abuse. Many experience chronic or frequent unemployment. Many of them do not graduate from high school and have low levels of literacy. Many are exposed to violence in their households and communities. Poverty causes stress not only from economic hardship but also because many of its victims *are* and *feel* marginalized as they see more affluent Americans in their daily lives, as well as on the mass media. Millions of families live on the edge of deep poverty—and fall into it when losing only a single paycheck.

Many safety-net programs have been remarkably successful in helping people meet their basic needs in contemporary society. When a measure of poverty was used that counted not just income derived from TANF and employment, but also income from SNAP, rent subsidies, the EITC, and some other safety-net programs—a broader measure of poverty recommended by an expert panel of the National Academy of Sciences and several poverty measures used by the Census Bureau—the poverty rate stood at 15.5% in 2010, as compared to 29% when income from these safety-net programs was not included. This means that safety-net programs "cut poverty nearly in half compared to what it would otherwise be" (Greenstein, 2012).

The positive effects of safety-net programs were demonstrated during the Great Recession of 2007 to 2009 and beyond. We would have expected sharp increases in poverty rates when unemployment rose to more than 12% during the early part of this Recession, yet poverty rates remained stable at 15.3% for 2007, 15.7% for 2009, and 15.5% for 2010, according to a poverty measure of the Bureau of Census (Greenstein, 2012). Safety-net programs are automatically triggered during economic downturns as people's income declines and makes them eligible for means-tested programs—and as *all* unemployed people become eligible for unemployment insurance. Moreover, the time-limited American Recovery and Reinvestment Act (the Stimulus Program) temporarily or permanently augmented benefits of some safety-net programs, helping them to keep people above the poverty line of the Census Bureau in 2009. These programs included unemployment insurance (4.8 million people), the child tax credit and the EITC (9.4 million people), and SNAP (4.3 million people). The American Recovery and Reinvestment Act also established a Making Work Pay Tax Credit that lifted 1.6 million people from poverty. These are accomplishments on a massive scale (Sherman, 2011). The U.S. Census Bureau estimates that the EITC, the Child Tax Credit, and SNAP respectively lifted 9 million, 5 million, and 4 million low-income working families out of poverty (Greenstein, 2012).

Even when we lack data that demonstrate the effectiveness of safety-net programs, such as the impact on people lifted from poverty, we can support them on ethical grounds. For centuries, we have lauded Good Samaritans who help people obtain food, shelter, and income when they might otherwise suffer malnutrition, illness, and exposure—and who relieve parents of angst on account of their inability to meet their children's needs. Liberals have used this ethical rationale on many occasions.

The safety-net sector is rife, however, with problems. Tens of millions of Americans remain in poverty and many experience hunger. Nor have safety-net programs redressed the economic inequality that has been growing in the United States since the late 1970s. More robust safety-net programs would give low- and moderate-income people more income or income substitutes, like food and subsidized shelter. The American tax system is inequitable, as many affluent Americans pay income taxes at rates of 15% or lower, unlike in many other industrialized nations, which require affluent people to pay income taxes at 50% or higher. Many of these nations have far more munificent safety-net programs as well. Their higher income taxes and more liberal safety-net programs cause them to have less economic inequality than the United States.

These positive benefits would be even larger if eligible individuals used specific safety-net programs. For example, roughly half of people eligible for SNAP (food stamps) and the Earned Income Tax Credit (EITC) do not use them. Many single heads of households are sufficiently intimidated by restrictions on use of TANF that they do not even apply for it, even though some of them resort to illegal activities, doubling up, and selling blood to afford the survival needs of themselves and their children. Many people with permanent and total disabilities do not apply for Social Security Disability Insurance (SSDI) or SSI. Many people do not update their eligibility for specific safety-net programs because of the complexity of application forms.

ANALYZING THE POLITICAL ECONOMY OF THE SAFETY-NET SECTOR

The safety-net sector has been associated with a great debate ever since the Great Depression. Many experts have lauded the positive economic effects of the safety-net sector, including Presidents Franklin Roosevelt, Harry Truman, Lyndon Johnson, Bill Clinton, and Barack Obama. These experts have disproportionately been liberals. While some conservatives have supported specific safety-net programs, such as nutritional ones, most conservatives have viewed safety-net programs in relatively negative terms. They have blamed them for increasing budget deficits at the federal and state levels, even as they have traditionally supported other fiscal programs that have increased deficits, such as military spending and low levels of taxation on affluent Americans. They have often argued that safety-net programs erode the work ethic of many Americans, even as experts from the National Bureau of Economic Research contend that the safety net has little impact on decisions about whether to work (Ben-Shalom, Moffitt, & Scholz, 2011).

As Republicans and Democrats sparred over the details of federal budgets in 2011 and 2012, it became clear just how wide the ideological gulf between the parties had become with respect to safety-net programs. The Democratic Party had become somewhat more liberal, but the Republican Party had become considerably more conservative, with only several Republican moderates remaining in the House and Senate. Leaders of the two parties developed divergent proposals for cutting the nation's unsustainable debt that had been caused by two wars, huge tax cuts in the Bush Jr. presidency, and diminished tax revenues due to the Great Recession. Republicans wanted to cut taxes even further, even for individuals in the top 1% of the income distribution who had already benefited disproportionately from the Bush tax cuts. Democrats wanted to raise taxes on couples earning more than $250,000. Republicans mostly did not want to cut military spending, whereas Democrats wanted to slash it considerably, as Obama was withdrawing most troops from Iraq and had started scaling back American forces in Afghanistan. Republicans wanted to end Medicare and replace it with tax incentives to encourage Americans to develop savings accounts that would pay for their medical expenses. Republicans wanted to turn Medicaid back to the states and remove its entitlement status, even as Democrats wanted to expand it to meet the needs of many people who lacked health coverage. Republicans wanted to slash spending on education, job training, and vocational education, while Democrats wanted to increase funding for these programs (see Policy Advocacy Learning Challenge 9.1). Leaders of both political parties realized that the aging of the baby boomers would hugely contribute to federal and state spending in coming decades.

The divide between liberals and conservatives was dramatically exposed during the presidential campaign of 2012. Romney told a roomful of affluent supporters in May 2012 that

> 47 percent of the people will vote for (Obama) no matter what . . . who are dependent upon government, who believe they are victims, who believe that government has a responsibility to care for them, who believe they are entitled to health care, to food, to housing, to you name it . . . these are people who pay no income tax. So our message of low taxes doesn't connect. (Corn, 2013)

Unbeknownst to Romney, someone videotaped his remarks and placed them on YouTube. These remarks were discovered months later by Jason Carter (the grandson of former president Jimmy Carter), who divulged them to David Corn, who published them in *Mother Jones*. Romney later admitted that these remarks were a devastating blow to his campaign. Already viewed as unsympathetic to ordinary people, they suggested that he viewed *anyone* who used programs widely needed by many Americans to survive harsh economic realities as a lazy person dependent on government programs—and as supporting Obama only because he gave them government benefits. Critics promptly noted that although many working Americans had such low wages that they did not pay federal income taxes, they paid payroll taxes and sales taxes in amounts that usually exceeded Romney's federal tax rate of 14%. Many other Americans did not pay federal taxes because they were retired, and many disabled veterans and unemployed people did not pay income taxes because they could not work. Romney compounded his comments by saying, "My job is not to worry about those people." (He later said that he had misspoken, but soon attributed the Democrats' and Obama's electoral victory to their "gifts" to poor people, college students, and others, including food stamps and college scholarships.)

Join this great debate between liberals and conservatives by reading Policy Advocacy Learning Challenge 9.1.

POLICY ADVOCACY LEARNING CHALLENGE 9.1

Connecting Micro, Mezzo, and Macro Policy Advocacy

Divergent Views About People Seeking Welfare

The State of Florida enacted a law that required applicants for welfare to obtain drug tests. Its backers believed it would reduce applications and catch significant numbers

(Continued)

(Continued)

of drug users. State data revealed that it accomplished neither of these goals, as only 2.6% of welfare applicants failed the drug test during a four-month period (Alvarez, 2012). In fact, Florida may have *lost* money on this experiment because it reimbursed passing applicants $30 each for the cost of their test, for a total of $118,140. Advocates of the law insisted that it be retained because it "was really meant to make sure that kids were protected (and that) our money wasn't going to addicts, that taxpayer generosity was being used on diapers and Wheaties and food and clothing." The American Civil Liberties Union (ACLU) of Florida sued the state for unconstitutional invasion of applicants' privacy as protected by the Fourth Amendment to the U.S. Constitution. On December 8, 2014, the 11th Circuit Court struck down the Florida law, finding it to be unconstitutional, in a unanimous ruling by a bipartisan panel of judges. The Court decided that Florida failed to show any evidence that it was necessary to force applicants seeking TANF to surrender their constitutional rights to receive aid (see Mataconis, 2014).

LEARNING EXERCISE

1. Discuss why backers of this law in Florida were confident that it *would* catch many drug offenders.
2. Can you think of public programs used by middle- and upper-income families that would require drug tests?
3. Do similar views exist with respect to users of SNAP, the EITC, Section 8 housing, or other safety-net programs?
4. Is the Florida law consonant with social workers' values as stated in the National Association of Social Workers Code of Ethics?

USING AMERICAN SAFETY-NET PROGRAMS TO IMPROVE CONSUMERS' WELL-BEING

You will now analyze the safety-net programs in Table 9.1. Remember this: Even though it can be tedious to learn about these many programs and policies, you can remarkably improve the well-being of specific people and families by using micro policy advocacy to connect them with these programs—and you can engage in mezzo policy advocacy and macro policy advocacy to improve them. Many technical details are discussed because the policies that you and your clients will navigate *are* detailed in nature—and you sometimes will advocate for clients who are wrongly declared to be ineligible. You can use the websites of key advocacy groups that support these programs, such as those listed in Table 9.2.

Table 9.2 Advocacy Groups That Support Income-Enhancing Programs

The **Center on Budget and Policy Priorities (CBPP)** conducts wide-ranging research on a wide variety of safety-net programs. It has been rated as the most effective lobbying group in its area of specialty in Washington, DC. It has close links with similar groups in many states in the United States as well as in other nations.

The **Urban Institute (UI)** conducts research on welfare, health, nutritional, housing, and many other domestic programs.

The **Brookings Institution (BI)** conducts research on a wide range of domestic programs.

Fellows of the **Center for American Progress** engage in wide-ranging research on safety-net programs.

Income-Enhancing Programs

Temporary Assistance for Needy Families (TANF)

TANF, which President Clinton and the Congress approved in 1996 as the replacement for AFDC, is the nation's major welfare program for families. Under pressure from Republicans to live up to his campaign promise of 1992 "to end welfare as we know it," Clinton decided to enact welfare reform with many provisions that Republicans supported in return for some concessions from them. While Clinton got Republicans to keep Medicaid as an entitlement, he signed the legislation over the vehement opposition of some cabinet members and top civil servants, who produced data that predicted it would cast millions of children into poverty. TANF consists of nine titles or sets of provisions that cover welfare, SSI, immigrants, childcare, child nutrition, and food stamps (now SNAP).

TANF replaced AFDC as a block grant to be funded until 2002 at roughly the annual level of federal expenditures for AFDC in the year preceding the enactment of TANF—but Congress could fund it at any level it desired after 2002. Liberals feared that conservative Congresses would slash federal funding and involvement considerably or entirely in future years, leaving welfare entirely in the hands of states. They feared a "race to the bottom" would then occur as generous states would fear that their high welfare benefits would be a magnet to destitute low-income individuals—saddling them with higher welfare costs and forcing them to raise their individuals' and corporations' tax rates higher as they left low-benefit states.

TANF stipulated that the states must ensure that adult recipients participate in work or work-related activities after receiving two years of cumulative benefits, with 25% of the single-parent family caseload participating by 1997 and 50% by 2002. It stated that recipients could receive cash assistance for a maximum of five years over a lifetime, with limited exceptions for no more than 20% of caseloads. It prohibited the use of federal funds for minor parents under 18 not participating in school activities or living in an adult-supervised setting.

The legislation gave states far more latitude than the defunct AFDC program. They could eliminate cash aid entirely if they chose, replacing it with any combination of cash and in-kind benefits; deny assistance to teen parents or other kinds of recipients; establish even more severe time limits; provide benefits to new residents at the same level as the state from which they emigrated for up to one year; or deny aid to persons convicted of a drug felony after August 1996 unless they participated in a rehabilitation program. Nor did the legislation require uniform statewide standards. The legislation gave local welfare workers enormous discretion in deciding who to cut off the rolls as recipients faced time limits and as they tried to comply with work requirements—discretion that had been greatly reduced in the AFDC program by legislation and court rulings. TANF families were no longer automatically eligible for Medicaid, even though those meeting the old AFDC income standards could often receive it based on income. Food stamp benefits were reduced by not allowing families to deduct more than 50% of their rent or housing costs from their income to determine the amount of stamps they could receive. The maximum food stamp benefit level was reduced by 3%—and severe restrictions were placed on benefits of childless able-bodied individuals.

TANF initiated other harsh policies. The welfare reform legislation restricted eligibility for SSI for children with behavioral disorders, even though Congress agreed in 1997 to continue Medicaid benefits to children who lost their SSI eligibility. (It also disqualified adults whose primary disability was substance abuse or alcoholism.) It decreased funding for meals for children in family day-care homes, as well as cut reimbursements for summer food programs—and eliminated start-up and expansion funding of the School Breakfast Program. The welfare reform legislation eliminated the *guarantee* of childcare for welfare recipients trying to move into employment, leaving it to individual states to determine whether and for how long former recipients would receive subsidized childcare. It did, however, consolidate federal childcare programs into the existing Child Care and Development Block Grant and increase funding through a new childcare block grant. It also allowed states to transfer up to 30% of their TANF block grant funds to the Child Care and Development Block Grant and the Title XX Social Services Block Grant.

The intent of the legislation was to move the nation toward a work-based safety net by making TANF sufficiently harsh that many recipients would migrate to the labor force. Many of them assumed that TANF recipients would earn sufficient monies to make them as affluent as they had been on AFDC. They assumed that TANF would decrease childhood poverty.

When coupled with an incentive to work spurred by marked expansion of EITC eligibility and benefits, as well as rapid economic growth in the 1990s, TANF appeared not to harm former welfare recipients. Vast numbers of them entered the workforce and increased their income (Grogger, 2003). While rolls declined by two thirds or more in 32 states in the decade after enactment of TANF, most families remained "near poor," and few social or educational benefits were given to children in these families (DeParle, 2012).

TANF met its most stringent test during the Great Recession from 2007 to 2009 and beyond. Cash rolls barely rose from 2007 through 2011 despite the most severe economic downturn since the Great Depression (DeParle, 2012). Only one in five poor children received cash aid—or the lowest level in 50 years. Sixteen states *cut* TANF rolls after 2007, often using the TANF grants they received from the federal government for *other* programs such as foster care or adoptions—or using cuts in TANF to cut their budget deficits (DeParle, 2012).

This near-absence of cash relief for single heads of households, when coupled with the economic downturn, caused unwarranted distress for these families. One in four of these women were jobless and without cash aid. While many of them received SNAP and/or Medicaid, as well as some help from relatives, charity, and food banks, they had no regular source of cash. It is not surprising that women often resorted to desperate, and sometimes illegal, measures. Some sold SNAP coupons, sold blood, skipped meals, doubled up with friends, scavenged trash cans, and shoplifted. Some of them returned to violent partners who had abused them and their children (DeParle, 2012). Researchers discovered that 4% (twice as many as in 1996) of households with children lived on less than $2 per day (DeParle, 2012). The Bureau of the Census discovered that 10% of households headed by women lived in "deep poverty" with less than $9,000 per year—the highest level in 18 years.

Few called for rethinking TANF, even though these outcomes of TANF, when coupled with the Great Recession, were "even worse" than predicted by Peter Edelman, a high-level official who resigned from the Clinton Administration to protest TANF's enactment. Top Republicans, such as Congressman Paul Ryan, called TANF an "unprecedented success," while Republican presidential contender Mitt Romney pledged to "place similar restrictions on all these federal programs" (DeParle, 2012). As Robert Greenstein, president of the Center on Budget and Policy Priorities contends, if the goal is *both* to promote work *and* to maintain an adequate safety net for those lacking well-paying jobs . . . then it would be a serious mistake to convert Medicaid and SNAP to block grants . . . and to shrink their funding [which would] magnify TANF's weaknesses and would substantially increase the ranks of the uninsured and deeply poor. (Greenstein, 2012)

General Relief (GR)

While providing welfare assistance to children in destitute families (ADC) and one or both of their parents (AFDC), to elderly destitute individuals (OAA), and to blind and then deaf persons (AB), the Social Security Act failed to enact welfare provisions for destitute individuals *not* attached to a family unit, such as single nonelderly men or women, in 1935. It left welfare for these individuals to local units of government or, in some cases, to those states that provided this assistance. This decision reflected widespread animus toward these persons because they were not seen as "deserving" as children, caregivers, and elderly adults.

Nor have local units of governments and states been benevolent toward people who receive GR (called General Assistance or GA in some jurisdictions). It was inevitable that these governments would fund GR benefits at lower levels than AFDC, OAA, or AB, because they received no matching federal funds. The offices that serve GR clients are often harsh, such as those with bulletproof windows and security staff. Many recipients of GR grants are single men and women who have been recently released from prison—people who often find it difficult to find work because of their prison records. Others are single homeless individuals and single veterans. Still others are married couples with no children.

Supplemental Security Income (SSI)

President Nixon developed the idea of joining means-tested programs for elderly and disabled persons funded by the Social Security Act into a single means-tested program in 1969, which soon was enacted as Supplementary Security Income (SSI). The federal government funded its benefits and administered it through the federal Social Security Administration.

Applicants to SSI must meet specific qualifications. They gain access due to blindness if vision in their best eye is no better than 20/200 with glasses, or if they have tunnel vision of 20% or less. People with other disabilities can qualify for SSI only if their medical records and/or a physician chosen by the state documents that they have been unable to work, or can be expected to be unable to work, for 12 continuous months or if they possess a disability that is likely to lead to death. Children under 18 can qualify for SSI if they have a medically validated "marked or severe" physical or mental disability that would disallow work if they were adults or that significantly interferes with their daily activities. Individuals cannot obtain SSI for alcohol or drug dependence. They cannot get SSI for any month when they are in prison, in violation of parole or probation, or a fugitive from felony charges (Los Angeles Coalition to End Hunger and Homelessness, 2010). Some states fund their own cash assistance programs for people with short-term disabilities, such as injuries caused by automobile accidents or other physical trauma and mental distress caused by traumatic events.

Five million adults received SSI in 2011, with payments of $33 billion and Medicaid services of $110 billion (Porter, 2012).

Some states offer State Disability Insurance (SDI) for people with temporary disability. In California, for example, individuals may be eligible for SDI if they cannot work for eight consecutive days and if they have lost wages due to their disability. They must be looking for work (Los Angeles Coalition to End Hunger and Homelessness, 2010).

Social Security Disability Insurance (SSDI)

Unlike the means-tested SSI program, SSDI is a universal entitlement for people with medical certification of lasting and permanent disabilities of the mind or body. They must be under age 65 and have disabling conditions of the body or mind that prevent them from "substantial gainful activity" for at least 12 months or that will result in death. They need specific numbers of social security credits to qualify—credits achieved by paying payroll taxes into Social Security—though this work requirement is waived if they became disabled at or before age 22. They need medical evidence to determine their eligibility. Many individuals use third-party disability representatives to make their applications and to appeal adverse eligibility decisions, whether from companies with trained specialists in filing and appealing claims or from law firms from their communities. These representatives screen applicants and may decline to represent them if they believe they will not meet SSDI eligibility requirements. (They are paid from 25% of retroactive awards made to applicants, not to exceed $6,000.) The Social Security Administration sometimes requires that people with mental disabilities assign someone to disburse their benefits to them or to landlords and others—usually a relative or friends at no fee (Office of the Inspector General, 2010).

SSDI is a huge program, having paid $128.9 billion in insurance payments to 10.6 million disabled workers and their family members in 2011, as well as $90 billion in Medicare benefits. Disability payments now constitute almost 20% of total Social Security benefits, as compared to 10% in 1990 (Porter, 2012). People must often wait eight months to complete the application process due to backlogs—and sometimes more than a year to get an appeals hearing. Roughly 39% of SSDI applications were approved at the state level in 2005.

SSDI has grown rapidly due to the increase in numbers of elderly persons, along with their inability to find jobs due to their low skill and education levels, as well as because many jobs have moved abroad or been supplanted with technology such as robots. People with back pain or depression often opt to work when they can find well-paying jobs, but otherwise seek SSDI—and they find it easier to obtain SSDI after Congress softened the eligibility criteria in the 1980s and gave more weight to pain and mental problems like anxiety (Porter, 2012). Moreover, they can appeal adverse decisions before administrative judges without testimony from personnel from Social Security who have rejected them (Porter, 2012). Once people receive SSDI, they rarely return to work—and they receive no assistance in terms of work accommodations that might enable them to rejoin the labor force.

Beneficiaries receive only roughly $1,100 per month as well as Medicare coverage. They can earn $1,000 extra per month, but only 10% of them make any additional money.

The Earned Income Tax Credit (EITC) and Other Tax Benefits

The United States did not have a broad-based federal income tax until the nation was forced to enact one to finance the huge costs of World War II. President Franklin Roosevelt enacted a *progressive tax system* based on multiple levels of income. Everyone paid the same rate of 19% for the first level of income (up to $2,000) in 1943, for example, but rates were increased for each succeeding level up to the top marginal tax rate of 88% for taxable income over $200,000. This progressive system of taxation remained mostly intact through the 1950s and early 1960s, with the top marginal rate of 70% existing even as late as 1980. It promoted a relatively equal distribution of income by exempting very poor people from any income taxes while levying successively higher marginal rates on individuals as they moved up the economic ladder.

This progressivity of the tax system was diminished over the ensuing six decades by regressive reforms. President Ronald Reagan cut the top marginal rate substantially to 28% in 1988. After this rate rose to 39.6% in the Clinton presidency, it descended to 35% by 2003, in the presidency of George Bush Jr.—and Republican presidential contender Mitt Romney proposed in 2012 that it be reduced to 28%. Large numbers of tax loopholes were enacted over many decades that disproportionately favored affluent Americans, such as lower capital gains taxes, lower taxes on dividends, and lower taxes on income kept in foreign nations. The estate tax on affluent Americans was also drastically reduced over many decades—and even eliminated by President George W. Bush. The net result was that many millionaires and some billionaires paid federal income taxes of 15% or less—including Mitt Romney, who had an estimated wealth of more than

$200 million—as compared to federal tax rates of 30% or more for many people who earned less than $100,000.

The federal tax code helps low- and moderate-income people in several ways. Roughly half of American taxpayers are exempted from federal income taxes for four major reasons. There are couples with two children who earn less than $26,400, then have their standard deduction of $11,600 and four exemptions of $3,700. (Sixty percent of households who owed no federal income tax in 2011 had incomes under $20,000.) There are elderly people who pay no federal income taxes because their Social Security benefits are not taxed. There are people who receive tax benefits back from the Internal Revenue Service in the form of the EITC, the child credit, and the childcare credit account. There are students. Roughly 40% of households did not pay federal income taxes in 2007—a percentage that rose to roughly 50% by 2009 due to the individuals' loss of income during the Great Recession.

Some conservatives suggest that the many people who do not pay federal income taxes are freeloaders. Virtually all employed people *do* pay payroll taxes for Social Security and Medicare, however, so that even the poorest fifth of households paid an average of 4% of their incomes in federal taxes in 2007, even when they had average income of only $18,400 (Marr & Huang, 2012.) Households with income between $20,500 and $34,000 paid 10.6% of their income in federal taxes. Even these figures are misleading, however, because these households pay state and local taxes—so the poorest fifth of households paid 12.3% of their incomes in state and local taxes in 2011 (Marr & Huang, 2012). State and local taxes are not progressive, moreover, because the sales tax, as well as the excise tax on gasoline, lands hardest on low-income individuals who spend a high proportion of their income on food and other purchases.

Moderate-income individuals benefit from various provisions in the federal tax code. They can deduct their mortgage payments, costs of seeking work, costs of obtaining job training, and work-related costs. They pay lower taxes than some people with higher incomes.

Many states exempt low-income individuals, seniors, renters, disabled people, and veterans from various taxes, such as state income taxes and property taxes. Some give low-income persons tax benefits like the federal EITC.

The enactment of the federal EITC helped low- and moderate-income working individuals in 1975, soon becoming the nation's largest anti-poverty program, with successive expansions in succeeding decades. Individuals and couples who care for qualified children receive a *tax refund* when they qualify for a tax credit that exceeds the amount of taxes they owe. A married-couple family with three or more qualified children and income less than $43,279 can receive a tax refund of as much as $5,657 when they fill out a W-5 tax form during the year. Qualified children include those who are 18 or younger, those who are 23 or younger and are also full-time students for five calendar months, and those of any age who are found by physicians to be permanently and totally disabled. (Benefit tables show maximum amounts available for individuals with fewer children, as well as for married couples ages 25 to 64 with no children.) Sixteen states supplement the federal EITC with their own tax refund programs for low-wage workers. The EITC lifted 6.5 million persons, including 3.3 million children, from poverty in 2009 (Williams & Johnson, 2010). The EITC provides an incentive to work and off-sets Social Security payroll taxes that are otherwise onerous for many low-income individuals. People can obtain help in getting the EITC by calling its hotline at 1–800–601–5552.

Research shows that cutting the EITC would discourage work, since people have to work to obtain its benefit. Cuts would also increase poverty. The EITC decreases use of welfare (Marr & Huang, 2012). Yet many conservatives favor cutting the EITC.

Many advocates seek changes to make federal, state, and local taxes more help-ful to low- and moderate-income people. For example, when John Kerry was a U.S. senator (D.-Mass.), he proposed reforming the EITC to allow people to earn more money before they have to pay taxes—and simplifying its eligibility rules (O'Connor, 2011). Some advocates want to reduce payroll taxes for Social Secu-rity for low-income individuals, such as by creating a refundable payroll tax credit. The federal income tax code is unfair to renters, who cannot deduct all or part of their rents from their taxable income, unlike homeowners, who can deduct their mortgage interest. These tax concessions could be funded by increases in taxes on more affluent Americans, which would have the added benefit of decreasing eco-nomic inequality in the United States.

Unemployment Insurance

Many people lose employment even during periods of economic growth, but mil-lions lose it during recessions, such as those that began in 1991, 2001, and 2007. Low- and moderate-income persons are particularly harmed by unemployment, since loss of even a single paycheck can push them into poverty—or, in the case of impoverished persons, extreme poverty. National unemployment rates exceeded 12% in 2008, remained above 8% in 2012, and receded to 7% in 2014.

While many people who lost employment in prior recessions regained it rela-tively rapidly as the economy improved, many—disproportionately those who were less than 25 years of age, persons of color, and unskilled workers—did not obtain reemployment within a year during the Great Recession and its aftermath. People who are unemployed long term suffer multiple hardships beyond their loss of wages. Their job skills erode. They lose confidence that they can find reemployment. They often develop mental problems such as anxiety and depression. They often develop health problems. Roughly 50% of college graduates under age 25 were unable to find full-time work in 2012, forcing many of them to move back into the homes of their parents, as they also had an average of $20,000 in college debt.

The United States has relied heavily on its Unemployment Insurance (UI) program, a joint federal–state program. UI is financed by payroll taxes of employers, with each state determining its tax rates. (The federal government maintains an Unemployment Trust Fund with accounts for each state within it.) Each state runs its own UI programs, such as determining eligibility and benefits. Most states make benefits available for a maximum of 26 weeks, but Congress often extends benefits during economic recessions, such as when it gave extended benefits to 2.3 million Americans in 2008—even extending maximum lengths to 99 weeks in 2010 and in 2012. However, people with relatively low wages receive far lower benefits than those with relatively high wages.

Unemployed individuals must meet specific requirements to receive UI benefits that equal roughly 36% of their average weekly wage. They must be actively seeking work. They must be able to work. They must have lost their work because their employer terminated them, although they can still obtain UI if they left work for good cause. They are not usually eligible if they were discharged for misconduct or a labor dispute. They must usually have worked full time for four of the last five calendar quarters before a claim is filed.

Applicants apply for benefits through their state unemployment agency and must usually wait two weeks to receive their benefits. They can often apply on the Internet or via an automated telephone call. Many states ask individuals to regularly verify that the conditions of benefits are still being met. Disqualified or discontinued applicants can appeal these decisions within a specified time.

Unemployed individuals are often eligible for other safety-net programs simultaneously with UI, including SNAP, Section 8 subsidized housing, Medicaid, and public housing. People who exhaust their UI benefits are eligible for other safety-net programs and must often rely on others, such as parents or relatives; apply for TANF or GR; or obtain one or more part-time jobs. Unemployed persons can appeal denials of UI benefits and receive a hearing before administrative law judges; roughly half of appellants win.

Workers' Compensation

Every state has a workers' compensation program that helps workers who have been injured on the job. Claims are paid by the state or private insurance company of specific states, whose premiums are paid by employers in those states. Workers' compensation is a no-fault program, so injured employees do not have to prove that their injury was someone else's fault (Los Angeles Coalition to End Hunger and Homelessness, 2010). People who have been injured at work file claims at workers' compensation offices in their region or hire a private attorney whose fees are set by law. Cases are often heard in a special administrative agency where administrative court judges preside, but appeals can be made to an appeals board and to the state's court system. Successful claimants may receive medical benefits for medical care of their work-related injury, which may be treated by the employer's physician of choice or the worker's own physician if treatment extends beyond 30 days. They may receive temporary disability benefits of up to two thirds of wages lost because of the injury. They may receive permanent disability benefits for life. They may receive permanent partial disability. They may receive vocational rehabilitation services if they cannot return to the kind of work they performed prior to their injury. Their dependents may receive death benefits if a worker is fatally injured (Los Angeles Coalition to End Hunger and Homelessness, 2010).

Minimum Wage and Living Wage Policies

A federal minimum wage was established in 1938 and has been increased by Congress periodically in ensuing years. Critics contend that the federal minimum wage has never been adequate to cover workers' costs—including at its level in 2014 of $7.25. Some employees are exempt from it, including persons reimbursed solely through tips (although their tips must add up to the minimum wage), the employees of some seasonal employers like summer camps, youth under age 18 for periods up to 90 days, and some nonprofit institutions and colleges if they obtain certificates. Many states have their own minimum wages that supersede the federal one if they are higher than it, such as $9.00 in California in 2014—and President Obama signed an executive order in 2014 to raise the minimum wage for federal contractors to $10.10. (See www.dol.gov/whd/minwage/america.htm to see your state's minimum wage.) Barack Obama sought an increase in the minimum wage to $15 in early 2014 in hopes it would decrease poverty, but was unable to persuade Congress to enact it because many conservatives believed this increase would lead employers to decrease their workforces.

A *living wage* is set at a level needed for workers to meet basic needs—to keep a decent standard of living in workers' communities *and* to be able to save for future needs and goals. A living wage movement took place, leading 140 states, cities, local governments, and universities to enact living wages by 2007 including Boston, Los Angeles, and St. Louis—usually $3 to $7 above the federal minimum wage (Wicks-Lim, 2009). States can establish their own minimum wage laws that can exceed the federal level.

Credit- and Loan-Providing Agencies

The finances of low- and moderate-income individuals are often jeopardized by victimization by credit- and loan-providing agencies. Before the Great Recession, millions of families obtained mortgages whose terms were not clearly revealed to them by lending officers who profited as they sold more of them. Many purchasers did not realize that their interest would balloon in coming years to place them beyond their means, even as the price of their homes plummeted during the Great Recession. Many middle-class families fall prey to these predatory practices when they purchase relatively expensive houses in highly regarded school districts at prices they can barely afford, even when both parents are employed. When either parent loses his or her job or when a family member develops a health problem not covered by their health insurance, such families must often foreclose on their home or enter bankruptcy.

Table 9.3 Advocacy Groups That Support Consumer-Friendly Regulations Over Credit- and Loan-Providing Businesses

Consumer Advocacy Group of America

Federal Bureau of Financial Protection

Predatory lenders and credit card companies devastate the finances of many families as well. Needing cash to keep financially solvent, many families obtain loans with interest rates exceeding 20%, only to find collection agencies pursuing them when they cannot repay their loans or their credit card debt.

Congressional Democrats and President Obama enacted the Dodd-Frank Wall Street Reform and Consumer Protection Act of 2010, the most sweeping overhaul of the financial services industry since the 1930s. It outlawed mortgage practices that entice consumers to take loans that they cannot afford or whose rates balloon excessively. It created the Bureau of Financial Protection to regulate the terms and pricing of financial products, as well as requiring the elimination of complex fine print in financial contracts that consumers cannot understand. It established regulations over payday lenders, check cashers, and other predatory nonbank financial services. It required greater transparency by issuers of credit cards.

The Bureau of Financial Protection became enmeshed in partisan conflict when Republicans refused to ratify the formal appointment of Elizabeth Warren, the Harvard professor who had proposed its establishment years earlier. Nor would they approve Obama's second nominee for the post, even though he was the highly regarded Republican treasurer for the state of Ohio—who nonetheless remained in the post pending the presidential election of 2012, when he was replaced by Richard Cordray. Consumers are now able to report violations by banks, lenders, and credit card issuers to a single federal agency for the first time in U.S. history at www.consumerfinance.gov.

The Obama administration proved unable to stem millions of foreclosures during and after the Great Recession of 2007 to 2009 due to these predatory lending practices that were exacerbated by high unemployment. Critics were disappointed that the administration only gave some homeowners temporary assistance to make housing payments and only urged banks to make temporary modifications of mortgages, unlike the state of Kansas that cut foreclosures by 90% by *requiring* mediators to work with banks and homeowners to prevent foreclosures by lowering interest payments.

Job-Related Programs

Various job-related programs help unemployed individuals, train students and welfare recipients, provide job placement and job-seeking skills for unemployed individuals or people who want to change their careers, create jobs, and give workers childcare, transportation, and social service aids to make it possible for them to work. (See Table 9.4 for advocacy groups seeking expansion of job-related programs and protections.)

Table 9.4 Advocacy Groups for Improving Job-Related Programs and Protections

Wider Opportunities for Women (WOW) seeks increased funding for the Workforce Investment Act, the Carl T. Perkins Technical Education Act, Pell Grants, the Women's Bureau, and the Women in Apprenticeship and Nontraditional Occupations Program (WANTO)

The **Military Family Employment Advocacy Program** helps military spouses and dependents find jobs.

Global Policy and Advocacy Jobs is funded by the Bill and Melinda Gates Foundation.

The **Federal Equal Opportunity Employment Commission** works to curtail discrimination in employment.

Training Students,
Welfare Recipients, and Displaced Workers for Jobs

Many employment experts worry that large numbers of Americans will suffer from unemployment even when the American economy returns to normalcy because they lack skills needed for a "new economy" in which workers need technical skills. Recall that many unskilled jobs and semi-skilled jobs were lost in the American economy as industries moved factories to emerging nations in preceding decades and as factories replaced workers with technology, such as robots on assembly lines.

Many employment experts contend that the United States was not prepared to address these problems. The Carl D. Perkins Career and Technical Education Act was enacted in 1984 and reauthorized in 1998 when it used the term "career and technical education" (CTE) instead of "vocational education." It provided $1.3 billion in grants to states to link academic and technical content in high schools, junior colleges, and colleges. In light of the magnitude of training needs, however, this was a paltry annual sum that had *declined* to $1.16 billion by 2012 despite the Great Recession's impact on job prospects. Compared to Germany and Japan, American career and technical education often prepared students for relatively unskilled jobs, such as offering them internships in fast-food restaurants rather than in industrial positions where they could become certified to perform specific technical tasks. Many secondary students refrained from engaging in vocational education because it had a low reputation.

President Obama proposed sweeping reforms of the Perkins Act in 2012 (U.S. Department of Education, 2012). He wanted to require states to work with workforce and economic development agencies to identify areas of focus for CTE programs. He wanted strong collaboration between schools and colleges, employers, and industry partners. He wanted the private sector to contribute funds to CTE programs to strengthen its participation. He wanted to reward local recipients that exceeded performance standards in placement rates and earnings of graduates. He wanted to retain CTE funding of $1.1 billion but align it with other administration initiatives "to align classroom teaching and learning with real-world business needs," including $2 billion in Trade Adjustment Assistance grants to strengthen community college programs and workforce partnerships, as well as $8 billion for the Community College to Career Fund that seeks to train 2 million workers for high-growth industries and $1 billion to help 500,000 high school students participate in career academies.

The Job Corps

The Job Corps provides vocational and academic training for low-income youth ages 16 to 24—and currently serves 60,000 youth at 125 residential centers throughout the United States. Applicants must meet income requirements; must be willing to participate in an educational environment; must agree to adhere to a no-violence, no-drug policy; and must agree to dormitory inspection rules. The Job

Corps provides multiple kinds of services, including career planning, on-the-job training, job placement, driver's education, basic health and dental services, and a biweekly living and clothing allowance. Some centers provide childcare for single parents. The Job Corps provides vocational training in advanced manufacturing, automatic and machine repair, construction, finance and business, healthcare and allied health professions, homeland security, hospitality, information technology, renewable resources and energy, retail sales and services, and transportation fields. Youth create a personal career development plan in their first 60 days with the help of Job Corps staff before entering a career development phase that links vocational and academic training. They complete their training with a career transition period where they obtain their first jobs.

Providing People With Tools to Find Jobs

The Workforce Investment Act (WIA) of 1998 streamlined federal and state job services by creating a one-stop delivery system to co-locate programs and providers in local workforce investment areas. Workforce investment boards (WIBs), chaired by a member of the private sector and with a majority of businesspeople, developed workforce education and career pathways programs for vulnerable populations. WIA provides youth opportunity grants to youth from high-poverty areas, as well as universal access to its one-stop system and its core employment-related services. It allows consumers to select the training program that meets their career needs from certified training providers that bestow certificates upon trainees to help them obtain jobs. WIA programs are funded by federal grants to states, but funding is inadequate so that only a fraction of persons who need them receive them.

President Obama proposed reforms of WIA services. He hoped to convert federal employment offices into reemployment programs to help workers who lose their jobs as corporations downsize, automate, outsource, or move their operations abroad. He strengthened the links of WIA to other federal training programs and unemployed populations, such as the Job Corps, TANF and GR recipients, returning veterans, and graduates of CTE programs in high school, junior colleges, and colleges.

WIA training programs often are not effective with TANF recipients, because many of them have mental health and substance abuse problems for which they do not receive specialized help. Many TANF recipients have children with mental health problems or physical disabilities. A survey of job training programs for these TANF recipients suggests that a planned strategy does not exist. Some of them run afoul of TANF time limits and lose their grants. Some receive job training from WIA, but it lacks social services to meet their needs. Some remain on TANF when TANF administrators waive time limits for them (Zedlewski, Holcomb, & Loprest, 2007).

Providing Childcare, Transportation, and Services

Many people need childcare, transportation, and services to be able to work. TANF and GR welfare programs require welfare recipients to search for employment. They can get help with job training and placement by visiting WIB-run one-stop worksource centers that provide computers, faxes, copiers, and job listings. These offices are also required to provide career counseling, funds for transportation and childcare, and sometimes quality job training. Recipients can visit community colleges. They can seek high school diplomas for GEDs, learn English as a second language (ESL), and attend job readiness classes and some certificate courses and local public schools.

State departments of rehabilitation provide services for people with physical or mental disabilities, including substance-abuse problems. These services can including vocational counseling and training, medical treatment, funds for tuition and books, funds for transportation and car modification, and reader and interpreter services (Los Angeles Coalition to End Homelessness and Hunger, 2010).

States' TANF programs usually provide childcare benefits to welfare recipients who have children. Considerable variation exists in the length of the childcare benefit. Many low-income individuals cannot afford transportation to places of employment, particularly when these workplaces are geographically distant from their residences. They can receive transportation subsidies from some TANF programs and from some transit agencies. Some nonprofit agencies donate or sell used automobiles to low-income individuals at reduced prices.

States' ability to fund childcare and training has been impeded by loose federal regulations that allow them to use TANF funds for *other* programs. Some of them have "raided" TANF funds to help finance state budgetary deficits. Those TANF recipients who *do* obtain jobs may receive TANF childcare and transportation subsidies, but only for limited periods so that they find it difficult to maintain their employment.

Programs to Protect Workers' Rights

We have already discussed federal and state minimum wages, as well as living wage ordinances in some local and state units of government, but these ordinances are sometimes not monitored or enforced. Employers may take improper deductions from pay checks, not pay owed wages, pay wages with checks that bounce, fail to give rest breaks, or fail to promptly pay all wages due to workers when they terminate their employment. Workers can obtain advice from their state's labor commissioner or from the U.S. Department of Labor—and use this information to decide whether to file grievances. They can file a wage claim in small claims court for up to $5,000 in California. They can contest discrimination on the basis of race, sex, religion, national origin, citizenship, age, disability, political affiliation, or sexual orientation, as well as sexual harassment, by filing a complaint with the Federal Equal Employment Opportunity Commission (FEEOC). The FEEOC will investigate complaints and give complainants letters authorizing them to file lawsuits if warranted. Workers can also contact their states' fair employment department for any of these problems (Los Angeles Coalition to End Hunger and Homelessness, 2010).

Nutrition-Enhancing Programs

People need sufficient nutrition, yet large numbers of Americans have inadequate diets. The U.S. Department of Agriculture (USDA) identifies four levels of "food security":

1. *High food security*, where households have no reported indications of food-access problems or limitations

2. *Marginal food security*, where household members report anxiety over food sufficiency or a shortage of food in the house—but with no or little indication of changes in diet or food intake

3. *Low food security without hunger*, where reports suggest reduced quality, variety, or desirability of diet, but little or no indication of reduced food intake

4. *Food insecurity with hunger*, with reports of multiple indications of disrupted eating patterns and reduced food intake

The USDA discovered that almost one in seven households (or 17.2 million of them) were in Groups 3 and 4 in 2010—and 3.9 million of these households had children in them. Roughly 6.7 million of these families were in Group 4. *The median food-secure families in Groups 1 and 2 spent 27% more on food than the median food-insecure family of the same size and household composition* (Coleman-Jensen, Nord, Andrews, & Carlson, 2010). Fifty-five percent of the households in Groups 3 and 4 had used SNAP, school lunch programs, or WIC during the month preceding the survey—but roughly 45% did *not* use any of these programs despite their food insecurity. (See Table 9.5 for advocacy groups that support nutrition-enhancing programs.)

Supplemental Nutrition Assistance Program (SNAP, formerly Food Stamps)

SNAP is the largest program in the U.S. to help low- and moderate-income people meet their basic food needs. It served 46.5 million in January 2012. It is a federal/state program administered by the states but wholly funded by the federal government.

Table 9.5 Advocacy Groups That Support Nutrition-Enhancing Programs

The **Food Research and Action Center (FRAC)** is the leading nonprofit organization seeking to eradicate hunger in the United States. It conducts research, monitors programs, coordinates and trains different nutrition programs and advocates, and conducts public information campaigns.

Feeding America coordinates a nationwide network of member food banks that serve 37 million Americans each year, including 14 million children and 3 million seniors. It also engages in advocacy with respect to public policy concerning hunger among children, rural residents, the working poor, and seniors.

It is reauthorized every five years as part of the Farm Bill. Households must meet resource eligibility standards: They cannot have more than $2,000 in countable resources, such as bank accounts, or $3,520 if at least one person is age 60 or older or is disabled. (Income from most retirement plans is not counted.) Households' net monthly income cannot exceed 100% of poverty, or $1,863 for a family of four. Households on TANF and SSI recipients automatically qualify. Able-bodied adults without dependents between 18 and 50 can get SNAP benefits only for three months in a 36-month period if they do not work or participate in a training program. (Go to www.fns.usda.gov/snap/ to find detailed eligibility requirements.)

SNAP benefits are very modest, averaging only $1.44 per person per meal. Enrollees are limited to food items; exclusions include alcoholic beverages, tobacco, soap, cleaning supplies, pet food, and paper products. SNAP benefits are increasingly obtained through Electronic Benefit Transfer using plastic electronic cards obtained from local state or county offices. Almost all food stores are authorized to accept these cards, which work like bank debit cards as the cost of groceries is subtracted from a household's account automatically. Congress made major cuts in SNAP in 2014 over the objections of the Obama Administration and many Congressional Democrats.

The Special Supplemental Nutrition Program for Women, Infants, and Children (WIC)

WIC provides food to pregnant women, postpartum women up to six months after the birth of an infant or the end of the pregnancy, and breastfeeding women up to the infant's first birthday. It serves infants up to their first birthday and children up to their fifth birthday. No residency requirement exists, but some states require applicants to apply to a WIC clinic that serves the area where they live. States' eligibility requirements cannot exceed 185% of federal poverty levels. Recipients of Medicaid and TANF are automatically eligible.

Applicants must be screened by a health professional—whether their own physician or a WIC health professional—to determine if they are at nutritional risk. They must have at least one of the medical or dietary conditions on their state's list of WIC nutrition risk criteria, such as anemia, underweight, a history of poor pregnancy outcome, or poor diet (www.fns.usda.gov/wic/). More than 9.1 million women, infants, and children used the WIC program each month in 2010. WIC provides food packages designed to meet the special nutritional needs of low-income pregnant and breastfeeding and nonbreastfeeding postpartum women, infants, and children who are at nutritional risk. These packages contain a wide variety of foods, including fruits, vegetables, and whole grains, and can accommodate cultural food preferences and allergies. They include infant formula.

Federal School Breakfast and Lunch Programs, Child and Adult Care Programs, and Summer Nutrition Programs

The Child Nutrition Act of 1966 authorized the School Breakfast Program. All children in participating schools and residential institutions are eligible for these federally subsidized meals, no matter their income, but only children from families at less than 130% of the federal poverty level can obtain free meals, and only children with family incomes between 130% and 185% of the poverty level can obtain reduced-price meals. The federal government funds these meals under the administration of the USDA Food and Nutrition Service, which subsidizes recipient schools with $1.51 per free breakfast, $1.21 per reduced-price breakfast, and $0.27 per paid breakfast. More than 87,000 schools and institutions participate, and in 2010–2011, 11.7 million children were served, with 83.4% of them receiving free or reduced-price breakfasts. Yet many children do not receive school breakfast even when they would qualify, such as 1 million low-income children in California in 2009, when the state ranked 33rd in participation by low-income students (Macvean, 2009).

The National School Lunch Program (NSLP) served 31.6 million children in almost 100,000 schools and residential institutions, with nearly 20 million children receiving free or reduced-price lunches in 2009–2010. The federal government spent $9.7 billion for the NSLP in fiscal year 2010. Like school breakfasts, school lunches meet nutritional standards and upgrade the nutritional intake of many children and youth. Eighty-eight percent of schools participating in NSLP also serve school breakfast.

Enactment of the Healthy Hunger-Free Kids Act of 2010 allows the federal government to improve the school lunch and breakfast programs. Nutritional standards will be upgraded for school meals. The USDA will set nutritional standards for food sold by vending machines at schools. It will connect 115,000 new children to the school programs by using Medicaid data to directly certify their eligibility. Twenty-one million at-risk children will receive food from nonprofits who receive federally subsidized food for the Child and Adult Care Food Program (CACFP) that gives meals to at-risk children after school, whether at dinnertime or at after-school programs.

The federal government also subsidizes summer nutrition programs, often at educational enrichment and recreational programs, with 2.8 million children participating each weekday. (These programs reached only one in seven low-income children with school lunches in 2009–2010.) These programs are often administered by a nonprofit organization or a local government agency.

Meals on Wheels

We discussed this program in Chapter 8.

Nonprofit Food Banks and the USDA

A huge network of food banks, food pantries, and soup kitchens exist in the United States that distribute or provide food to hungry persons. Some are non-profit community-based organizations. Some are faith-based organizations. Some are associated with shelters for the homeless. They obtain food from grocery stores, restaurants, and private donations. They also obtain food from the USDA's Emergency Food Assistance Program (TEFAP) and the Commodity Supplemental Food Program (CSFP) that distribute food commodities to the states, which supervise their distribution to public or nonprofit organizations. The USDA's Senior Farmers' Market Nutrition Program (SFMNP) selects local government agencies or private nonprofit organizations to provide low-income individuals over age 60 with coupons or checks to purchase fresh fruits and vegetables at authorized farmers' markets, roadside stands, and community-supported agriculture programs.

Shelter-Enhancing Programs

People need secure and adequate shelter, yet roughly 170,000 families with children lived in temporary shelters in 2010, according to the Department of Housing and Urban Development (HUD). Roughly four times as many families "doubled up" or occupied other unstable home situations, according to the U.S. Department of Education. Considerable research documents the negative effects of housing instability on children's mental health and school performance, as well as on their health (Price, 2011).

Estimates of the numbers of homeless people have been collected for specific jurisdictions. In New York City, for example, the Coalition for the Homeless estimated that 41,200 persons were homeless in October 2011, including 10,000 homeless families with 17,000 homeless children. The Coalition estimates that 113,553 persons slept in the New York City municipal shelter system in fiscal year 2010. A large majority of "street homeless people" are individuals with mental illness or other health problems—and 80% are men. Families often experience episodes of homelessness due to eviction, doubling up or overcrowding, domestic violence, and hazardous housing conditions. The Los Angeles Homeless Services Authority estimated that roughly 43,000 persons were homeless in Los Angeles County on any given day in 2009. (See Table 9.6 for advocacy groups that seek adequate shelter.)

Table 9.6 Advocacy Groups That Seek Adequate Shelter

National Coalition for the Homeless

National Law Center on Homelessness and Poverty

Section 8 Rental Housing Subsidies

Shelter-enhancing programs include public housing, Section 8 rent subsidies for privately owned rental units, senior citizen housing, subsidized housing units owned by the government with sliding rates of monthly rent or mortgage payments, and housing constructed by nonprofit or religious groups such as Habitat for Humanity. They include shelters for temporary stays for homeless individuals that are financed by nonprofit or religious groups or by local, state, and federal governments.

Continuum of Care Systems (COC)

The McKinney-Vento Homeless Assistance Act provides funds for competitive grants provided by HUD to local jurisdictions for a coordinated community-based process of identifying needs and building a system to address them. Coordinated programs require the development of shelters, including use of a supportive housing program, rental assistance for homeless individuals with disabilities, and single-room occupancy programs (SROs) that give rental assistance to homeless persons. Strategies must be developed to address the physical, economic, and social unmet needs of homeless persons. HUD funds, as well, an Emergency Solutions Grant Program (ESG) to provide street outreach and emergency shelter services, as well as rapid-rehousing assistance that helps homeless individuals and families obtain permanent housing quickly. All of these programs are inadequately funded to address homelessness—and need to be supplemented with funding from localities and states. Information about housing resources in local areas is found on the HUD website at the home page of the Homelessness Resource Exchange (HRE).

Shelter-Enhancing Programs: Public Housing

Federally funded public housing programs were initiated in the New Deal for low-income persons, including seniors. They developed a poor reputation in subsequent decades because they often contained many units that were located in low-income areas. Some of them have been demolished—and others have been gradually converted into units owned by their residents. They remain an important source of housing for low-income persons.

Asset-Creating Programs

People not only need current income to meet their basic needs, but they need *assets*, that is, backup resources for when they face adversities, such as loss of work or uninsured medical costs; want education for themselves or family members; want to care for parents and relatives; or want to purchase homes. They can use assets as collateral to obtain loans or mortgages. Assets allow people to take risks, such as leaving a specific job to find a better one. Low- and moderate-income persons usually have no or few assets as compared to more affluent persons, making them less able to meet these contingencies. (See Table 9.7 for advocacy groups that help members of vulnerable populations obtain assets.)

Table 9.7   Advocacy Groups That Enhance Asset Creation by Vulnerable Populations

The **American Association of Retired Persons (AARP)** advocates maintaining Social Security. However, some critics view the organization as being excessively accommodating to groups that favor benefit cuts.

The **National Academy of Social Insurance (NASI)** seeks to retain the benefits of Social Security by expanding taxes on employers and employees.

The **National Committee to Preserve Social Security and Medicare** has assumed a leading role in fighting efforts to privatize Social Security and Medicare.

The **Center for Enterprise Development (CFED)** engages in policy advocacy at the federal, state, and local levels to enable low-income families to increase their savings, start businesses, attend college, obtain health insurance, and increase economic mobility.

Social Security and Private Pensions

Many people need economic assistance after they retire because they no longer receive their work-related income. Moreover, many elderly persons retire with no assets, such as homes, and in debt.

Social Security is not a generous program. It replaces, on average, roughly 40% of workers' earnings before they retired, with an average benefit of $12,530 in 2007. The United States ranks low among 30 nations with advanced economies in the generosity of its public pensions. Even with its modest payments, it keeps 20 million Americans out of poverty. (Roughly half of retirees have no assets, including houses, when they retire—and they often have credit card and other kinds of debt.) Social Security helps stabilize the American economy by giving people spendable resources. It provided benefits to 55 million persons in 2012.

Social security has become even more important because seniors have found that two other sources of income during retirement have become less reliable: employer-funded pensions and personal savings. Many employers have cut back or eliminated their contributions to employees' private pension plans, such as 401(k) or 403(b) plans, without paying taxes on these savings until employees receive them in annual payments after they retire. (Relatively affluent workers disproportionately receive private pensions, because their employers are more likely than employers of less affluent workers to match their contributions.)

Many conservatives say they want to save Social Security from bankruptcy by cutting its benefits, but many people argue that its benefits should be expanded (Hiltzik, 2012). Benefits are "indexed" annually for inflation, but not sufficiently to reflect seniors' actual living costs, such as medical care and the goods and services they consume. Social Security's formula for computing benefits discriminates against women because they currently spend only an average of 27 years in the labor force due to their caregiving with children, disabled family members, and parents. (Benefits are calculated on the best-paid 35 years of workers' working lives.) Terry O'Neill, president of the National Organization of Women, wants a "caregiver credit" for women where Social Security would count caregiver years at a value equivalent to half the median wage for full-time work, which is $41,000 (Hiltzik, 2012).

Benefits might be expanded and the solvency of the Trust Fund protected, some contend, if the payroll tax were expanded to include *all* of workers' income rather than only their income to the current cap of $110,000.

Survivors' Benefits

Benefits for survivors of Social Security beneficiaries were added to Social Security in the 1950s and 1960s. The following persons receive specific percentages of the benefit amounts of deceased workers, up to a family limit of 150% to 180% of the basic benefit rate:

- Widows or widowers can receive 100% at full retirement age or older.
- Widows or widowers can receive 71.5% to 99% of the deceased worker's basic amount at age 60.
- Disabled widows or widowers, aged 50 through 59, receive 71.5%.
- Widows or widowers of any age who care for a child under age 16 receive 75%.
- Children under age 18 (or up to age 19 if they are still in elementary or secondary school) or disabled receive 71%.
- Dependent parent(s) of the deceased worker, if age 62 or older, receive 82.5% (for one surviving parent) or 75% each (for two surviving parents).

The survivors' benefits for children should be expanded to cover part or all of their college tuition costs, which *had* been added to their benefits in 1965 by Congress through age 21, but were removed by President Reagan in a cost-cutting move in 1981. This benefit would pay for itself, because college graduates pay far higher payroll taxes than nongraduates, as they earn 60% to 70% higher wages than high school graduates (Hiltzik, 2012).

Home Ownership Programs

HUD has a variety of programs geared toward helping people own their own homes. It provides subsidies to nonprofit agencies to construct homes to be purchased by low- and moderate-income persons. The Federal Housing Agency (FHA), Fannie Mae, and Freddie Mac issue many of the nation's mortgages along with private banks. The federal government has several programs geared toward helping people who are "under water" (whose mortgages exceed the market value of their homes) to avoid foreclosure, even if they have been relatively ineffective.

Individual Development Accounts (IDAs)

We have discussed how low-income people often lack assets, such as houses and savings accounts that they can invest or use as economic backups. IDAs are savings accounts where people receive an additional deposit, called a match, every time they place their own funds in them. These plans are usually sponsored by nonprofit agencies that recruit members and offer them financial counseling. They target low-income populations to help them obtain resources to purchase houses, send children to college, and make other personal investments. The Personal Responsibility and Work Opportunity Reconciliation Act of 1996 authorized states to fund IDAs with the use of federal grants. The location of IDAs in specific jurisdictions can be discovered at the website of the nonprofit Corporation for Enterprise Development (CFED; cfed.org) by clicking on "Find an IDA Program Near You!"

UNDERSTANDING HOW SEVEN CORE PROBLEMS EXIST IN THE SAFETY-NET SECTOR

Core Problem 1: Engaging in Advocacy to Protect People's Ethical Rights, Human Rights, and Economic Justice—With Some Red Flag Alerts

- **Red Flag Alert 9.1.** A client is not getting his basic needs met and has not applied to programs for which he may qualify.
- **Red Flag Alert 9.2.** A decision by a local, state, or federal official appears incorrect or discriminatory.
- **Red Flag Alert 9.3.** A client believes she has been discriminated against on the basis of gender, race, disability, age, or any other personal characteristic.
- **Red Flag Alert 9.4.** An applicant to a safety-net program believes that intake or service staff have inadequate information or are making erroneous decisions.
- **Red Flag Alert 9.5.** A client is confused about how to obtain legal assistance.
- **Red Flag Alert 9.6.** A client needs specialized advocacy.

Many people do not apply to specific safety-net programs that might help them meet their basic needs. They may be unaware of the programs. They may falsely believe they do not qualify. They may believe they will be stigmatized as others learn about their enrollment—not realizing that many safety-net programs require them to maintain strict confidentiality. They may not know where to go. They may fear they cannot fill out forms because they have limited literacy or because they speak another language. They may fear they cannot locate needed pay stubs and the many documents that need to be assembled. They may fear they will have to wait for many weeks to receive benefits or services due to bureaucratic delays. These nonenrolled persons and families sacrifice billions of dollars of income and nutrition in aggregate.

Social workers should sometimes consider macro policy interventions. Perhaps application procedures for specific programs can be simplified to make them more consumer friendly. Perhaps long waits can be shortened. Perhaps brief videos can be developed to educate people about how to apply for a program.

Specific appeal procedures are defined for each safety-net program. Clients should be encouraged to file appeals whenever they believe that they have not received benefits or services to which they have been entitled. They should be encouraged to file appeals when they believe that staff have discriminated against them. Social workers engage in micro advocacy when they inform applicants that they have a right to request a hearing to appeal a specific decision. They may get a favorable decision by an agency *just* by asking for a hearing. Applicants should insist on a hearing even when told it will be fruitless. They should retain all documents and obtain copies of documents they receive or bring. They have a right to see relevant statutes and regulations. They should keep good records. They have a right to see their case file and to copy any documents from it. People who believe they have been treated unfairly because they are disabled or have health problems can send a letter to the Civil Rights Division of the Department of Justice, PO Box 66118, Washington, DC 20035-6118. In the case of TANF, applicants should complain to their worker's supervisor when they are not satisfied with any decision or call the helpline for their welfare office. If this fails, they should ask to speak to the deputy director and then the director of their welfare office. If they are still dissatisfied, they should file for a fair hearing by writing to the appeals office in their region or by calling a designated toll-free number, possibly seeking assistance from an advocate, legal aid, local government official, or local legislator. (The request for a fair hearing should take place before the date that their benefits will be reduced or stopped, as explained in a special notice that the public agency is required to send to them that explains why the action was taken and when it will occur.) The state sends a notice to the applicant that tells them when the hearing will occur and where, usually in three or four weeks—but the applicant can request a delay to prepare for it. An appeals hearing specialist is assigned to the case to represent the public agency's position. Hearings for disabled or homebound people can be held by phone if requested. An applicant can file a lawsuit to contest rulings at these hearings. Applicants can get free legal help from federally funded legal aid programs if their income roughly qualifies them for TANF.

Social workers can help people appeal decisions or obtain information from supervisors. Applicants to safety-net programs should ask to talk with supervisors when they believe that intake or service staff have inadequate information or are making erroneous decisions.

Advocates can also help people obtain legal and related assistance. Legal aid programs provide invaluable assistance to social workers and clients who want to know if they have been wrongly denied benefits or services from safety-net programs, such as the state programs that implement TANF. An inquiry from an attorney may lead eligibility and other public personnel to reconsider their decisions.

Social workers may refer people to specialized advocacy groups. In many cases, they can refer specific clients to nonprofit advocacy organizations that specialize in income, housing, nutrition, and other human needs in their communities. Not only will the staff be familiar with existing eligibility and service policies, but they may act as intermediaries with specific public organizations. In Los Angeles County, for example, these organizations include the Bus Riders Union, California Food Policy Advocates, the California Partnership, the Coalition for Humane Immigrant Rights of Los Angeles, the Community Coalition, Hunger Action LA, the L.A. Alliance for a New Economy, the L.A. Community Action Network, the Legal Aid Foundation of Los Angeles, the Maternal and Child Health Access Project, and Neighborhood Legal Services of Los Angeles.

Social workers engage in policy advocacy in a polarized context as they seek to raise the eligibility and benefit levels for many safety-net programs. An important question to consider is, does social justice require expansion of these levels in a society with marked economic inequality?

Barriers

Widespread animus in the United States toward people who need or use many safety-net programs makes it difficult to obtain sufficient resources, shelter, and benefits for low- and moderate-income persons. Current policies are sometimes punitive in nature, such as federal laws that preclude people with prison records from using TANF—even women exiting prison for minor drug offenses who must house, feed, and cloth their children. Some staff in local welfare offices are themselves hostile to their clients. It is difficult for many people to understand the complex rules and accounting procedures of safety-net programs such as TANF.

Many Americans believe that poor people turn to safety-net programs unnecessarily, sometimes using words like *lazy*, *immoral*, *welfare queens*, and *parasites* to describe them. Develop your own position with respect to Policy Advocacy Learning Challenge 9.2.

POLICY ADVOCACY LEARNING CHALLENGE 9.2

Connecting Micro, Mezzo, and Macro Policy Advocacy

Do the Math to Decide What a Family Needs to Survive

Some contend that eligibility levels for many safety-net programs are excessively high, allowing people to gain benefits from them when they do not truly need them. Using the Internet, find the eligibility level of the food stamps program (now called SNAP) for a single mother with two dependent children. The eligibility level of TANF varies by state. Find the eligibility level for your state on the Internet for a mother with two children.

Determine likely expenditures for the single mother and her two dependent children, including rent, living expenses like utilities and heat, food, transportation, clothing, necessary personal items, entertainment, medical and dental expenses, and miscellaneous expenditures. Use your personal experience to make your estimates.

Compare the eligibility level of SNAP and TANF with your calculations. Are they excessively high? Compare the actual benefits this woman and her children would receive under SNAP and TANF. Are they excessively high?

Now assume that the mother finds work at the minimum wage in your state (i.e., the federal minimum wage or the minimum wage established by your state, whichever is higher; find these figures on the Internet). Her working hours are from 8 a.m. to 5 p.m. with one hour's release time for lunch. Assume she has to travel 15 miles to get to work, or 30 miles round trip. Assume she has to use childcare for both children from 3 p.m. (when preschool ends) to 5:45 (when she returns from work). Select a probable rent level for this woman and her family in a relatively safe neighborhood. Would SNAP and TANF suffice to meet the family's expenses?

Where do you position yourself in the debate about whether safety-net programs are excessively generous or punitive? Would you support or oppose political candidates who want to markedly cut or markedly increase the eligibility levels and benefits of SNAP?

Core Problem 2: Engaging in Advocacy to Promote the Quality of Safety-Net Programs—With a Red Flag Alert

- **Red Flag Alert 9.7.** Members of low-income and other vulnerable populations need benefits from one or more safety-net programs, yet they lack personal knowledge of them.
- **Red Flag Alert 9.8.** A client fails to complete an application for a safety-net program.
- **Red Flag Alert 9.9.** A client in an urgent situation (as well as the agency staff member she has consulted) is unaware of circumstantial exceptions in a safety-net program that will allow her to obtain benefits she would otherwise be ineligible for.
- **Red Flag Alert 9.10.** A client depending on a certain safety-net program fails to renew his eligibility.
- **Red Flag Alert 9.11.** A client benefiting from one safety-net program fails to apply to complementary safety-net programs for which he is eligible.

Social workers should routinely conduct assessments of their clients' need for the benefits and services of safety-net programs to which they may be entitled. They can hand them, for example, a list of safety-net programs with their rough income or other eligibility requirements clearly stated—and ask them to identify which ones might help them meet their basic needs. They can provide them with handouts about relevant programs or give them (if they are computer savvy) websites to locate relevant information. When specific clients urgently need specific benefits and services, they can monitor their progress in seeking and obtaining them.

Social workers should participate in local publicity campaigns in liaison with the mass media so that people learn about specific safety-net programs—possibly in collaboration with state or federal campaigns, such as those publicizing WIC or SNAP. (See Policy Advocacy Learning Challenge 9.3.)

POLICY ADVOCACY LEARNING CHALLENGE 9.3

Connecting Micro, Mezzo, and Macro Policy Advocacy

Initiating a Community Outreach Campaign

A social worker was worried because many of her clients from low- and moderate-income families were not using SNAP, to the detriment of their food intake as well as their family finances. She discovered a tendency of many of them to curtail food expenses, such as by organizing their meals around low-cost items like macaroni and cheese instead of eating vegetables, fish, fruit, chicken, and low-fat meat. She discovered on a website established by the Food and Nutrition Service of the U.S. Department of Agriculture (FNS) that federal officials welcomed collaboration with state and local agencies, advocates, employers, and community- and faith-based organizations in reaching out to eligible low-income people *not* using SNAP. Go to their website at www.fns.usda.gov/snap/outreach/ and develop some ideas for an outreach strategy in your local area or region.

Many people fail to complete the application process for specific safety-net programs. They may disagree with a staff person about certain conditions. They may lack important documents. They may not understand the staff worker. They may believe that they have an emergency that will not be addressed by bureaucratic procedures that don't allow them to obtain SNAP, TANF, Medicaid, or other benefits for weeks or even months. Or they may become frustrated with the laborious application process and leave. Social workers should coach clients prior to their visits, such as highlighting situations where they could ask to see a supervisor, ask for a translator, and ask permission to bring certain documents at a later date but without delaying the likely date they will receive benefits.

Applicants to some safety-net programs are unaware that specific *exceptions* exist in the regulations, depending on the circumstances of the applicant. For

TANF, for example, individuals may be able to obtain cash immediately when they are being evicted from an apartment, when they are subject to intimate partner violence, and when they have specific medical needs. Agency staff may not understand these exceptions or may direct an applicant elsewhere. An applicant may have to talk with a supervisor or call legal aid if they persist in failing to honor exceptions.

Many people who use safety-net programs fail to renew their eligibility. Perhaps they have changed locations or jobs and wrongly believe that it will be difficult to renew their services or benefits. Perhaps they had bad experiences when they applied on a prior occasion, such as long waits in an office, hostile treatment from staff, or long waits to obtain benefits or services. Micro advocates need to help these individuals understand that, by not renewing their eligibility, they may cause themselves or their families harm, such as poorer nutrition, lack of needed resources, and evictions that could have been forestalled if they'd had additional funds to pay rent. Advocates can work with public agencies to make it less difficult to reapply for specific benefits or services. People who have already qualified on one or more prior occasions might receive, for example, expedited service, simpler application forms, and mail-in options.

Many people do not apply for *complementary* programs. Someone who receives TANF may be eligible for Medicaid, SNAP, housing assistance, temporary shelter, rent subsidies, help with the cost of moving, special payments for evictions, extra money for higher food costs due to a medical condition or breastfeeding, welfare-to-work services like counseling and job training, additional funds for pregnancy, a monetary bonus for being a woman who receives child support, and a higher payment for children who qualify for foster care payments. People who use combinations of programs improve their economic condition more dramatically than those who use only single programs. Social workers should ask agencies to inform their clients of complementary programs for which they are eligible and give them fact sheets, referrals, and other assistance to use them. A macro advocate could attempt to promote formal linkages between these programs at higher levels of administration by asking them to form partnerships of outreach in communities with large numbers of poor people.

Core Problem 3: Engaging in Advocacy to Promote Culturally Competent Safety-Net Programs—With Some Red Flag Alerts

- **Red Flag Alert 9.12.** Clients are denied benefits or services based on the discriminatory actions of service personnel, even though civil rights statutes and regulations at federal, state, and local levels of government protect people who use safety-net programs from discrimination.

- **Red Flag Alert 9.13.** People with limited English proficiency are not given translation services under Title VI of the 1964 federal Civil Rights Act, which declares that "no persons in the United States shall, on the ground of race, color, or national origin, be excluded from participation in, be denied the benefits of, or be subjected to discrimination under any program or activity receiving financial assistance."
- **Red Flag Alert 9.14.** People with disabilities are not given special assistance in filling out forms, gaining access to offices, obtaining forms, or using benefits or services, even though the Americans with Disabilities Act (ADA), as well as other federal, local and state legislation, requires that they be given this assistance.
- **Red Flag Alert 9.15.** The cultural preferences of certain individuals are not heeded in the provision of services and benefits in specific safety-net programs. (The federally funded school breakfast and lunch programs, as well as WIC, have increasingly honored the food preferences of people from specific ethnic groups.)

Core Problem 4: Engaging in Advocacy to Promote Preventive Safety-Net Programs—With Some Red Flag Alerts

- **Red Flag Alert 9.16.** A single head of household manages to hold three part-time jobs to support her two children, including funding their childcare, medical bills, dentist bills, and survival needs. When she loses one of the jobs and her income plummets, she can no longer fund an adequate diet for her children and has to foreclose on her house. Even though SNAP helps her, her remaining income disqualifies her from TANF—and she cannot receive unemployment insurance because she still holds two part-time jobs. When the bank moves aggressively to evict her from her home, she loses her shelter—and the family resorts to living in their car.
- **Red Flag Alert 9.17.** It is obvious that a particular safety-net program creates dependency and needs to be reformed.

Social workers need skills in predicting when individuals and families are likely to experience adverse cascading events. Low-income families and single heads of households are particularly vulnerable to *adverse cascading events* that precipitate a downward cycle. Advocates may arrest adverse cascading events by helping clients obtain job training and placement services, gain eligibility for one or more safety-net programs, find (and keep) affordable housing, avoid foreclosure, find shelter if they are homeless, improve their management of personal finances, and find social and mental health services for depression and anxiety.

Some safety-net programs foster excessive dependency and need to be reformed. TANF creates excessive dependency when it fails to provide effective job training and childcare services to recipients—benefits that have been cut by many states due to deficits arising in the Great Recession and beyond. Social Security encourages people to leave the workforce prematurely and at great cost to the broader society (see Policy Advocacy Learning Challenge 9.4).

POLICY ADVOCACY LEARNING CHALLENGE 9.4

Connecting Micro, Mezzo, and Macro Policy Advocacy

Reforming SSDI to Encourage Work

Even as the health of the American population has markedly improved since 1990, annual SSDI disability payments to Social Security recipients have increased from roughly $200 billion to more than $700 billion—or from 10% to 18% of total Social Security benefits (Porter, 2012). This change partly occurred because Congress relaxed eligibility criteria by giving more weight to subjective factors like pain, anxiety, back pain, and other muscular problems as compared to traditional medical diagnoses. Rejected applicants were allowed to appeal before administrative judges—and 50% to 60% of them were successful.

Many SSDI recipients are relatively young people who are harmed by leaving the workforce prematurely. Policy advocates should seek reforms that help workers stay in the workforce. They could avoid the current either/or situation by allowing workers to apply for SSDI benefits while still working to encourage them to take less demanding jobs at lower wages. They could penalize employers who send many workers into disability programs by asking them to pay more into the system. They could increase EITC payments to adults with no dependents to encourage disabled people to work. They could seek job training to help disabled people obtain positions that require less physical effort.

Core Problem 5: Engaging in Advocacy to Promote Affordable and Accessible Safety-Net Programs—With a Red Flag Alert

- **Red Flag Alert 9.18.** People who use safety-net programs must endure significant nonmonetary costs.

Many safety-net programs impose excessive nonmonetary costs on persons who use them, such as long waits for Section-8 subsidized rental housing, public housing, SSI, SSDI, and TANF as well as excessively complex applications. Policy advocates should seek to diminish these nonmonetary costs. They should also work to reduce fees and deductibles associated with many other public programs.

Core Problem 6: Engaging in Advocacy for Services to Help Reduce the Mental Distress of Consumers Using Safety-Net Programs—With a Red Flag Alert

- **Red Flag Alert 9.19.** People who use many safety-net programs experience disproportionate levels of health and mental health problems, whether because they are often poverty stricken or because they experience cascading adverse events (Barr, 2008).

The 2005/2006 National Health Interview Survey discovered that "anywhere from 10 to 40 percent of TANF recipients have a disability and almost one-fifth have a family member with a disability"—and SNAP recipients have similar disability rates (Loprest & Maag, 2009). Residents of public housing often have unaddressed mental health, substance abuse, and other problems. Safety-net programs should hire staff or contract with mental health agencies who can screen enrollees and provide mental health assistance to those who need it.

POLICY ADVOCACY LEARNING CHALLENGE 9.5

Connecting Micro, Mezzo, and Macro Policy Advocacy

Advocacy to Promote Mental Health for TANF Recipients

Discuss how a social worker might engage in micro policy advocacy to obtain mental health or substance abuse services for a specific TANF recipient. How might she use mezzo policy advocacy to place mental health services within TANF offices or offices that take applications for SNAP? How might she use macro policy advocacy to change local or state TANF regulations related to specialized services for recipients with mental health or substance abuse challenges?

Core Problem 7: Engaging in Advocacy to Link Safety-Net Programs to Communities—With a Red Flag Alert

- **Red Flag Alert 9.20.** Safety-net programs distribute benefits and services to applicants without analyzing *why* they make disproportionate use of their benefits and services in specific communities. Nor do staff in safety-net programs work in tandem to improve economic and social conditions in these communities.

"THINKING BIG" AS POLICY ADVOCATES IN THE SAFETY-NET SECTOR

With renewed interest in the sheer level of economic inequality in the United States in the aftermath of the Great Recession, new impetus for reforms of safety-net programs has developed—and could come to fruition if congressional gridlock abates. For the first time in decades, public interest in reducing economic inequality has increased. Discuss the following reforms:

1. Marked expansion of eligibility and benefits for SNAP and many other safety-net programs (select one of them for particular emphasis)

2. Replacing TANF with a national guaranteed income that places an economic floor under all citizens

3. Marked increase of taxes on affluent Americans—and use of these funds to buttress safety-net programs or to fund a national guaranteed income

4. Establishment of a public jobs program that guarantees work for people who are unemployed long term, placing particular priority on younger persons

LEARNING OUTCOMES

You are now equipped to:

- Identify an array of safety-net programs that are needed by vulnerable populations
- Analyze how these safety-net programs began and evolved in the United States
- Place these safety-net programs in the American cultural and political context
- State the strengths and weaknesses of specific safety-net programs after critically analyzing them
- Describe possible micro, mezzo, and macro policy advocacy initiatives in the safety-net sector that might help consumers of service
- Identify and discuss policy reforms in the safety-net system

REFERENCES

Alvarez, L. (2012, April 18). No savings are found from welfare drug tests. *New York Times*, p. A14.
Barr, D. (2008). *Disparities in the United States: Social class, race and ethnicity.* Baltimore, MD: Johns Hopkins University Press.
Ben-Shalom, Y., Moffitt, R. A., & Scholz, J. K. (2011). *An assessment of the effectiveness of anti-poverty programs in the United States* (No. w17042). National Bureau of Economic Research.

Coleman-Jensen, A., Nord, M., Andrews, M., & Carlson, S. (2010). *Household food security in the United States in 2010* (ERR-125). U.S. Department of Agriculture. Retrieved January 10, 2013, from http://www.ers.usda.gov/Publications/err125/

Corn, D. (2013, March 4). Mitt Romney's "twisted" defense of his 47 percent rant. *Mother Jones*. Retrieved from http://www.motherjones.com/mojo/2013/03/mitt-romneys-twisted-defense -his-47-percent-rant

DeParle, J. (2012, April 7). Welfare limits left poor adrift as recession hit. *New York Times*, p. 1.

Greenstein, R. (2012, April 17). *Testimony before the House Budget Committee hearing on strengthening the safety net*. Center on Budget and Policy Priorities. Retrieved January 10, 2013, from http://www.cbpp.org/cms/index.cfm?fa=view&id=3745.

Grogger, J. (2003). The effects of time limits, the EITC, and other policy changes on welfare use, work, and income among female-headed families. *Review of Economics and Statistics, 85*(2), 394–408.

Hiltzik, M. (2012, April 25). Let's *expand* social security benefits. *Los Angeles Times*, pp. B1, B5.

Loprest, P., & Maag, E. (2009, May). *Disabilities among TANF recipients: Evidence from NHIS*. Urban Institute.

Los Angeles Coalition to End Hunger and Homelessness. (2010). *The people's guide to welfare, health, and other services* (33rd ed.). Retrieved January 10, 2013, from http://cfpa.net/ LosAngeles/ExternalPublications/LACEHH-PeoplesGuideEnglish-2010.pdf

Macvean, M. (2009, December 12). California students underutilize School Breakfast Program. *Los Angeles Times*. Retrieved January 10, 2013, from www.latimes.com

Marr, C., & Huang, C. (2012). *Misconceptions and realities about who pays taxes*. Center on Budget and Policy Priorities. Retrieved January 10, 2013, from http://www.cbpp .org/cms/index.cfm?fa=view&id=3505

Mataconis, D. (2014, December 8). 11th Circuit strikes down Floriday law mandating drug tests for welfare recipients. *Outside the Beltway*. Retrieved from http://www.outsidethebeltway .com/11th-circuit-strikes-down-florida-law-mandating-drug-tests-for-welfare-recipients/

O'Connor, K. (2011, March 3). Sen. John Kerry proposes tax relief to low-income families. *Herald News*. Retrieved January 10, 2013, from http://www.heraldnews.com/news /x1174965957/Sen-John-Kerry-proposes-tax-relief-to-low-income-families

Office of the Inspector General. (2010). *Social Security Administration: Disability impair-ments on cases most frequently denied by disability determination services and subse-quently allowed by administrative law judges*. Retrieved January 10, 2013, from http://oig.ssa.gov/disability-impairments-cases-most-frequently-denied-disability-determi nation-services-and

Porter, E. (2012, April 25). Disability insurance causes pain. *New York Times*, pp. B1, B10.

Price, D. (2011). *Off the charts: Hardship in America: Part 3. homelessness growing among families with children*. Center on Budget and Policy Priorities.

Sherman, A. (2011, October 13). The 2009 Recovery Act—Even better in preventing poverty than we thought. *Off the Charts Blog*. Center on Budget and Policy Priorities. Retrieved January 10, 2013, from http://www.offthechartsblog.org/the-2009-recovery-act-—-even-better-in -preventing-poverty-than-we-thought/

U.S. Department of Education. (2012). *Investing in America's future: A blueprint for transforming career and technical education.* Retrieved April 30, 2012, from http://www2.ed.gov/about/offices/list/ovae/pi/cte/transforming-career-technical-education.pdf

Wicks-Lim, J. (2009). Should we be talking about living wages now? *Monthly Review Press.* Retrieved January 10, 2013, from http://www.peri.umass.edu/fileadmin/pdf/other_publication _types/magazine___journal_articles/0309wicks-lim.pdf

Williams, E., & Johnson, N. (2010). *How much would a state earned income tax credit cost in fiscal year 2012?* Center on Budget and Policy Priorities. Retrieved January 10, 2013, from http://www.cbpp.org/files/11-12-09sfp.pdf

Zedlewski, S., Holcomb, P., & Loprest, P. (2007). *Hard-to-employ parents: A review of their characteristics and the programs designed to serve their needs* (Low-Income Working Families, Paper 9). Urban Institute.

Chapter 10

BECOMING POLICY ADVOCATES IN THE MENTAL HEALTH SECTOR

Bruce S. Jansson, Judith A. DeBonis, and Eri Nakagami

LEARNING OBJECTIVES

In this chapter, you will learn about:

1. The evolution of the mental health sector in the United States

2. The sheer magnitude of mental disorders in the United States

3. Effects of income inequality on mental health

4. The political economy of mental health services

5. Ways to engage in micro, mezzo, and macro policy advocacy to redress seven core recurring problems in the mental health sector

6. How to apply the eight challenges in the multilevel policy advocacy framework

The severity of mental health symptoms and mental disorders, like that of other medical illnesses, can fall along a continuum ranging from "normal" to severe; some of the most severe and persistent mental disorders include major depression, schizophrenia, bipolar disorder, and posttraumatic stress disorder. Even with treatment, people with mental disorders often experience distress, disability, death or the loss of freedom as a direct result of their condition (Morrison, 1995). Mental health services help people with a wide array of mental trauma, mental illnesses, and mental distress. Historically, mental health services have been greatly underfunded in the United States. Social workers assume a major role in these services and can improve services for millions of people through policy advocacy.

ANALYZING THE EVOLUTION
OF THE MENTAL HEALTH SECTOR

▶

VIDEO LINK 10.1
Advocacy for
Persons With
Mental Illness

Grob (1994, 2008) points out that throughout history, mental health policy goals have been shaped and transformed by the shifting of funding responsibility between the local, state, and federal sectors of government. The following timeline (Figure 10.1) depicts the evolution of the American mental healthcare system from the colonial era to the present:

Figure 10.1 Timeline of the Evolution of the American Mental Healthcare System.

- **Mental illness in colonial times:** Low incidence of mental illness reported; not defined as a medical problem or a matter of social concern. There were no effective treatments; families were responsible for providing care to members unable to work (Deutsch, 1937; Grob, 1973, 1994).
- **By the late 17th century:** As numbers grew, the mentally ill were housed with other dependent populations (the aged, infirm, or criminals) in local workhouses or almshouses (Grob, 1983) or in the basements of early private hospitals (Grob, 1973).
- **The Moral Age**: Progressive communities applied Christian principles and established well-ordered asylums to cure the effects of the outer world (Grob, 1983; Jansson, 2015).
- **The Public Mental Hospital Movement:** In 1848, social reformer Dorothea Dix advocated more humane treatment and state financing for building 95 asylums (Jansson, 2015).
- **By the late 1800s:** Optimism diminished as state hospitals offered custodial care but little hope of cure, and costs for care became the largest piece of the budget; state regulations pressed for a scientific basis for provisions (Deutsch, 1937; Grob, 1983; Mechanic, 1989).
- **The mental hygiene movement: The Progressive Era:** Following institutional care failures, many medical treatments shifted to an outpatient services focus (Grob, 1994). Explorations in neurology and psychiatry, including Freudian insights into the mind, created hope that understanding and cures were possible (Grob, 1983). Treatment innovations became supplements to institutional care rather than a substitute for it; by 1940, admissions to state hospitals increased to 455,000 (Grob, 1973, 1983).
- **The Great Depression, World War I, and World War II:** This era brought increased public awareness that given sufficient stress, anyone could develop psychiatric symptoms (Grob, 1983); America's involvement in wars exposed the need for crisis-oriented and group treatments (Grob, 1973). New laws and the creation of the National Institute of Mental Health (NIMH) provided the impetus for research to develop preventive and therapeutic services (Grob, 1994).
- **The deinstitutionalization movement:** In the early 1940s, public reports of state hospital overcrowding and mistreatment of patients, combined with evidence of the debilitating effects of institutionalization (Grob, 1991), made deinstitutionalization an appealing opportunity to shift costs to the federal government (LaFond & Durham, 1992).
- **The late 1950s:** The introduction and use of antipsychotic drugs in the treatment of the mentally ill was credited with the successful release of large numbers of patients from state hospitals (Deutsch, 1937; Grob, 1994).
- **The liberal era: The Great Society and community mental health:** In 1963, the federal budget allocated to creating community mental health treatment centers (Jansson, 2015; Kennedy, 1990; Kiesler et al., 1983; Koyanagi & Goldman, 1991) resulted in fewer hospitalized patients but failed to produce positive treatment outcomes. By the early

1970s, many former hospital patients had been abandoned to psychiatric ghettos and jails or had become homeless (Dear & Wolch, 1987; LaFond & Durham, 1992).

- **The Carters:** In 1978, the Carter administration increased funding for community-based services and Rosalynn Carter made mental health her major domestic issue (Grob, 2005; Jansson, 2015) in response to sharp criticism of care provided for serious mental illness (Koyanagi & Goldman, 1991). Unfortunately, funding was inadequate to implement real reform (Jansson, 2015).
- **The Neoconservative Era:** Between 1980 and 1993, the Reagan administration relinquished federal responsibility for the mentally ill and slashed state block funding and support of the national institutes (NIAAA, NIDA, and NIMH). States were allowed to ignore mental health issues (Mechanic, 1989), and the numbers of mentally ill who became homeless, incarcerated, or confined to nursing homes increased (Jimenez, 2009). Public outcry and grassroots advocacy and public education efforts were organized by the newly formed National Alliance on Mental Illness (NAMI).
- **Social reform in a polarized context: President Bill Clinton and Vice President Al Gore:** By the 1990s, Medicaid and Medicare became the source of most mental health funding, helping to restore state authority for mental health services policy while the federal government covered more of the costs (Grob, 2008).
- **The Mental Health Parity Act (1996):** This act aimed to improve mental health reimbursement for private insurance recipients (Mental Health America, 2012) but failed to require employers to offer mental health coverage, and many employers dropped coverage completely (Jimenez, 2009).
- **The George W. Bush Era:** The New Freedom Commission on Mental Health (2003) committed to promoting early treatment of mental disabilities and confronting barriers to reform (stigma, treatment limitations, delivery system fragmentation).
- **The Paul Wellstone and Pete Domenici Mental Health Parity and Addiction Equity Act** (2008; Substance Abuse and Mental Health Services Administration, 2012a): This act required that large insurance plans provide parity of coverage for behavioral health. Plans could be exempt from the law if they excluded mental health and substance health coverage and were allowed to retain higher premiums/copays for use of those services (Substance Abuse and Mental Health Services Administration, 2012a).
- **Barack Obama and the "audacity of hope":** The Affordable Care Act (ACA) was signed into law in 2010, expanding coverage to 32 million uninsured Americans. The ACA reformed the parity law to integrate the care and managing of physical health and mental health conditions and disorders, as well as requiring them to be equally funded in the hope of lessening or removing the historic barriers (U.S. Department of Health and Human Services, 2011).

Table 10.1   Some Advocacy Groups for Individuals With Mental Health or Substance Use Disorders

The **American Psychiatric Association** (APA) is a leading advocate for mental health services. **www .psychiatry.org**

The **American Psychological Association** (APA) adopts a variety of policy statements. **www.apa.org**

The **National Alliance on Mental Illness** (NAMI) mobilizes people with mental illness to improve mental health services. **www.nami.org**

Table 10.1   (Continued)

The **National Council for Behavioral Health** (NCBH) is a leading advocate for improved mental health services. **www.thenationalcouncil.org**

The **National Association of Social Workers** (NASW) injects social workers' policy preferences into public arenas. **www.socialworkers.org**

UNDERSTANDING THE PREVALENCE OF MENTAL HEALTH DISORDERS

Reports of the prevalence of mental disorders in the United States raise our awareness about how common mental illness is and how likely we are to personally experience it or to have it impact people we know and care about (Carter, Golant, & Kade, 2010). In the following box, we present statistics about mental illness that highlight the need for social workers to serve as advocates for people with mental disorders:

MENTAL HEALTH IN AMERICA AT A GLANCE

- In any given year, approximately 57.7 million Americans will experience a mental disorder.
- One in 17 people lives with a serious mental illness (Shirk, 2008).
- There are 2.4 million Americans, or 1.1% of the adult population, living with schizophrenia (National Institute of Mental Health, n.d.).
- More than 350 million people worldwide are living with depression (World Health Organization, 2012).
- Anxiety disorders, such as panic disorder, obsessive-compulsive disorder, posttraumatic stress disorder, generalized anxiety disorder, and phobias, affect an estimated 40 million individuals (or 18.7% of adults; National Institute of Mental Health, n.d.).
- Among adults diagnosed with a mental illness, 20% or 9.2 million are diagnosed with substance dependence or abuse (Substance Abuse and Mental Health Services Administration, 2012b).
- Thirty percent of those with a combination of conditions will be more likely to use homeless services (Burt, 2001).
- Individuals with serious mental illness are more likely to have a chronic medical condition (Colton & Manderscheid, 2006) and are likely to die 25 years earlier than other Americans, largely due to treatable medical conditions that go untreated (Manderscheid, Druss, & Freeman, 2007).
- More than 90% of those who die by suicide have a diagnosable mental disorder (Centers for Disease Control and Prevention, National Center for Injury Prevention and Control, n.d.; National Institute of Mental Health, n.d.).

- Suicide is the third leading cause of death for people ages 10 to 24, which is the age group that coincides with the onset of mental illness (half of mental disorders are diagnosed by age 14 and three quarters by age 25; Wang et al., 2005).
- In any year, less than one third of adults with a diagnosable mental disorder receive mental health services (U.S. Department of Health and Human Services, 1999).
- In one study, while nearly two thirds of all prison inmates met the criteria for a mental health problem, fewer than half of the inmates had ever received treatment for their problem and one third or fewer had received mental health treatment after admission (James & Glaze, 2006).

ANALYZING THE IMPACT OF INCOME INEQUALITY ON MENTAL HEALTH

The direct and indirect financial costs of mental illness are estimated to be $79 billion in the United States; most of that amount—approximately $63 billion—reflects the loss of productivity as a result of illness (U.S. Department of Health and Human Services, 1999). When combined with national spending for substance abuse treatment, mental health costs totaled $121 billion in 2003, or 7.5% of all health spending—27% for hospital-based services, including inpatient and outpatient care, and 22% for payments to physicians and other professionals (Organization for Economic Co-operation and Development, 2008). The human costs in terms of pain and suffering cannot be calculated. The impact of mental illness on the individual with the disorder and his or her family is devastating.

All people, regardless of age, race, religion, or income, are vulnerable to mental illness. While the exact causes are unknown, most mental illnesses are believed to be brain disorders impacted by both biological and genetic vulnerabilities and environmental stressors (Nuechterlein & Dawson, 1984). Although it is known that mental illnesses are not the result of personal weakness, lack of character, or poor upbringing and cannot be managed with a person's will or determination, many myths associated with mental illness persist, as does universal stigma against people with mental disorders. Despite efforts to educate the public, the enormous stigma associated with mental illness continues to devalue people suffering from the disorders, resulting in discrimination and hopelessness about recovery. This stigma also serves as an obstacle to those who might seek or utilize treatment.

Low-income people have markedly higher rates of anxiety, depression, and many other forms of mental illness than relatively affluent individuals. They die by suicide at higher rates than affluent individuals. Yet they have far poorer access to mental health services than other people, whether medications or counseling. They have higher rates of mental illness that stem from multiple causes. Some researchers contend that stress that is induced by poverty, as well as the turmoil in low-income neighborhoods, causes physiological changes that lead to various kinds of mental illness (Barr, 2008). Low-income people are far more likely than affluent individuals to experience personal danger in their neighborhoods, such as from gangs. Their mental illness is less likely than that of affluent persons to be effectively addressed by mental health services because they have poorer access to counseling and medications. People with chronic health conditions and substance abuse are far more likely to be poor than other people—and these conditions themselves cause depression, anxiety, and other kinds of mental illness (Barr, 2008).

ANALYZING THE POLITICAL ECONOMY OF MENTAL HEALTH

Mental health services have traditionally been viewed as a stepchild of the medical system. Until relatively recently, mental health was given poorer coverage than physical health conditions. Psychiatrists have lower status in the medical profession than surgeons. Primary care physicians, who often have little training in counseling and who often rely excessively on medications, provide most mental health services within the medical system.

Pharmaceutical companies have been highly successful in marketing medications for an array of mental health conditions to physicians as well as consumers. Many experts have wondered whether children and adolescents are overmedicated in the United States for such conditions as attention deficit hyperactivity disorder as well as a variety of mental health conditions on the autism spectrum. Many adults may be overmedicated for a variety of disorders, including sleep problems and anxiety. Yet many medications provide positive benefits.

Mental health services are highly affected by state and local budget shortages. As patients have been deinstitutionalized from mental hospitals, they have often resided on the streets or in substandard neighborhoods because local, state, and federal governments have failed to fund supervised group homes and shared apartments as substitutes. Over 280,000 people with mental conditions are placed in prisons each year, where they seldom receive quality mental health services (Jansson, 2015). Funding by states for mental health services has declined by 30% since the mid-1950s when adjusted for inflation (Jansson, 2015). People who need counseling for substance abuse must often wait for months before they are seen by counselors.

Yet advocacy groups for the mentally ill, as well as prominent people who have experienced mental health problems themselves, have often had surprising success in enacting state and federal legislation, which we discuss subsequently in this chapter. The massacre of children in 2012 at Sandy Hook Elementary School in Newtown, Connecticut, stimulated widespread demands for increased spending on mental health.

ADDRESSING SEVEN CORE PROBLEMS IN THE MENTAL HEALTH SECTOR WITH ADVOCACY

Core Problem 1: Engaging in Advocacy to Promote Ethical Rights, Human Rights, and Economic Justice—With Some Red Flag Alerts

- **Red Flag Alert 10.1.** Ethical features associated with a patient's care are violated because healthcare staff are not aware of the individual's rights to confidentiality, self-determination, informed consent to treatments and medication, accurate information, and safety related to danger to oneself or others.
- **Red Flag Alert 10.2.** Patients experience a lack of empathy from providers because of differences in life experiences, attitudes, personal values, and culture.
- **Red Flag Alert 10.3.** Patients experience negative stereotyping and nontherapeutic attitudes and behavior from providers.
- **Red Flag Alert 10.4.** Patients are misdiagnosed or experience diminished expectations for improvement due to clinicians' negative bias or inaccurate stereotypes, such as the belief that individuals with mental illness are not intelligent and cannot change or that older adults are all frail, ill, or inflexible.
- **Red Flag Alert 10.5.** Patients work with healthcare providers who are not transparent about their lack of clinical expertise in mental health conditions.
- **Red Flag Alert 10.6.** Some patients do not have "conservators" appointed through special court proceedings even though they cannot provide for their basic needs, cannot engage in treatment voluntarily, or engage in hostile or disruptive behaviors at a high level.
- **Red Flag Alert 10.7.** Insufficient numbers of mental health staff exist in specific settings, neighborhoods, regions, or states to help people with mental health or substance use problems.

Background

According to the Code of Ethics of the National Association of Social Workers (NASW; www.naswdc.org/pubs/code/code.asp), mental health consumers have the right to access service, resources, and other needed information; the right to be treated with dignity and respect and as having worth; and the right to self-determination, including the right to refuse treatment. Mental health consumers also have the right to receive care from providers who are competent and committed to them, act responsibly and honestly, acknowledge the importance of human relationships, and act respectfully with regard to lifestyle choices.

Power disparities during treatment can create difficulties for consumers. Mental health providers tend to be placed in the expert role, which creates a power imbalance (McCubbin, 1994; Sullivan, 1992; Ware, Tugenberg, & Dickey, 2004). Tarrier and Barrowclough (2003) affirm that "without an equality and collaboration between those who provide and those who use professional mental health services there is always a risk of paternalism, stigmatization, and coercion" (p. 240).

Contrary to the goal of effective patient–provider partnerships, consumers may be undervalued and underestimated in their capacity to think and speak for themselves. These commonly held negative beliefs, perceptions, and attitudes about people with mental illness can lead providers to a type of "self-fulfilling prophesy" about the potential for the person to participate fully in treatment or to recover (Rosenhan, 1973).

Resources for Advocates

Mental health advocates can draw upon many existing policies to protect patients' ethical rights at the micro level. These include professional ethical values and standards of accreditation agencies that license health professionals.

The Patient Self-Determination Act (PSDA) of 1991 mandated that healthcare facilities receiving Medicare or Medicaid reimbursement inform individuals of their right to engage in treatment decisions (Bradley, Wetle, & Horwitz, 1998). The ability of individuals with mental illness to participate in shared decision-making about treatment choices and goals or to complete advance directives is an important matter for clients, families, and their providers.

Each state has a board of behavioral sciences (BBS) that serves as a consumer protection agency, with the goal of protecting consumers by determining and upholding standards for competent and ethical behavior by the professionals under its jurisdiction. For example, the BBS in California has adopted guidelines that identify the types of violations and range of penalties or disciplinary actions that may be imposed on practitioners. Detailed information about the violations of statutes and regulations under the jurisdiction of the BBS and the appropriate scope of penalties for each violation can be found at http://www.bbs.ca.gov/pdf/publications/dispguid.pdf.

Historically, the lack of mental health awareness and supportive services for the mentally ill has contributed to unnecessary deaths and injuries in hospitals, in prisons, and in the community. Further, community agencies, services, and other professionals who have interactions with people with mental health symptoms or disorders may require additional training and protocol to act in an ethical and safe way.

In 2011, Kelly Thomas, a homeless 37-year-old man with schizophrenia, was beaten to death by two California police officers (Lopez, 2011). While some law enforcement agencies have provided training to their officers and staff so that they can safely and appropriately communicate with people who are homeless or mentally ill, training is not as extensive as the training offered to mental health professionals. In addition, staff may not be able to learn and implement specific techniques and approaches for responding to certain populations in particular settings, such as with people who have psychotic symptoms and are unmedicated and homeless.

Public officials have historically responded to problems or disruption in the community related to mental health by proposing additional laws to enforce mandatory treatment of individuals with mental disorders, particularly in the wake of publicized violent incidents where either the victim or perpetrator is mentally ill. For example, Andrew Goldstein, a 29-year-old man with schizophrenia, pushed Kendra Webdale into a subway train, leading to her death. Reports of Mr. Goldstein's refusal of treatment and medicine noncompliance resulted in Kendra's Law in New York State (1999), which gives judges the authority to mandate that individuals with severe mental illness receive outpatient psychiatric treatment or be subjected to involuntary inpatient state hospitalization. Opponents to involuntary treatment argue that the notion that individuals with mental and substance use disorders are "dangerous" is an exaggerated bias and unsubstantiated fact that has influenced public policy (Stuart & Arboleda-Flórez, 2001). Statistics show that only 3% of violent, incarcerated offenders have committed crimes that are attributable to a primary non-substance-use-related disorder (Stuart & Arboleda-Flórez, 2001) and that individuals diagnosed with a serious mental illness are 14 times more likely to be a victim of a violent crime than to be arrested as the perpetrator of one (Brekke, Prindle, Bae, & Long, 2001).

Conservators are often appointed through special court proceedings for people with mental illness that leads them not to be able to care for their basic needs or leads to disruptive behaviors (Jansson, 2011).

POLICY ADVOCACY LEARNING CHALLENGE 10.1

Connecting Micro, Mezzo,
and Macro Policy Advocacy to Protect Patients' Ethical Rights

The following case story is quoted directly from Barrio and Yamada (2005).

Josie Mora, a 35 year-old woman, was diagnosed with schizophrenia (disorganized type) at the age of 22. Despite large doses of psychotropic medication, Josie exhibited disruptive and bizarre behavior, disorganized speech, inappropriate affect, and daily auditory hallucinations. For example, she called out to people using derogatory language, often falsely accusing them of trying to harm her. At home, she required constant limit setting as she would drink continuous pots of coffee and large amounts of soft drinks unless stopped. During the night she would get up several times to pace and clang pots and pans in the kitchen. As a result, she required ongoing supervision and was unable to participate in any psychiatric rehabilitation program activities offered at the mental health center.

The Mora family lived in the same community since they emigrated from Mexico over thirty years ago. The parents preferred to speak in Spanish, although

(Continued)

(Continued)

they understood and spoke limited English. Josie preferred English, although Spanish was her first language. Josie lived at home and her parents were her primary caretakers. Several adult siblings and other extended family members lived in the same city and participated in Josie's care. Mrs. Mora had not worked outside the home since the onset of Josie's illness. During the day while Mr. Mora was at work, Mrs. Mora relied on a network of family and friends to help her with Josie, particularly whenever Mrs. Mora had her own medical appointments or needed to run certain errands. Eventually, Mr. Mora opted for early retirement from his factory job because he wanted to help his wife with Josie's care.

Both parents always accompanied Josie to her medication management appointments and monthly meetings with a social worker. The Moras took turns sharing the highlights of the month regarding Josie's behavioral outbursts, which generally involved family members, friends, and neighbors. Often they shared certain successful outcomes, like going to the park for a family gathering where Josie was able to tolerate being around many people without causing much disruption. Because of her severe impairment and her extensive need for supervision, on several occasions the social worker gently raised the option of a board-and-care facility or other supervised residential care for Josie. The Moras considered the various options presented, but always expressed their willingness to accept their parental responsibility for Josie's caregiving, and their great "hope" that Josie would get better. The Mora family wanted to raise enough money for a trip to Mexico City. They hoped to take Josie to a special church to receive a holy blessing that would lead to healing and possibly a miracle. Several years later Josie was prescribed a new atypical antipsychotic medication, and with additional rehabilitation she made a substantial improvement in her social functioning. The Moras expressed that this progress was more than they had "hoped" Josie would achieve.

LEARNING EXERCISE

1. How does the social work value of "self-determination" apply to this case example?
2. Does the social worker respect the values of interdependence and the family's sense of hope?
3. What other advocacy actions could a social worker take to protect the patient's ethical rights at the micro, mezzo, and macro levels? For example, do the laws of your state allow judges, under specific circumstances and safeguards, to require specific patients to take antipsychotic medications—and would you agree that this is ethical in these specified circumstances?

Core Problem 2: Engaging in Advocacy to Promote Quality Care—With Some Red Flag Alerts

- **Red Flag Alert 10.8.** Clients receive one eclectic or generic treatment from an agency or practitioner that is used for all clients.
- **Red Flag Alert 10.9.** Clients are treated by practitioners who are not fully trained to implement evidence-based practices (EBPs).
- **Red Flag Alert 10.10.** Clients are offered treatments that are provided by clinicians who do not have access to ongoing supervision or training and thus are not up to date on the empirically supported treatments.
- **Red Flag Alert 10.11.** Clients are treated by clinical staff or at agencies with negative attitudes about EBPs or new interventions.
- **Red Flag Alert 10.12.** Clients are recommended for treatment interventions without attention to their individual preferences.
- **Red Flag Alert 10.13.** Clients are treated with EBPs that have not been adequately researched, such as with specific ethnic/racial populations.
- **Red Flag Alert 10.14.** Social workers' distinctive focus on diagnoses and treatments based on a biopsychosocial model are not sufficiently recognized in settings that rely on EBPs (see Policy Advocacy Learning Challenge 10.2).

Background

As the emphasis on implementing evidence-based practices (EBPs) and empirically supported treatments (ESTs) has gained stronger literature support, mental health providers are expected to choose and implement the best possible services and EBPs that target the client's specific needs and desired health outcomes. Treatments need to be implemented with fidelity (sometimes called adherence or integrity) in order to preserve the components that made the original practice effective.

Despite extensive evidence of EBPs' effectiveness, mental health practitioners and programs often underutilize them with the majority of clients with mental health disorders (Kirk, 1990; Mullen & Bacon, 2000; Weissman & Sanderson, 2001). This often results from lack of training in the EBP process, insufficient provider education on implementing specific ESTs, limited resources, lack of support for EBPs in community practice settings (Bellamy, Bledsoe, Mullen, Fang, & Manuel, 2008; Bledsoe et al., 2007; Brekke, Ell, & Palinkas, 2007), lack of reimbursement from Medicaid and other health insurance (Ganju, 2003), competing organizational demands, insufficient length of client visits or number of sessions, excessive reliance on existing treatments (Cohen et al., 2008), and inadequate preparation to interpret research findings (Bellamy et al., 2008; Murray, 2009).

It must be acknowledged that considerable controversy exists about the science of mental health. Some mental health experts questioned the validity of some diagnostic information provided in the fourth edition of the *Diagnostic and Statistical Manual of Mental Disorders*. Bryan King, director of the Seattle Children's Autism Center, who served on the task force of the American Psychiatric Association, influenced the decision in the fifth edition of this manual to eliminate many autism spectrum diagnoses such as Asperger's syndrome, pervasive developmental disorder, and childhood disintegrative disorder and to consolidate them in a single diagnosis of autism spectrum disorder. It must also be acknowledged that some medications produce side effects that offset their positive effects for some patients, including recently developed antipsychotic medications. It is often difficult to diagnose patients with borderline or multiple conditions.

Resources for Advocates

Current CSWE Educational Policy and Accreditation Standards (EPAs; Council on Social Work Education [CSWE], 2008) have established 10 professional social work competencies that specify that social workers in accredited MSW programs learn to use research to inform practice and their practice to inform research (e.g., EPA 2.1.6; CSWE, 2011). Despite this preparatory educational training, social work practitioners may have had little opportunity to gain experience in translating research to practice or may lack confidence in translating research findings.

Table 10.2 Websites That Provide Evidence-Based Practices for Mental Health and Substance Abuse

1. SAMHSA: A Guide to Evidence-Based Practices (EBP) (http://www.samhsa.gov/ebp -web-guide):
   Information and research on specific evidence-based practices for prevention and treatment of mental and substance use disorders.

2. National Guideline Clearinghouse™ (NGC) (www.guideline.gov).

3. Suicide Prevention Research Center: Best Practice Registry (http://www.sprc.org/ featured_resources/bpr/index.asp): Information about best practices that address the specific objectives of the *National Strategy for Suicide Prevention*.

4. *Diagnostic and Statistical Manual of Mental Disorders*, 5th edition (www.dsm5.org).

POLICY ADVOCACY LEARNING CHALLENGE 10.2

Connecting Micro, Mezzo, and Macro Policy Advocacy to Advance Quality of Care

Adams, LeCroy, and Matto (2009) believe that social workers do not share the medical model philosophy of treatment (focusing on symptoms and diseases) that typically underlies an EBP model because it may not reflect a sufficient focus on the individual and environmental factors that social workers view as essential to quality care. Consider an example of a discouraged and caring family who presents in treatment with a family member who has previously been diagnosed and treated for major depressive disorder and despite treatment motivation and adherence is currently so seriously depressed that he or she is unable to work or care for personal daily needs. The potential complexity in the case may not fit neatly into an EBP model.

LEARNING EXERCISE

Discuss the following questions posed by Adams, LeCroy, and Matto (2009):

1. How would a social work frame of reference—which includes the biopsychosocial model; the developmental stage of the person; cultural, spiritual and community factors; and the ecosystems context—assess and choose an EBP?
2. How might a social work frame of reference impact the assessment and treatment planning for this case?
3. How does the social work emphasis on the alliance or therapeutic relationship get incorporated into the treatment response?
4. What mezzo and macro policy advocacy interventions might social workers consider in these circumstances?

Core Problem 3: Engaging in Advocacy to Promote Culturally Competent Care—With Some Red Flag Alerts

- **Red Flag Alert 10.15.** A diagnosis of a mental health disorder is made based on the presentation of one or more symptoms taken out of context of the person's situation.
- **Red Flag Alert 10.16.** A person is judged incompetent based on his/her failure to respond in the language and rules of the predominant culture.

- **Red Flag Alert 10.17.** A practitioner assumes that a person has certain mental health problems or a diagnosis based on demographic characteristics (education level, age, gender).
- **Red Flag Alert 10.18.** A practitioner fails to consider the importance of cultural values and beliefs and include them in the assessment or treatment of a patient's mental health.
- **Red Flag Alert 10.19.** Insufficient numbers of personnel, members of boards of directors, and public officials exist to engender multicultural services in specific programs or agencies.

Background

Access to healthcare is a leading health indicator, and barriers to access include cost, language differences, lack of information about mental health services, the scarce presence of mental health services in the consumer's native country, the stigma attached to mental health services, and competing cultural practices (Betancourt, Green, Carrillo, & Ananeh-Firempong, 2003). Lack of interpreter services or culturally/linguistically appropriate health education materials is associated with patient dissatisfaction, poor comprehension and compliance, and ineffective or lower-quality care. Bureaucratic intake processes and long waiting times for appointments have also been particularly cited by ethnic minorities as major obstacles to obtaining healthcare (Phillips, Mayer, & Aday, 2000).

Resources for Advocates

In response to the surgeon general's report, the President's New Freedom Commission on Mental Health was established in 2002 (New Freedom Commission on Mental Health, 2003), and a call for the elimination of disparities in health services due to cultural or geographic factors was identified.

The National Center for Cultural Competence (2007) reported that California, New Jersey, and Washington had passed laws mandating the integration of cultural and/or linguistic competence into curricula, continuing education, and licensure requirements for health and mental healthcare professionals.

POLICY ADVOCACY LEARNING CHALLENGE 10.3

Connecting Micro, Mezzo, and Macro Policy Advocacy

Ensuring Culturally Competent Care

An 80-year-old Italian immigrant woman named Maria, who had lived in the United States for 60 years, arrived at an emergency room of a local hospital with her Italian friend and neighbor. She had fallen from her chair as she tried to pick up something that she had dropped, and as a result she cut her eyebrow on the edge of an end table. Her family was called, and when her daughter-in-law and adult granddaughter arrived, the daughter-in-law went with a nurse to fill out some paperwork and the granddaughter stood in the waiting room anxious to find out where her grandmother was and how she was doing. A resident emerged and told the granddaughter in a matter-of-fact tone that he did not have good news.

"Your grandmother has blood collecting in the sinus cavity above her eye, and it will eventually go to her brain and kill her."

"Isn't there anything that can be done?"

"Well, she's very old and likely has a type of dementia, so I'm sure your family will not want to put her through surgery; her quality of life is already poor. What medical conditions does she have? How old is she?"

The granddaughter knew that her grandmother had no medical conditions and that the day before she had planted her garden and had eaten dinner with the family, as was usual for a Sunday, and she had seemed fine. "Demented? How did you assess that?"

The resident went on to say that when the patient was first seen in the hospital, she was unable to answer any questions they asked and wasn't making sense.

"Did they have someone speak to her in Italian?"

At that moment, the women's son arrived, and the resident repeated to him that he was sorry that there was nothing to be done for his mother. Hearing what had happened, the son requested that before the resident decide that it was his mother's time to die, he tell the family what he would do for this type of problem if his mother were 50 years old instead of 80.

"I'd do a CAT scan to see the full extent of the trouble, and then likely surgery to remove the blood and repair the bleed."

The son suggested he do the CAT scan. He then went to talk to his mother in her dialect and ask how she felt. She spoke to him normally, apologizing for taking him away from his workday. Clearly, as the son suggested later to the resident, his assessment was that his mother's "mental faculties" were working as usual. The resident was surprised to see the patient was able to respond to her son when he translated questions for her and to laugh when he joked with her about how she looked as if she had been in a brawl (her eye was swollen from the fall, but this was a very petite and mild-mannered woman who hardly ever raised her voice above a whisper). After the CAT scan, the resident returned and reported in astonishment that the woman had no sinus cavity on the right side of her head (where she had sustained the injury), and therefore the black area that had shown up on the x-ray that was thought to be blood was really only the absence of the sinus cavity (a condition that patient had been born with but had not caused any problem). The woman received five stitches over her right eye and left the hospital with her family. She lived happily and independently on her own for another 17 years. This was her first and only trip to a hospital in her entire life. A week after her visit, she removed her own stitches, reporting to her son that she was feeling fine and didn't need them anymore.

LEARNING EXERCISE

1. Which of the problems encountered by this patient could benefit from micro, mezzo, and/or macro policy interventions?
2. What assumptions were made by the practitioner? How did those shape the assessment?
3. What advocacy skills do families need when a member of the family is determined to be "incompetent"?

Core Problem 4: Engaging in Advocacy to Promote Prevention of Mental Distress—With Some Red Flag Alerts

- **Red Flag Alert 10.20.** Prevention screenings are not universal but are offered based on selection criteria in hospitals, schools, places of employment, and elsewhere.
- **Red Flag Alert 10.21.** Clients in medical settings, schools, places of employment, or elsewhere are not screened for behavioral health risks or problems that were not included as the presenting problem due to practitioner discomfort.
- **Red Flag Alert 10.22.** Clients have insufficient insurance coverage for behavioral health screenings.

Background

The lack of knowledge about the etiology and causes of mental illness and the absence of a formalized test (such as a blood test) to detect or confirm the presence of the illness is a serious barrier to preventive services. While it is currently believed that many genetic and environmental factors contribute to mental health problems, there is no certainty or understanding as to the exact mechanisms of mental illnesses, and therefore scientific support for the creation of prevention programs is lacking. There has been a lack of funding from private insurance companies, Medicare, and Medicaid for services intended to prevent illness. There also has been less money allocated for research to show the efficacy of preventive interventions, in part because of the expense of conducting the longitudinal studies necessary to show positive results (research and interventions related to prevention may appear to be more costly in that they do not provide cost savings immediately). Finally, the stigma associated with mental illness continues to stand as a barrier to prevention.

Resources for Advocates

Primary care providers (PCPs) are often the first point of contact for many people as they enter the healthcare system. This offers PCPs an opportunity to identify mental health concerns early, to educate individuals and families about behavioral health, and to help facilitate referrals where necessary. Recognition of the need for PCPs to participate more fully in early screening and intervention has led to new models of "integrated health," which focus on the impact of all health conditions on the person. These efforts encourage healthcare practitioners to view the person as a whole and to consider mental health, physical health, substance use, and behavioral health as essential components of health. Screenings to treat all known risks and manage existing conditions can improve the person's health status, reduce the need for additional healthcare services, and reduce financial and human costs (www.samhsa.gov/About/strategy.aspx). It is essential for mental health providers to collaborate and coordinate with primary care providers to screen for physical illness and substance abuse.

Examples of the integration of health, mental health, and behavioral health services that aim to implement more screening, brief interventions, and referrals for all clients can be found in numerous federal and state agencies. Readers are referred to the following website for innovative prevention practices: http://www.nami.org/Content/ContentGroups/CAAC/Online_Resource_List.htm.

As part of the ACA, a new Prevention and Public Health Fund was created to expand the infrastructure needed to prevent disease through early detection and support the management of existing health conditions at the lowest severity level possible. Inclusion of additional prevention measures (the Prevention and Public Health Fund and the National Prevention Strategy) signals a significant shift in the focus of the ACA and movement in our country "from a focus on sick care towards a system that advances health and health equity, saving money and lives" (Prevention Institute, n.d.).

POLICY ADVOCACY LEARNING CHALLENGE 10.4

Connecting Micro, Mezzo, and Macro Policy Advocacy

Benefits and Risks of Prevention

The *Diagnostic and Statistical Manual of Mental Disorders* (DSM) was recently revised. During the revision process, the inclusion of a "category" or disorder that would reflect a prediagnosis risk group was considered, specifically for individuals presenting with psychosis-like or attenuated symptoms that might convert and eventually meet the criteria for a DSM disorder. While supporters of the risk category highlighted

(Continued)

(Continued)

the fact that "early intervention may help delay or prevent exacerbation into psychosis," others felt that distinguishing between "ill and non-ill persons is difficult," which would make the likelihood of false positive diagnosis higher (Carpenter, 2009, p. 841).

Given the controversy surrounding screening for psychotic risk and treating individuals before they have a diagnosis, Carpenter (2009) suggested that we consider whether the benefits of early intervention intended to help prevent a psychotic exacerbation outweigh the negative damage of "labeling" individuals with a mental health disorder when it is not certain that it will develop. Further, Carpenter (2009) asked practitioners to consider whether placing a person in a diagnostic risk category could "do more harm than good because of stigma or the unwarranted administration of treatment with a poor benefit/risk ratio" (p. 841). Yet screening for mental health problems is widely practiced in health settings, such as by asking patients to respond to several questions that have proven effective in diagnosing depression.

LEARNING EXERCISE

1. What are your thoughts about this controversy?
2. As an advocate, what direction would you recommend? Why?
3. Do other efforts to prevent problems associated with mental health serve to educate the public or to reinforce the stigma?
4. How do you think that early detection efforts in schools, hospitals, and other public settings would help to lower risks of suicide and incidence of violence? To be effective, what other changes would be required in the various settings?

Core Problem 5: Engaging in Advocacy to Promote Affordable and Accessible Mental Health Services—With Some Red Flag Alerts

- **Red Flag Alert 10.23.** People who do not have health insurance, including immigrants, cannot get coverage for mental health treatments.
- **Red Flag Alert 10.24.** People have health insurance but their coverage offers inadequate coverage of mental health services, including the appropriate amount, duration, and coverage of certain types of services.
- **Red Flag Alert 10.25.** Insurance deductibles or co-insurance for mental health services and medications places financial burdens on people seeking treatment.
- **Red Flag Alert 10.26.** People with limited resources (lower socioeconomic status or fixed income) give priority to treating health conditions (such as

life-threatening conditions or chronic medical conditions) over treating mental health concerns.

- **Red Flag Alert 10.27.** Patients are not compliant with mental health treatment recommendations due to costs rather than personal motivation issues or health beliefs.

Background

The financial structure of the healthcare system in the United States has presented as one of the primary barriers to addressing the healthcare needs of individuals with mental illness:

- Healthcare systems lack reimbursement for coordinated care across service systems, including health education and supportive services; lack adequate case management services to promote self-management and linkage to services; have poor coordination between physical and mental healthcare systems; and lack integrated treatment for dual diagnoses.
- Many individuals with mental health problems are uninsured or underinsured, putting them at a disadvantage as far as receiving integrated healthcare.
- The majority of individuals who seek services in community mental health centers have healthcare insurance through Medicaid. To be effective in serving patients in the public mental health system, Medicaid and Medicare must become partners in designing and implementing new strategies to improve access to care.
- Community mental health centers (CMHCs) are not nationally required to serve the uninsured. A decrease in non-Medicaid funding to CMHCs at the state level has led more patients to choose community health centers (CHCs), thereby giving them a lower quality of mental healthcare.
- Medicare has a large gap between mental health and physical healthcare coverage. Much larger copays are required for mental health visits than physical health visits. These cost differences force many individuals to pay high prices for mental healthcare or seek mental health diagnosis and treatment through their physical healthcare providers.

Resources for Advocates

Since the 1996 Mental Health Parity Act did not offer coverage for substance use/abuse disorders and increased insurance premiums for some, California voters enacted Proposition 63 (SB1136) to increase resources and access to mental health services to underserved or uninsured persons. Proposition 63, or the Mental Health Services Act 2004, was funded by a 1% tax on those individuals with incomes of over $1 million; the associated funding has established full-service partnerships across California and allowed for service expansion, innovation, and outreach programs addressing the concern for the rising numbers of those with mental illness who are also homeless. Unfortunately, similar legislation was not enacted in most other states.

While the federal parity law of 2008 provided necessary coverage to people with private insurance, millions of Americans remained uninsured and did not qualify for federal Medicaid or Medicare programs. The ACA attempts to close the service gap, or the loopholes created under the federal parity law, with new rules added to the parity law that require mental health coverage levels to be the same as standard medical and surgical coverage in terms of out-of-pocket costs, benefit limits, and practices such as prior authorization and utilization review. These practices must be based on the same level of scientific evidence used by the insurer for medical and surgical benefits. The ACA's provisions are outlined in the following bullets:

- The ACA creates additional incentives to coordinate primary care, mental health, and addiction services.

Grants and Medicaid reimbursement are available for the creation of health homes for individuals with chronic health conditions, including mental illness and substance use disorders. Studies demonstrate that integrated and coordinated care is ultimately beneficial, as it can help to detect health problems before they become more serious concerns. It can also ensure that if a person gets a life-threatening diagnosis, he or she is seen by a psychiatric professional to address any emotional health needs.

- The ACA provides improved coverage of mental health and substance abuse conditions.

Mental health parity law prohibits insurers and/or healthcare service plans from discriminating between coverage offered for mental illness, serious mental illness, substance abuse, and other physical disorders and diseases. The ACA carries forward and considerably expands the requirements set forth in the parity law.

- The ACA prioritizes services in the home and community instead of within institutions.

To promote the coordination of care, the ACA provides Medicaid payments for "medical homes" or "health homes" that coordinate care for people with chronic physical and/or behavioral health conditions.

POLICY ADVOCACY LEARNING CHALLENGE 10.5

Connecting Micro, Mezzo, and Macro Policy Advocacy

The ACA Cuts Consumers' Mental Health Costs

The ACA has greatly decreased disparities between the cost of care for patients of health-care and patients of mental healthcare. For example, a patient who was treated for diabetes and bipolar disorder prior to the ACA's implementation paid a 20% copay for his diabetes care but a 50% copay for his bipolar disorder. The new healthcare law changes this so that there is parity in copays. Think about some policy implications of this major shift in policy:

LEARNING EXERCISE

1. Are patients aware that mental health treatment is now much cheaper for them? If not, what kinds of community outreach and education might be considered?
2. Have health providers added sufficient mental health personnel, including social workers, to their rosters to provide the increased levels of mental health services needed by patients who will now receive them?
3. See Silberner (2008) to find how one patient advocate sees this issue.

Core Problem 6: Engaging in Advocacy to Promote Mental Health Services for Underserved Populations—With Some Red Flag Alerts

We discuss in this section two specific underserved populations: people in places of employment and current and retired military personnel and their families.

- **Red Flag Alert 10.28.** Employees report that they fear that their mental health problems, if known by colleagues, will lead to adverse repercussions such as termination.
- **Red Flag Alert 10.29.** High rates of absenteeism, dropout, resignation, and discharge as well as poor performance stem from untreated mental conditions.
- **Red Flag Alert 10.30.** People currently in military service, as well as veterans, often fail to receive services for PTSD, traumatic brain injuries, substance abuse, and family violence.

Background

Stigma, as well as lack of mental health personnel, interferes with mental health services in many institutional settings, such as schools and universities, military units, prison systems, nursing homes, and workplaces (Carter et al., 2010). The U.S. National Comorbidity Survey of Americans ages 15 to 54 found that 18% of those who were employed reported that they had experienced symptoms of a mental health disorder in the previous month. In 1990, mental health disorders cost the U.S. economy almost $79 billion in lost productivity (Rice & Miller, 1996, as cited in U.S. Department of Health and Human Services, 1999). Mood disorders cost more than an estimated $50 billion per year in lost productivity and result in 321.2 million lost workdays (Kessler et al., 2006). In addition, serious mental illnesses, which afflict about 6% of American adults, cost society $193.2 billion in lost earnings per year (Insel, 2008).

The failure of the Veterans Administration to provide timely and effective mental health services to military personnel and veterans has received extraordinary publicity as veterans have returned from the wars in Afghanistan and Iraq during the past 10 years. The toll on these veterans has been particularly linked to the sheer prevalence of traumatic brain injury from improvised explosive devices (IEDs) in these wars. Veterans from Korean and Vietnam wars have also complained about lack of treatment for long-standing cases of PTSD. A new head of the VA, Robert McDonald, was appointed in the summer of 2014 with the mandate to cut delays in mental health and medical services that have been experienced by tens of thousands of veterans in recent years.

Resources for Advocates

We have already discussed augmented health insurance for mental healthcare by the ACA, but the ACA also benefits veterans' mental healthcare because the ACA counts Veterans Administration healthcare as insurance coverage along with TRICARE, other military health plans, Medicaid, and Medicare. President Obama signed an executive order in 2012 authorizing additional funding to improve access to mental health services for veterans, service members, and military families (White House, Office of the Press Secretary, 2012), including expansion of crisis services, additional staffing for the VA healthcare system, improved research on PTSD, and care for traumatic brain injuries (O'Gorman, 2012). These services remained grossly inadequate, however, in 2014 and into 2015. Military personnel and veterans were also underserved in areas of substance abuse and family violence. It remained to be seen if services would be dramatically increased in coming years. Automatic access to medical care is provided to all veterans.

Mental health services are inadequately provided in many places of employment. Some corporations possess relatively large human resource departments with Employee Assistance Programs (EAPs) that offer free or low-cost mental health services. They provide short-term counseling, either with their own hired staff or through contracts with external providers. Some employees are reluctant to seek help for mental problems because of stigma or because they fear that their diagnoses will be disclosed to their employers even when EAPs pledge confidentiality.

POLICY ADVOCACY LEARNING CHALLENGE 10.6

Connecting Micro, Mezzo, and Macro Policy Advocacy

The Impact of Support From Fellow Employees

Without the insistence of her colleagues, who knew that this episode of psychotic symptoms was somehow "different" from previous episodes that they had observed, Elyn Saks, an accomplished law professor at the University of Southern California and recipient of the MacArthur Foundation genius award, might have died of encephalitis. Brought to the emergency room by her colleagues due to worsening psychosis, she was immediately assessed to be psychotic and might have been dismissed by the hospital with additional antipsychotic medications except that her work colleagues strongly requested that doctors check her for something other than psychosis. They knew the symptoms that Dr. Saks usually experienced when her mental illness worsened, and believed that her current behavior was different. Dr. Saks, whose symptoms and mental illness and treatment resulted in hospitalization, forced treatment, isolation, and restraints (Carter et al., 2010), has reported that one of the "pillars" that offered her support was her workplace and doing work that she loved. Saks and other tenured college professors with mental illness, including depression, have spoken openly about their decision to disclose information about their diagnosis due to fear that they might be looked upon as unstable or less competent or be ostracized by peers.

LEARNING EXERCISE

1. What micro, mezzo, and macro policy actions would you promote in specific employment settings to address employees' mental health problems, such as help from Employment Assistance Programs? Should social workers be central to EAPs in light of their biopsychosocial orientation?
2. What mezzo and micro policy advocacy initiatives might social workers lead to obtain more responsive care by the VA and other health systems for military personnel and veterans?

Core Problem 7: Engaging in Advocacy to Promote Care Linked to Communities—With a Red Flag Alert

- **Red Flag Alert 10.31.** A national network of mental health agencies that are based in communities and that also help people with substance abuse does not currently exist. Many patients who are discharged from hospitals, particularly in low-income areas, cannot obtain mental health or substance abuse services because of this problem.

Background

Historically, the care for mental illnesses has been offered by separate facilities, programs, and systems of care. Even as there is increasing evidence that a person-centered approach, which integrates services for health, mental health, and substance use disorders can improve health outcomes, the need for more effective and collaborative community-based services, including outreach and transitional programs, exists. Philosophies of care, missions, and mandates that are not complementary and also separate funding sources act as barriers to collaboration.

Resources for Advocates

Many common mental illnesses are similar to the common physical chronic illnesses (e.g., diabetes, asthma, and cardiovascular disease) in that they are unlikely to be "cured" but with proper care can effectively be managed over a person's lifetime. To successfully manage any chronic illness, patients will require treatment that is integrated and collaborative so that all aspects of their health are considered (i.e., that they are treated as a "whole" person). Members of their healthcare team also need to be able to communicate effectively about ongoing treatment planning and decisions. Access to community care that is integrated and collaborative will allow for smooth transitions from one type of treatment to another, when and if necessary, to manage the person's condition. For example, hospitalization to stabilize a person on a new medication may be necessary in a crisis, but having outreach services and an emergency on-call staff member available to the person may help him or her to return home sooner with family support. Continuity of care between healthcare institutions and community agencies is essential in providing patients the best and safest care in the least restrictive environment, which is cost-effective as well as being more desirable for the patient.

The ACA has begun to implement changes that will promote collaborative care. The ACA provides new flexibility in existing Medicaid state plan options for covering home- and community-based services. Outreach services, which began in 2014, will help enroll vulnerable and underserved populations in Medicaid and will target individuals living with mental illness (Mental Health America, 2012). Unfortunately, in many medically underserved areas, Americans may also lack access to mental health services. We subsequently discuss a policy initiative (The Excellence in Mental Health Act) that would fund neighborhood centers.

POLICY ADVOCACY LEARNING CHALLENGE 10.7

Connecting Micro, Mezzo, and Macro Policy Advocacy

Fragmented Care

The *Los Angeles Times* (Morocco, 2007) reported on a story that highlights the negative impact created by a fragmented system of care. The story tells of the struggle to find a way to respond to the complex needs of a woman who was homeless, 22 weeks pregnant, and mentally ill, who had been brought to the hospital ER by two good Samaritans who found her mumbling and wandering the street naked. Her physical exam and lab tests were normal except for her mental status. After hours of trying to locate a place for this unnamed person ("Jane Doe"), she was refused admission to the psychiatric unit in the hospital (they didn't treat women more than eight weeks pregnant), was deemed to have no medical reason for being admitted to the hospital, and was refused by a county psychiatric center who never called back after reading her faxed record. Even after almost a day of effort on the part of the ER staff and after locating the name of a brother (who would not take responsibility for his sister), the hospital failed to find any possible support for the woman and started the process of re-making every call they had previously made in the hope of eventually being successful.

LEARNING EXERCISE

1. What failures in the current healthcare system are identified in this case?
2. How would you advocate, and at what level, to assist this woman in getting the help that she needs?
3. Which of her needs would you prioritize? Her medical needs? Her psychiatric needs? Her situational needs?

"THINKING BIG" AS POLICY ADVOCATES IN THE MENTAL HEALTH SECTOR

The nation witnessed the tragedy of the massacre of 20 children and 6 adults at the Sandy Hook Elementary School in Newtown, Connecticut, on December 14, 2012. The assailant was Adam Lanza, a person who had lived with his mother—who he had killed shortly before the massacre. Lanza later killed himself as police entered the school after the massacre. It was widely speculated that Lanza was mentally ill, even if his diagnosis had not been established. Within a month, President Barack Obama established a task force to develop recommendations to address gun control, mental health, and school security issues—issues that had surfaced at prior massacres in schools, universities, and movie theatres.

A knotty issue soon emerged with respect to mental health services that pitted the confidentiality of mental health patients against the wishes of government authorities to obtain mental health information from mental health professionals about specific patients. Mental health professionals have long championed the confidentiality of mental health information about specific patients. They have argued that many people will not use counseling services *unless* they are certain that personal information will not be released to others because they fear that they will lose (or not obtain) jobs or suffer adverse repercussions from friends, spouses, or other individuals. Yet the massacre at Newtown led many public officials to *want* information about the mental health problems of people so that they could place relevant names in a database to be circulated to gun dealers and prevent mentally ill individuals from acquiring guns that might be used to harm others (Carey & Hartocollis, 2013). New York State enacted a gun bill on January 15, 2013, that required therapists to divulge the names of clients who were "likely to engage in" violent behavior so that police could take weapons from them. This New York law went farther than preceding state laws, which only required therapists to divulge the names of clients who had made direct threats against one or more other people or who had been involuntarily committed.

Advocates of confidentiality noted, however, that warning signs of violent acts are often unclear to therapists unless clients make direct threats. Dr. Michael Stone, a forensic psychiatrist, notes that "most mass murders are done by working-class men who've been jilted, fired, or otherwise humiliated." Serious mental illness is not, per se, a predictor of violent acts; indeed, only 4% of violent crimes are committed by people with such illnesses, according to Dr. Paul Appelbaum, director of the Division of Law, Ethics, and Psychiatry at Columbia University—and only 20% of mass murderers have a serious mental illness, according to Dr. Stone (Carey & Hartocollis, 2013).

Perhaps another strategy should be considered that would make mental health and substance abuse services more available to tens of millions of Americans, particularly in underserved areas. The Excellence in Mental Health Act (HR 1263) was introduced by Congresswoman Doris Matsui D.-CA, and Congressman Leonard Lance, R.-NJ, on March 13, 2013. This bill would support the nation's community mental health and substance use systems by instituting national standards and implementing federal qualification of community behavioral health centers in order to ensure that the centers cover a range of mental health services, including 24-hour crisis care; increased integration of physical, mental, and substance abuse treatment so that persons with dual disorders are treated simultaneously rather than separately for these conditions.

This bill would enhance Medicaid funding for community mental health centers that offer evidence-based treatment and support for millions of vulnerable individuals with mental health disorders. The Excellence in Mental Health Act amends the Public Health Service Act to authorize the Secretary of Health and Human Services to award matching grants to states or Indian tribes to expend funds for the construction or modernization of facilities used to provide community-based mental health and substance abuse services to individuals.

The certified behavioral health clinics providing this care could get reimbursed from the government as traditional health centers.

The Excellence in Mental Health Act has been referred to a congressional committee, which will consider the bill before sending it on to the House or Senate as a whole. This bill is cosponsored by a bipartisan group of 41 senators and is also supported by over 50 mental health organizations, veterans organizations, and law enforcement organizations, including the National Association of Police Organizations, the National Sheriffs' Association, the American Psychiatric Association, the American Psychological Association, the National Alliance on Mental Illness, and the National Council for Behavioral Health, among many others.

LEARNING OUTCOMES

You are now equipped to:

- Describe the numbers of Americans with specific mental problems
- Analyze the impact of poverty and income inequality on mental health
- Identify how mental health policies evolved in the United States
- Identify and analyze seven problems in the mental health sector

REFERENCES

Adams, K. B., LeCroy, C. W., & Matto, H. C. (2009). Limitations of evidence-based practice for social work education: Unpacking the complexity. *Journal of Social Work Education, 45,* 165–186.

Barr, D. (2008). *Health disparities in the United States: Social class, race, ethnicity, and health.* Baltimore, MD: Johns Hopkins University Press.

Barrio, C., & Yamada, A. M. (2005). Chapter 5: Serious mental illness among Mexican immigrant families. *Journal of Immigrant and Refugee Services, 3*(1–2), 87–106.

Bellamy, J., Bledsoe, S. E., Mullen, E. J., Fang, L., & Manuel, J. (2008). Agency–university partnership for evidence-based practice in social work. *Journal of Social Work Education, 44*(3), 55–75.

Betancourt, J. R., Green, A. R., Carrillo, J. E., & Ananeh-Firempong, O. (2003). Defining cultural competence: A practical framework for addressing racial/ethnic disparities in health and health care. *Public Health Reports, 118,* 293–302.

Bledsoe, S. E., Weissman, M. M., Mullen, E. J., Ponniah, K., Gameroff, M., Verdeli, H., . . . Wickramaratne, P. (2007). Empirically supported psychotherapy in social work training programs: Does the definition of evidence matter? *Research on Social Work Practice, 17,* 449–455. doi: 10.1177/1049731506299014

Bradley, E. H., Wetle, T., & Horwitz, S. M. (1998). The Patient Self-Determination Act and advance directive completion in nursing homes. *Archives of Family Medicine, 7,* 417–423.

Brekke, J. S., Ell, K., & Palinkas, L. A. (2007). Translational science at the National Institute of Mental Health: Can social work take its rightful place? *Research on Social Work Practice, 17,* 123–133.

Brekke, J. S., Prindle, C., Bae, S. W., & Long, J. D. (2001). Risk for individuals with schizophrenia who are living in the community. *Psychiatric Services, 53*(4), 485.

Burt, M. R. (2001). *What will it take to end homelessness?* Retrieved from www.urban.org/UploadedPDF/end_homelessness.pdf

Carey, B., & Hartocollis, A. (2013, January 16). Warning signs of violent acts often unclear. *New York Times,* pp. A1, A15.

Carpenter, W. T. (2009). Anticipating DSM-V: Should psychosis risk become a diagnostic class? *Schizophrenia Bulletin, 35*(5), 841–843.

Carter, R., Golant, S. K., & Cade, K. E. (2010). *Within our reach: Ending the mental health crisis.* Rodale Books.

Centers for Disease Control and Prevention, National Center for Injury Prevention and Control. (n.d.). *Web-based Injury Statistics Query and Reporting System (WISQARS).* Retrieved from www.cdc.gov/ncipc/wisqars

Cohen, D. J., Crabtree, B. F., Etz, R. S., Balasubramanian, B. A., Donahue, K. E., Leviton, L. C., . . . Green, L. W. (2008). Fidelity versus flexibility: Translating evidence-based research into practice. *American Journal of Preventive Medicine, 35,* S381–S389. doi: 10.1016/j.amepre.2008.08.005

Colton, C. W., & Manderscheid, R. W. (2006). Congruencies in increased mortality rates, years of potential life lost, and causes of death among public mental health clients in eight states. *Preventing Chronic Disease, 3*(2). Retrieved from www.pubmedcentral.nih.gov/articlerender.fcgi?tool=pubmed&pubmedid=16539783

Council on Social Work Education. (2008). *Educational policy and accreditation standards.* Retrieved from http://www.cswe.org/Accreditation/Reaffirmation/page2008EPAS.aspx

Council on Social Work Education. (2011). *Accreditation standards.* Alexandria, VA: Author.

Dear, M. J., & Wolch, J. R. (1987). *Landscapes of despair: From deinstitutionalization to homelessness.* Cambridge, UK: Polity Press.

Deutsch, A. (1937). *The mentally ill in America.* New York, NY: Columbia University Press.

Ganju, V. (2003). Implementation of evidence-based practices in state mental health systems: Implications for research and effectiveness studies. *Schizophrenia Bulletin, 29*(1), 125–131.

Grob, G. N. (1973). *Mental institutions in America: Social policy to 1875.* New York, NY: Free Press.

Grob, G. N. (1983). *Mental illness and American society, 1875–1940.* Princeton, NJ: Princeton University Press.

Grob, G. N. (1991). *From asylum to community: Mental health policy in modern America.* Princeton, NJ: Princeton University Press.

Grob, B. N. (1994). Government and mental health policy: A structural analysis. *Milbank Quarterly, 72*(3), 471–500.

Grob, B. N. (2005). Public policy and mental illness: Jimmy Carter's presidential commission on mental health. *Milbank Quarterly, 83*(3), 425–456.

Grob, B. N. (2008). Mental health policy in the liberal state: The example of the United States. *International Journal of Law and Psychiatry, 31,* 89–100. doi: 10.1016/j.ijlp.2008.02.003

Insel, T. R. (2008). Assessing the economic costs of serious mental illness. *American Journal of Psychiatry, 165*(6), 663–665. doi: 10.1176/appi.ajp.2008.08030366

James, D. J., & Glaze, L. E. (2006). *Mental health problems of prison and jail inmates* (p. 12). Washington, DC: US Department of Justice, Office of Justice Programs, Bureau of Justice Statistics.

Jansson, B. S. (2011). *Improving healthcare through advocacy: A guide for the health and helping professions.* Hoboken, NJ: Wiley.

Jansson, B.S. (2015). *The reluctant welfare state: Engaging history to advance social work practice in contemporary society.* Belmont, CA: Brooks/Cole Cengage Learning.

Jimenez, J. (2009). *Social policy and social change: Toward the creation of social and economic justice.* Thousand Oaks, CA: SAGE.

Kennedy, E. M. (1990). Community-based care for the mentally ill: Simple justice. *American Psychologist, 45*(11), 1238–1240.

Kessler, R. C., Akiskal, H. S., Ames, M., Birnbaum, H., Greenberg, P. A., Robert, M., . . . Wang, P. S. (2006). Prevalence and effects of mood disorders on work performance in a nationally representative sample of U.S. workers. *American Journal of Psychiatry, 163,* 1561–1568. Retrieved from http://ajp.psychiatryonline.org/cgi/reprint/163/9/1561

Kiesler, C. A., McGuire, T., Mechanic, D., Mosher, L. R., Nelson, S. H., Newman, F. L., . . . Schulberg, H. C. (1983, December). Federal mental health policymaking: An assessment of deinstitutionalization. *American Psychologist,* pp. 1292–1297.

Kirk, S. A. (1990). Research utilization: The substructure of belief. In L. Videka-Sherman & W. J. Reid (Eds.), *Advances in clinical social work research* (pp. 233–250). Washington, DC: National Association of Social Workers.

Koyanagi, C., & Goldman, H. H. (1991). The quiet success of the national plan for the chronically mentally ill. *Hospital and Community Psychiatry, 42*(9), 899–905.

LaFond, J. Q., & Durham, M. (1992). *Back to asylum.* New York, NY: Oxford University Press.

Lopez, S. R. (2011, September 21). Kelly Thomas death should be a call to action. *Los Angeles Times.*

Manderscheid, R., Druss, B., & Freeman, E. (2007). *Data to manage the mortality crisis: Recommendations to the Substance Abuse and Mental Health Services Administration.* Washington, DC.

McCubbin, M. (1994). Deinstitutionalization: The illusion of disillusion. *Journal of Mind and Behavior, 15,* 35–53.

Mechanic, D. (1989). *Mental health and social policy.* Englewood Cliffs, NJ: Prentice Hall.

Mental Health America. (2012, June 28). *Mental Health America hails ruling on ACA as a tremendous victory.* Retrieved July 7, 2012, from http://www.mentalhealthamerica.net/go /about-us/pressroom

Morocco, M. (2007). He's willing to be her safety net. *Los Angeles Times*. Retrieved from http://articles.latimes.com/2007/jul/09/health/he-inpractice9

Morrison, J. R. (1995). *DSM-IV made easy*. New York, NY: Guilford Press.

Mullen, E., & Bacon, W. (2000). *A survey of practitioner adoption and implementation of practice guidelines and evidence-based treatments*. Paper presented at Developing Practice Guidelines for Social Work Intervention: Issues, Methods, and Research Agenda, St. Louis, MO.

Murray, C. E. (2009). Diffusion of innovation theory: A bridge for the research–practice gap in counseling. *Journal of Counseling and Development, 87,* 108–116.

National Center for Cultural Competence. (2007). *A guide for advancing family-centered and culturally and linguistically competent care*. Retrieved from http://nccc.georgetown.edu /documents/fcclcguide.pdf

National Institute of Mental Health. (n.d.). *Suicide in the U.S.: Statistics and prevention*. Retrieved from www.nimh.nih.gov/publicat/harmsway.cfm

New Freedom Commission on Mental Health. (2003). *Achieving the promise: Transforming mental health care in America* (Final Report, DHHS Pub. No. SMA-03—3832). Rockville, MD: Department of Health and Human Services. Retrieved from http://govinfo.library.unt .edu/mentalhealthcommission/reports/FinalReport/downloads/Execsummary.pdf

Nuechterlein, K. H., & Dawson, M. E. (1984). A heuristic vulnerability/stress model of schizophrenic episodes. *Schizophrenia Bulletin, 10*(2), 300–312.

O'Gorman, K. (2012, August 18). The U.S. Army reports record high suicide rates for July. *Huffington Post*. Retrieved September 10, 2012, from http://www.huffingtonpost.com/kate -ogorman/army-suicides-veterans_b_1797199.html

Organization for Economic Co-operation and Development. (2008). *Policy brief: Mental health in OECD countries*. Retrieved February 12, 2012, from http://www.oecd.org/dataoecd /6/48/41686440.pdf

Phillips, K. A., Mayer, M. L., & Aday, L. A. (2000). Barriers to care among racial/ethnic groups under managed care. *Health Affairs, 19*(4), 65–75.

Prevention Institute. (n.d.). *A victory for health—Prevention Institute's statement on Supreme Court's Affordable Care Act decision*. Retrieved from http://www.preventioninstitute.org /press/press-releases/903-a-victory-for-health-prevention-institutes-statement-on-supreme -courts-affordable-care-act-decision-.html

Rice, D. P., & Miller, L. S. (1996). The economic burden of schizophrenia: Conceptual and methodological issues, and cost estimates. In M. Moscarelli, A. Rupp, & N. Sartorious (Eds.), *Handbook of mental health economics and health policy: Vol. 1. Schizophrenia* (pp. 321–324). New York, NY: Wiley.

Rosenhan, D. L. (1973). On being sane in insane places. *Clinical Social Work Journal, 2*(4), 237–256.

Shirk, C. (2008). Medicaid and mental health services. *Background Paper, 66.*

Silberner, J. (2008, July 21). Elderly to pay less for mental health care. *NPR News*. Retrieved from http://www.npr.org/templates/story/story.php?storyId=92751635

Stuart, H., & Arboleda-Florez, J. (2001). Community attitudes toward people with schizophrenia. *Canadian Journal of Psychiatry, 46*(3), 245–252.

Substance Abuse and Mental Health Services Administration. (2012a). *Mental Health and Addiction Parity Act*. Retrieved June 3, 2012, from http://www.samhsa.gov/healthreform/parity/

Substance Abuse and Mental Health Services Administration. (2012b). *Results from the 2010 National Survey on Drug Use and Health: Mental health findings* (NSDUH Series H-42, HHS Pub. No. [SMA] 11-4667). Rockville, MD: Author.

Sullivan, W.P. (1992). Reclaiming the community: A strengths perspective and deinstitutionalization. *Social Work, 37*(3), 204–209.

Tarrier, N., & Barrowclough, C. (2003). Professional attitudes to psychiatric patients: A time for change and an end to medical paternalism. *Epidemiologia e Psichiatria Sociale, 12*(4), 238–241.

U.S. Department of Health and Human Services. (1999). *Mental health: A report of the surgeon general* (pp. 408, 409, 411). Rockville, MD: U.S. Department of Health and Human Services, Substance Abuse and Mental Health Services Administration, Center for Mental Health Services.

Wang, P. S., Berglund, P., Olfson, M., Pincus, H. A., Wells, K. B., & Kessler, R. C. (2005). Failure and delay in initial treatment contact after first onset of mental disorders in the National Comorbidity Survey Replication. *Archives of General Psychiatry, 62*(6), 603.

Ware, N. C., Tugenberg, T., & Dickey, B. (2004). Practitioner relationships and quality of care for low-income persons with serious mental illness. *Psychiatric Services, 55*(5), 555–559.

Weissman, M. M., & Sanderson, W. C. (2001). *Promises and problems in modern psychotherapy: The need for increased training in evidence based treatments.* Prepared for the Josiah Macy Jr. Foundation conference "Modern Psychiatry: Challenges in Educating Health Professionals to Meet New Needs," Toronto, Canada.

White House, Office of the Press Secretary. (2012, August 31). *Executive order: Improving access to mental health services for veterans, service members, and military families.* Retrieved from http://www.whitehouse.gov/the-press-office/2012/08/31/executive-order-improving-access -mental-health-services-veterans-service.

World Health Organization. (2012, October). Depression. Retrieved from http://www.who.int /mediacentre/factsheets/fs369/en/

Chapter 11

BECOMING POLICY ADVOCATES IN THE CHILD AND FAMILY SECTOR

Bruce S. Jansson,
James David Simon, and Anamika Barman-Adhikari

LEARNING OBJECTIVES

In this chapter, you will learn how to:

1. Identify advocacy groups in the child and family sector

2. Analyze the evolution of the child and family sector and child welfare policies

3. Understand the scope of child abuse and where to find relevant statistics

4. Understand the political economy of the child and family sector

5. Recognize the impact of an inegalitarian nation on the child and family sector

6. Understand how seven core problems are often experienced by children and families

7. Apply the eight challenges in the multilevel policy advocacy framework to the child and family sector

The nation's child welfare system serves as the most important safety net for children who have been abused or neglected. This chapter focuses on micro, mezzo, and macro policy advocacy in the child and family sector in the United States.

IDENTIFYING ADVOCACY GROUPS IN THE CHILD AND FAMILY SECTOR

The website of the National Association of Social Workers (http://www.socialworkers .org/advocacy/grassroots/default.asp) offers different tools that encourage social work practitioners to get involved in the advocacy process.

Other sites that are helpful to policy advocates in child and family welfare include:

Alliance for Children and Families: www.alliance1.org

American Humane Society: www.americanhumane.org

Annie E. Casey Foundation: www.aecf.org

Child Welfare Information Gateway: www.childwelfare.gov

Child Welfare League of America: www.cwla.org

Children's Defense Fund: www.childrensdefense.org

Court Appointed Special Advocates for Children: www.casaforchildren.org

First 5 Los Angeles: www.first5la.org

First 5 California: www.ccfc.ca.gov

ANALYZING THE EVOLUTION OF THE CHILD AND FAMILY SECTOR

VIDEO LINK 11.1
Child Welfare
in the Inner City

We provide a brief chronology of the evolution of child welfare policies in the United States.

- The concept of *parens patriae*, which today has been expanded to justify the intervention of the court to protect minors, evolved in late-17th-century England—a power that allowed magistrates to remove children from their parents and place them with other families (Areen, 1975; Murray & Gesiriech, 2005; Myers, 2008).
- Many children in the 1800s were either abandoned or sent to live in almshouses with other poor families, sick adults, and people declared insane (as cited in Schene, 1998).
- Criticism of the horrible conditions of children living in almshouses gave rise to orphanages and children's asylums, where many children were subsequently moved in the 19th century. The Children's Aid Society sent upwards of 150,000 children on orphan trains to live in rural homes throughout the Midwest (Schene, 1998).

- The beginning of organized child protection started in 1874 with the formation of the New York Society for the Prevention of Cruelty to Children in response to the physical abuse and neglect of a child when there was no child protective services agency or juvenile court to intervene on her behalf (Myers, 2008).

- Anticruelty societies grew in numbers across the United States, which gradually led to the establishment of child protection legislation and juvenile courts toward the end of the 19th century (Fogarty, 2008).

- The federal government held the White House Conference on the Care of Dependent Children in 1909 and established the Children's Bureau in 1912 (Costin, Karger, & Stoesz, 1996).

- Although there were hundreds of anticruelty societies assisting needy families and intervening legally to protect abused children in the 1920s, government agencies slowly took over these responsibilities (Brittain & Hunt, 2004). In January 1921, the Child Welfare League of America was formed out of the Bureau for the Exchange of Information Among Child-Helping Agencies (Anderson, 1989).

- The federal government became a major funder of children's programs with the enactment of the Social Security Act, where programs under Title IV funded government child welfare agencies in the various states, survivors' benefits funded dependents of deceased workers, and Aid to Dependent Children—which became Aid to Families with Dependent Children (AFDC) in the 1950s—funded welfare for low-income families (Schott, 2009).

- In the 1950s, child protection became recognized as a profession that encompassed both social casework and child welfare services (Anderson, 1989).

- The Child Abuse Prevention and Treatment Act of 1974 was passed in response to the public outcry over *battered child syndrome* to provide fiscal aid to programs for the prevention, detection, and treatment of child abuse and neglect and to establish a National Center on Child Abuse and Neglect (Pecora, 2000).

- The Title XX amendment to the Social Security Act was enacted in 1975, which provided states with flexibility to fund social service programs for children and their families, provided funding for children in foster care who had special needs, and provided funding for foster parents to receive extra services that had not been provided earlier (Twiname, 1975).

- The Indian Child Welfare Act (ICWA), another landmark piece of legislation, was passed in 1978 to protect the integrity and support the continued existence of Native American children. The ICWA established a minimum federal standard for removal of Native American children from their homes and provided guidelines for placement in foster or adoptive homes. If out-of-home placement became necessary, then the preference for placement was with another Native American family (Pecora, 2000; Wilkins, 2004). Tribal courts were given the right to determine what is in the best interest of children in such cases.

- The Adoption Assistance and Child Welfare Act (AACWA) amended Title IV-A and Title IV-B of the Social Security Act in 1980 and created Title IV-E (Pecora, 2000). The AACWA provided federal subsidies for adoption of children from foster care and was instrumental in reducing the financial hurdles that deterred a lot of people from adopting children (Child Welfare Information Gateway [CWIG], 2011). It provided funds to help children with special needs. The act was the first to provide both state and federal assistance for children with special needs, which included help with medical care (CWIG, 2011).
- President Clinton enacted the Multi-Ethnic Placement Act in 1994, which eliminated policies that favored same-race placements and prohibited agencies that receive federal dollars from delaying or denying placements based on race or ethnicity.
- The Adoption and Safe Families Act (ASFA) was enacted in 1997. It established timelines to move foster children into permanency, provided bonuses to states for adoptions, and expanded funds available for time-limited reunification services, adoption promotion, and support services (Child Welfare League of America, n.d.).
- The Affordable Care Act (ACA) has provisions that have significant and far-reaching implications for children and youth who are a part of the child welfare system (Lehmann & Guyer, 2012). It allows former foster youth who have aged out of the system to continue to receive Medicaid coverage until the age of 26, with the federal government providing matching Medicaid funds to the states to fund this extended benefit (Lehmann & Guyer, 2012). It has established community-based "health homes" to provide integrated care for children and youth who have a chronic condition (Lehmann & Guyer, 2012).

UNDERSTANDING THE SCOPE OF CHILD ABUSE AND NEGLECT

The notion of child welfare has changed profoundly over the past 300 years. From the colonial period to the 19th century, childhood was not regarded as a special period for development and children were regarded as almost "miniature adults" (Trattner, 1999). Therefore, they were often thrust into work and family responsibilities pretty early in their life. However, as time passed, due to the work of a number of scholars and religious ministers, the trend that emerged was to view children as needing to be nurtured in order to grow into healthy and well-adjusted individuals later in their life (Trattner, 1999). The federal government first developed policies to deal with child abuse and neglect in 1935. Beginning in the 1970s, mandated reporting laws were passed. As soon as such mandatory laws were passed, the question that naturally emerged was, "How would one define child maltreatment/abuse and neglect for this and other purposes?" This definition until now has been subjective and subject to a number of controversies. While federal legislation sets minimum standards, each state is responsible for providing its own definition of maltreatment within civil and criminal contexts. According to the Child Welfare Information Gateway,

> federal legislation provides a foundation for States by identifying a minimum set of acts or behaviors that define child abuse and neglect. The Federal Child Abuse Prevention and Treatment Act (CAPTA) (42 U.S.C.A. §5106g), as amended by the Keeping Children and Families Safe Act of 2003, defines child abuse and neglect as, at minimum: Any recent act or failure to act on the part of a parent or caretaker which results in death, serious physical or emotional harm, sexual abuse or exploitation; or An act or failure to act which presents an imminent risk of serious harm. This definition of child abuse and neglect refers specifically to parents and other caregivers. A "child" under this definition generally means a person who is under the age of 18 or who is not an emancipated minor (CWIG, 2009).

More information and specific definitions of the various types of child abuse and neglect can be found at http://www.childhelp.org/page/-/pdfs/Child-Abuse -Definitions.pdf.

In order for policy advocates to do their job effectively, they need access to accurate and reliable data. Data are essential to establishing the scope, magnitude, and urgency of the problem. There are three main data sources of child abuse statistics in the United States ("Child Protective Services," n.d.; Wulczyn, 2009): the National Child Abuse and Neglect Data System (NCANDS), the National Incidence Study (NIS), and the National Survey of Child and Adolescent Well-Being (NSCAW). Established in 1974, both NCANDS and the NIS included suspected child abuse reports investigated by child protective services (CPS) agencies. The difference between the two is that NCANDS uses solely administrative data of all reports of suspected child abuse and neglect, whereas NIS uses data collected by CPS and other reporting sources, called community sentinels, to gather a more comprehensive picture of the incidence of child abuse and neglect. NSCAW was established in 1996 and includes only those reports of child abuse and neglect that are investigated by CPS, but adds clinical measures of child and family well-being ("Child Protective Services," n.d.; Wulczyn, 2009).

Using estimates from NCANDS, approximately 9.2 per 1,000 children were victims of abuse in 2012 (U.S. Department of Health and Human Services [USD-HHS], 2013). Using conservative estimates from the most recent NIS accounting for children who had been observed to have been harmed, 1.25 million children were abused or neglected between 2005 and 2006—7.5 per 1,000 were abused and 10.5 per 1,000 were neglected. Using less stringent estimates that account for children who were believed to be placed in harm's way, approximately 39.5 children per 1,000 were abused or neglected (Sedlak et al., 2010). In an economic impact study that looked at the direct and indirect costs of child maltreatment, the 2007 cost for child victims was an estimated $103.8 billion. The direct costs included hospitalization, mental health care, child welfare services, and law enforcement, whereas the indirect costs included special education, juvenile delinquency, mental health and medical care, use of the adult criminal justice system, and lost productivity to society (Wang & Holton, 2007).

A large discrepancy exists between reported cases and proven child abuse. Nearly 2.1 million reports of suspected child abuse were investigated by CPS agencies in 2012, of which nearly 60% were closed as unsubstantiated, meaning that there was not enough evidence to conclude that maltreatment occurred (USD-HHS, 2013). Given this high rate of unfounded allegations of child abuse, the current adversarial approach to investigating child abuse used by many CPS agencies across the country is being called into question (Schene, 2005). In its place, some CPS agencies are focusing on assessing families to identify problems and obtain services, rather than investigating them to substantiate allegations. This new way of responding to child abuse allegations, known as alternative response or differential response, has been accepted by several states and counties across the United States. To learn more about this discrepancy, explore the following links:

American Humane Association: http://www.americanhumane.org/children/ programs/differential-response/

Child Welfare Information Gateway: https://www.childwelfare.gov/pubs/issue -briefs/differential-response/

Quality Improvement Center on Differential Response: http://www.ucdenver .edu/academics/colleges/medicalschool/departments/pediatrics/subs/can/ QIC-DR/Pages/QIC-DR.aspx

UNDERSTANDING THE POLITICAL ECONOMY OF THE CHILD AND FAMILY SECTOR

VIDEO LINK 11.2
Policy Advocacy
for Children

Three principles govern child welfare policy: (1) reasonable efforts to prevent placement, (2) permanency planning for children in out-of-home care, and (3) placement in the least detrimental alternative. Child welfare programs are supported financially and shaped by national, state, and local laws and regulations.

A pendulum exists in child welfare that fluctuates between a cautious approach that emphasizes child protection through the removal of children and a more family-oriented approach that emphasizes family preservation (Gelles, 2001). When agencies focus on family preservation, specific instances of child abuse in families lead to protests that child welfare workers mistakenly keep children in unsafe situations. CPS agency directors and their staff are often held culpable and fired when a child under CPS supervision dies. When they focus upon removing children, however, other critics contend that they are usurping the roles of families as they remove children from their natural parents.

The child welfare system is unique because of its intricate relationship with the legal system. Specifically, *child abuse* and *neglect* are legal terms that only courts with appropriate jurisdiction can designate after complying with due process and the equal protection of law (Brittain & Hunt, 2004). There are three types of courts that handle legal matters dealing with child abuse and neglect: juvenile court, civil court (domestic relations courts), and criminal court. Juvenile courts, which encompass family courts with juvenile jurisdiction, typically use state statues to guide court procedures, and they can utilize state and federal case law when considering definitions of child abuse and neglect. State statutes that define child abuse and neglect guide civil courts, or domestic relations courts, and these courts often utilize case law when interpreting criminal and juvenile statutes. Criminal courts are the only courts where state criminal codes are applicable, and these courts use statutes that can apply to a person or to juveniles. If a perpetrator of child abuse and neglect is a relative or caregiver, the matter can be heard in criminal court, as well as juvenile court and domestic relations court. If a perpetrator of child abuse and neglect is not a relative or caregiver, the matter can be heard only in criminal court (Brittain & Hunt, 2004).

Child welfare is shaped by federal, state, and local policies. Federal legislation and regulations provide a national framework for the child welfare system. Within this framework, states have discretion to establish legal and administrative structures and programs within their jurisdictions. States differ in the manner that they have interpreted and implemented federal policy, resulting in a range of types and quality of services available to at-risk children and families (Lind, 2004).

The federal government frames and implements national policy by passing rules, monitoring state performance, and conducting compliance reviews. The Department of Health and Human Services (DHHS) is the principal federal agency that regulates and partially funds services to maltreated children and their families. The Administration for Children and Families and the Centers for Medicaid and Medicare Services within DHHS oversee services provided to children and families involved with the child welfare system (Reed & Karpilow, 2002).

State governments implement child welfare programs. California is an example of a child welfare services system that is organized into a continuum of programs and services aimed at safeguarding the well-being of children and families in ways that strengthen and preserve families, encourage personal responsibility, and foster independence. The California Department of Social Services (CDSS) is the principal agency responsible for the state's child welfare program. CDSS receives federal funding that provides partial support for state and county child welfare programs, develops and oversees programs and services for at-risk children and families, licenses out-of-home (foster) care providers, secures state and county funds for services to children in out-of-home (foster) care, provides direct-service adoption programs in some counties, and conducts research and provides oversight and evaluation of local and statewide demonstration projects and statewide best-practices training for social workers (Reed & Karpilow, 2002).

California is one of 11 states that operate a state-supervised/county-administered model of governance. Under this system, each of California's 58 individual counties administers its own child welfare program, and the CDSS monitors and provides support to counties through regulatory oversight, administration, and the development of program policies and laws (Reed & Karpilow, 2002). In other states, state governments operate child welfare agencies that they establish in different jurisdictions.

Child welfare agencies differ considerably. The effective functioning of service delivery systems requires what are known as "organizational components" (Pecora, 2000). These components include, among other things, a clear organizational mission, program capacity, careful personnel recruitment and training, reasonable caseloads, adequate clerical supports, supervision, performance data, and fiscal support that is consistent with the outcome requirements. Researchers have discovered that the organizational context greatly influences the effectiveness of the services of specific child welfare agencies. The organizational climate, broadly defined as employees' shared perceptions, for example, can affect the quality of service and child welfare outcomes (Glisson, 2009). In a study that looked at the emotional and behavioral outcomes of 1,640 children in 88 child welfare agencies, maltreated children served by investigative caseworkers from positive organizational climates (high in personal accomplishment and low in depersonalization) had made significant improvements in their psychosocial functioning 36 months later as opposed to the children served by investigative caseworkers from negative organizational climates (Glisson, 2009).

The funding system for child welfare services is complicated. The primary sources of funding for the child welfare system are within Title IV and Title XIX of the Social Security Act (Reed & Karpilow, 2002). These funds are passed through to the states, and in California they are further distributed to the counties. More than 80% of California's foster children are eligible for and receive partial funding from the federal government for board, care, and medical costs, with the balance covered by state and county funds. Foster children who are not eligible for federal funds are supported by state, county, and private funds. Schematically, this arrangement is best represented by Table 11.1.

Table 11.1 The Child Welfare Financing Structure

MAJOR FEDERAL CHILD WELFARE FUNDING STREAMS				
Funding Source	**Type of Funding**	**Authorized Services**	**Eligibility**	**Funding Level (in millions) Fiscal Year 2003**
Title IV-B of the Social Security Act				
Subpart 1	Discretionary	Broad array of prevention, family reunification, and permanency services	Defined by the state	$290
Subpart 2	Part capped state entitlement, part discretionary	Family support, family preservation, time-limited family reunification, and adoption promotion and support services	Defined by the state	$405
Title IV-E of the Social Security Act				
Foster Care	Open-ended entitlement	Maintenance payments to foster families, administration, and training	Based on old AFDC need standards	$4,600
Adoption Assistance	Open-ended entitlement	Maintenance payments to adoptive families, administration, and training	Based on old AFDC need standards	$1,500
Adoption Incentive Payments	Discretionary	Any allowable IV-B or IV-E service	Generally defined by the state	$43
Chafee Foster Care Independence Program	Part capped state entitlement, part discretionary	Broad array of independent living support services	Adolescent foster youth and former foster youth up to age 21	$182

Note: Adapted from *The Child Welfare Financing Structure* by K. N. Murray, 2000.

The mass media plays an influential role in bringing attention to issues of social significance, and it plays a pivotal role in not only shaping public opinion about child welfare services but also exposing cases of child abuse. The influence of the media on CPS was highlighted by an infamous sexual abuse scandal involving Jerry Sandusky, the revered former assistant football coach at Pennsylvania State University and founder of a charity for abused children. After news broke in 2011 that he had sexually abused eight young boys at the university and that university officials allegedly covered up or ignored the abuse, an investigation resulted in his conviction on 45 counts of child abuse and a life sentence in prison (Penn State, n.d.). Cases like this bring attention to child abuse that is suspected but not reported and raise questions about the responsibilities of several other employees at the university who may have been aware of the abuse. Another example of the role of the media comes from Los Angeles County. A Blue Ribbon Commission was formed to examine the child protection system in Los Angeles County after the widely publicized death of an eight-year-old boy, Gabriel Fernandez, who had been known by CPS and law enforcement agencies. Despite six investigations in which social workers were told that he had numerous bruises and despite a suicide note, five investigations were closed after the allegations were deemed to be unfounded, and Gabriel remained in his home. In May 2013, paramedics took Gabriel to the hospital, where he died of injuries related to severe physical abuse (Therolf, 2013). This tragedy sparked the formation of a Blue Ribbon Commission that declared a state of emergency and developed scores of reforms, such as establishing a single entity with sole responsibility for child protection that would collaborate with other public agencies, including the Department of Mental Health, Department of Public Social Services, law enforcement agencies, the Office of Education, and Dependency Court (Bluecommissionla.com, n.d.).

RECOGNIZING CHILD AND FAMILY PROBLEMS CREATED BY AN INEGALITARIAN NATION

Child poverty is a massive problem in the United States—and particularly among children from specific racial and ethnic groups, as can be seen in Table 11.2.

Children represent 22% of the total population, but they account for 36% of the total population living in poverty. Census figures indicate that there were nearly 16.5 million children living in poverty in 2010, most of whom were from ethnic minorities.

Children from racial and ethnic groups are disproportionately represented in child welfare systems (Hill, 2006). Nearly 60% of children in foster care are children from racial and ethnic minorities, although there is no evidence to suggest

Table 11.2 Children Younger Than 18 Living in Poverty, 2010

Category	Number (in thousands)	Percent
All children under 18	16,401	22.0
White only, non-Hispanic	5,002	12.4
Black	4,817	38.2
Hispanic	6,110	35.0
Asian	547	13.6

Note: Adapted from DeNavas-Walt, C., Proctor, B. D., & Smith, J. C. (2010). *Income, poverty, and health insurance coverage in the United States: 2010* (Report P60, No. 238). Retrieved from http://www.census.gov/prod/2010pubs/p60-238.pdf

that nonwhite children are at more risk of being subjected to abuse and neglect than white children. In 2008, 15% of children in the United States were African American children, but they represented a quarter of the children removed from their families and a third of children in foster care (American Humane Association, n.d.b).

The sheer number of low-income children in foster care stems from multiple factors. Poverty causes many stressors on families. It increases levels of neglect, since low-income parents lack resources for food and other necessities. Substance abuse is far higher among low-income persons than among more affluent individuals. Low-income persons are more likely to have disabilities and mental illness that make parenting more difficult. Relatively affluent families have legal and other resources that allow them to contest allegations of child abuse—and possibly to hide child abuse (Pecora, 2000).

UNDERSTANDING HOW SEVEN CORE PROBLEMS EXIST IN THE CHILD AND FAMILY SECTOR

Core Problem 1: Engaging in Advocacy to Protect Children's Ethical Rights, Human Rights, and Economic Justice—With Some Red Flag Alerts

- **Red Flag Alert 11.1.** Foster children are not made aware of their rights or these rights are not respected. This places social workers in the unique position of advocating for these children and ensuring that their rights are being protected.

- **Red Flag Alert 11.2.** Children do not receive the services they are entitled to. They are often not consulted on their case plans and are actually sidelined when it comes to making pivotal decisions that affect their lives.
- **Red Flag Alert 11.3.** Children in foster care are often *lost in the system*. They see their social workers rarely and often do not even know the lawyers who are representing them.

Background

The child welfare system is deluged with huge caseloads and high rates of worker burnout. Many serious problems continue to plague a service delivery system that is high on stress, short on resources, has high staff turnover, and deals with very difficult family situations (Arkansas Advocates, 2005). Given all these structural problems, ethical rights are sometimes not addressed or compromised. In addition, many clients in child welfare are often unaware of their ethical rights, especially clients in vulnerable populations such as foster youth, low socioeconomic status (SES) families, and undocumented families. Because social workers work with such vulnerable populations, extra care should be taken to ensure that these children and families are made aware of their rights (CWIG, n.d.a).

Many minority youth experience a violation of their basic civic and human rights simply because of the color of their skin. For example, youngsters in the inner city, city, and suburban lower- and middle-class who are of African American, Hispanic, or Asian descent are often suspected of being gang members and are subject to racial profiling (Morales, Sheafor, & Scott, 2011). The shooting of unarmed African American 17-year-old teenager Trayvon Martin by neighborhood watchman George Zimmerman grabbed the nation's attention as a prime example of the ethically dangerous practice of racial profiling. On February 26, 2012, George Zimmerman shot Trayvon Martin fatally after a brief altercation in a gated condominium complex in Sanford, Florida, where Trayvon was staying temporarily. It has been alleged that Trayvon was profiled primarily because of his race, which ultimately led to his death.

Ethical barriers also exist in the context of educating the country's children and youth. Education is a known indicator for the financial success people experience as they develop into adults; the higher the educational level attained, the smaller the difficulty experienced in finding employment and supporting one's family. However, because black and Hispanic children are more likely to live in poverty than their white and Asian counterparts, they are included in a snowball effect of circumstances that lead to negative outcomes. For example, ethnic minority children are more likely to attend worse schools, have poorer health and nutrition, experience violent crime, perform worse on standardized tests, and drop out of high school at higher rates (Fryer & Levitt, 2004; Harding, 2003; Lee, 2002; Menchik, 1993; Sampson & Wilson, 1995).

Resources for Advocates

Children in foster care are entitled to a bill of rights. The rights are legal, and it is illegal to violate these rights. A number of these rights are delineated in the Adoption and Safe Families Act of 1997. According to this act, the child's safety and well-being is of paramount concern when planning his or her case plan. In 2001, California enacted the following bill of rights, along with a provision to its Health and Safety Code, requiring that foster care providers give every school-age child and his or her authorized representative an age-appropriate orientation and an explanation of the child's rights (Doherty, 2005). Some of the most important rights are as follows:

1. To live in a safe, healthy, and comfortable home where one is treated with respect

2. To receive medical, dental, vision, and mental health services

3. To be free of the administration of medication or chemical substances, unless authorized by a physician

4. To contact family members, unless prohibited by court order, and social workers, attorneys, foster youth advocates and supporters, court-appointed special advocates, and probation officers

5. To visit and contact brothers and sisters unless prohibited by court order

6. To make and receive confidential telephone calls and send and receive unopened mail, unless prohibited by court order

7. To attend religious services and activities of one's choice

8. To attend school and participate in extracurricular, cultural, and personal enrichment activities, consistent with one's age and developmental level

9. To attend court hearings and speak to the judge

10. At 16 years of age or older, to have access to existing information regarding the educational options available, including but not limited to the course-work necessary for vocational and postsecondary educational programs and financial aid for postsecondary education

In 1997, the ASFA was enacted and modified many of the goals and policies set forth by the Adoption Assistance and Child Welfare Act. Some important modifications include the following policy requirements:

Enhancing the safety of the child—in home and in foster care. The law clarified the meaning of the "reasonable efforts" condition, which had appeared in the Family Preservation and Support Services Act (P.L. 96-272). This 1984

law had stated that the state must take reasonable measures to prevent or eliminate the need for removing a child from his or her home, or if the child had been removed, then the state must make reasonable efforts to reunify the child with his or her family within a suitable time frame (Welte, 1997). The new law emphasized that the child's well-being, safety, and security should be of paramount concern in arriving at a decision about a logical and rational plan of action. This law also allowed for dual planning, which is the process of looking at suitable prospective adoptive families while reunification services are still being provided (Welte, 1997).

Shortening the time frame for permanent placement. Services to reunify families funded under Title IV-B would not extend beyond 15 months (Welte, 1997). These services included counseling, substance abuse treatment services, domestic violence services, and temporary childcare and related services. A petition to terminate parental rights would be filed for parents whose child has been in foster care for 15 of the last 22 months, if a court had determined a child was an abandoned infant, or in the circumstances described under "reasonable efforts" above.

Providing incentives for adoptions or other permanency placements. The law provided states with cash incentives to find permanent homes for children in foster care. A state would receive $4,000 in federal funds for each foster child adoption exceeding a base number of foster care adoptions in a fiscal year, and an additional $2,000 for special needs adoptions (Welte, 1997).

Decreasing geographic barriers to adoptions. To facilitate timely adoptions for waiting children across state and county jurisdictions, states would be required to develop plans to utilize cross-jurisdictional resources. Title IV-E foster care and adoption assistance payments to the state would also be predicated upon a state's cooperation in processing a child's adoptive placement if an approved family was available outside the jurisdiction (Welte, 1997).

Establishing outcome measures to assess state performance. The secretary of health and human services, in discussion with public officials and child advocates, would develop outcome measures, as well as a rating system, to assess states' performance in child protection and child welfare programs. Measures would include length of stay in foster care, the number of placements, and the number of adoptions and, to the extent possible, use data available from the established Adoption and Foster Care Analysis and Reporting System. States would report their performance on each outcome measure, and the secretary of health and human services would provide an annual report to Congress (Welte, 1997).

Expanding health coverage for special needs children and independent living services. States would be required to provide health insurance coverage for any child with special needs for whom it would be hard to find placement without providing these services. States could provide health coverage, including mental health coverage, through the Medicaid option or another program at least equivalent to Medicaid. Independent living services were extended to young people whose assets did not exceed $5,000, rather than the current $1,000 cap. Services were designed to assist young people in preparing for living independently when they left foster care (Welte, 1997).

Defining legal and standby guardianship. The phrase "legal guardian" is defined in the statute as a permanent relationship between child and caretaker and transfers parental rights to the caretaker for the child's protection, education, care, custody, and decision making. The new law urged states to adopt laws and procedures to allow parents who were chronically ill or near death to designate a standby guardian for their children, without surrendering their parental rights (Welte, 1997).

POLICY ADVOCACY LEARNING CHALLENGE 11.1

Connecting Micro, Mezzo, and Macro Policy Advocacy

Who Will Uphold the Rights of a Native American Child?

A. J. is a four-year-old American Indian child in foster care within the purview of the Indian Child Welfare Act (ICWA). The newborn was considered a medically fragile child, experienced drug withdrawal symptoms, and exhibited signs of fetal alcohol syndrome. The mother denied serious drug use and did not want to participate in services or raise A. J., and his father wanted custody but was deemed unfit to raise a medically fragile child. It was under these circumstances and because no other family member offered to care for A. J. that he was detained in foster care, and dependency proceedings were initiated.

Based on the mother's membership in her tribe, the child welfare agency in that county notified the tribe of the dependency proceedings pursuant to ICWA. Meanwhile, A. J. was moved to a foster home at the age of one. Although A. J. presented with a flat affect and did not engage with his parents, A. J. engaged with his foster mother and used her as a reference base for most of his activities. According to the child's therapist, A. J. needed to be either reunited with his parents or placed in a permanent placement as soon as possible to reduce attachment difficulties and

(Continued)

(Continued)

avoid future mental health problems. The tribe, however, first wanted to explore options within the tribe, and A. J.'s grandmother was put forward as a possible option. The tribe's council approved a resolution-authorizing placement of A. J. with the grandmother for the purposes of legal guardianship.

In the meantime, the child protective services agency modified its recommended permanent plan for A. J. and alternatively recommended legal guardianship with the foster mother or adoption by the foster mother because A. J. had no relationship with the grandmother. In addition, A. J. had been in his current placement for two years and had developed a significant bond with his foster mother. In conflict with ICWA, the ASFA indicates that "the child's well-being, safety and security shall be of paramount concern in arriving at a decision regarding the child's permanency options." However, the social worker attached to this case discovered that ICWA has a provision that would allow ASFA to take precedence if she could prove that it was in the child's best interest for him to remain with his foster mom. The social worker was able to get expert testimony from bonding experts and ICWA experts, who testified that whereas the law prefers placement with an American Indian family, they could see how this could prove to be counterproductive to A. J.'s developmental goals and was, therefore, not in the right spirit of the ASFA.

The courts agreed with the testimony of the expert witnesses and the social worker and gave the following ruling:

> It is obvious that the grandmother has had very limited contact with A. J. and her failure to engage him in any meaningful way. Her lack of effort to visit, interact and develop a relationship with A. J. was striking. Although there was evidence that a child who has an attachment can attach to another care provider, it was undisputed a child's ability to attach also depended on the new care provider's skill. Under the circumstances of this case, the juvenile court reasonably could infer it was unlikely A. J. could develop a healthy attachment to the grandmother. (Fearnotlaw.com, n.d.)

LEARNING EXERCISE

1. How does this vignette illustrate the conflicting provisions of the two laws and the reasoning that the safety of the child needs to be of paramount concern?
2. Which skills came in handy for the social worker in this situation to advocate for this child?
3. Could the social worker have taken any other steps to resolve the situation?

Core Problem 2: Engaging in Advocacy to Improve Quality of Care—With Some Red Flag Alerts

- **Red Flag Alert 11.4.** High turnover of children and youth often exists in the child welfare system, leading, for example, to multiple foster homes for specific children and youth.
- **Red Flag Alert 11.5.** Lack of respect often exists between social workers and clients.
- **Red Flag Alert 11.6.** Many standard services are provided that do not meet the individual needs of clients.
- **Red Flag Alert 11.7.** Clients' unique needs are often not sufficiently assessed when determining what type of services to provide.
- **Red Flag Alert 11.8.** Some services are provided without any consideration of empirical evidence to back up their effectiveness.

Background

Funding for social welfare services is never enough, because the number of people who require those services expands enormously each year, yet the level of funding often remains constant. Because the resources are sparse, agencies should strive to use these resources in the most cost-efficient and effective manner to increase the likelihood of the accessibility of services. Patton and Sawicki (1993) state, "Efficiency is measured in dollars per unit of output (benefit)," which can be operationally defined by examining all program costs (i.e., direct, indirect, operation, maintenance, etc.), number of participants, the delivery of service, and what services will be provided. Effectiveness is based on whether the program or policy achieves the desired goals and objectives (Bardach, 1996). Accessibility can best be described as the availability of programs and services to the population being served.

At-risk children and families are typically poor and face multiple challenges, such as substance abuse, mental illness, domestic violence, and inadequate housing. Supports and services geared toward addressing these needs can help mitigate sources of stress and instability that may contribute to child abuse and neglect. By making a continuum of care available to at-risk children and families, states and counties can not only intervene, but they can also successfully prevent child abuse and neglect (Lind, 2004). Unfortunately, this is not the situation in many cases. The reality is that services are scattered, and there is little systematization or consolidation of these resources, so people are often left scrambling to find resources.

Adding to this complexity, many of the programs and practices in child welfare lack specific evidence about their effectiveness. To catch up with fields such as medicine and public health, child welfare has recently begun implementing more evidence-based practices and evidence-based policies. As the volume of research evidence grows, social workers will be able to complement their practice-based knowledge and clinical judgment to include practices that have been shown to be effective (CWIG, n.d.b).

For more information about evidence-based practice in child welfare, explore the following links:

Annie E. Casey Foundation: http://www.aecf.org/work/evidence-based-practice/

California Evidence-Based Clearinghouse: http://www.cebc4cw.org/

Child Welfare Information Gateway: https://www.childwelfare.gov/topics/management/practice-improvement/evidence/ebp/

Resources for Advocates

In accordance with the Child and Family Services Improvement Act of 2006 (P.L. 109-288), which came into effect on September 28, 2006, and amended the Social Security Act Title IV-B, a new purpose for child welfare services programs was established that allowed for an expansion of services and flexibility. With this expansion, different states could change their programs as needed to increase the breadth of services (CWIG, n.d.b). The act also allowed for competitive grants to regional partnerships that were able to provide collaborative, integrated services and programs to improve children's safety in out-of-home care and to meet the needs of children at risk of entering out-of-home care due to parent/caregiver substance use.

POLICY ADVOCACY LEARNING CHALLENGE 11.2

Connecting Micro, Mezzo, and Macro Policy
Advocacy to Address a Lack of Community Resources

Imagine that you are an emergency response social worker for the Los Angeles Department of Children and Family Services (DCFS). Your client needs a parenting class that caters to parents with children with developmental disabilities. After completing your child abuse investigation and finding no evidence of abuse, you have to close the case but need to find appropriate services to help the family, which is difficult because you are able to find only generic parenting classes. After reviewing the policy on community response and alternative response services (DCFS, 2014) and noting that the investigation should be closed once a family links to services, you decide to engage in micro advocacy. As a micro policy advocate, you should be detailed and specific when locating resources for the family so that the receiving agency can easily understand the identified problem. You contact the agency beforehand and explain the extent of the problem and see if they can cater their services to the client's need. It helps to ask the parenting class instructor to address particular issues. As part of mezzo policy advocacy, you discuss the lack of specialized classes with a supervisor and with an administrator, once given approval by a supervisor. If the problem appears to be common and affects many clients, you should inquire about the process of changing a policy within the agency. As a macro policy advocate, you might check into statewide regulations regarding parenting classes and advocate new legislation that permits such parenting groups to customize their services to the needs of particular clients. This legislation should also provide additional funding to design, implement, and evaluate those services.

LEARNING EXERCISE

1. How does this vignette illustrate the difficulties of finding resources that meet a client's need?
2. Why does the social worker call the agency beforehand instead of just providing the client with the telephone number for the agency?
3. When would it be appropriate for a social worker at DCFS to engage in mezzo or macro policy advocacy to address a limitation of services?

Core Problem 3: Engaging in Advocacy to Promote Culturally Competent Care—With Some Red Flag Alerts

- **Red Flag Alert 11.9.** Culture is not taken into consideration in case planning.
- **Red Flag Alert 11.10.** Cultural practices are misinterpreted to form the basis of neglect or abuse charges.
- **Red Flag Alert 11.11.** Lack of staff training on cultural sensitivity exists.
- **Red Flag Alert 11.12.** Clients express that their cultural needs are not being met.
- **Red Flag Alert 11.13.** Lack of consideration of cultural needs exists when staff try to engage clients.
- **Red Flag Alert 11.14.** There is lack of staff diversity to match a diverse client population.

Background

Children and families from ethnic minority groups are at considerable risk for developing several problems, such as substance abuse, low grades, delinquency, and poor self-esteem, and there is an increasing need for effective culturally sensitive interventions designed for this population (Jackson, 2009). Children and families who are from minority racial and ethnic backgrounds are also more likely to be poor. Family income has a substantial effect on child and adolescent well-being. Poor children experience emotional and behavioral problems more often than their more privileged counterparts, including emotional issues such as aggression, fighting, acting out, anxiety, social withdrawal, and depression, and the incidence of out-of-wedlock births among poor teens is nearly three times higher than the rate among nonpoor families (Brooks-Gunn & Duncan, 1997). In addition, poor children face higher rates of adverse health and developmental outcomes than their nonpoor counterparts, such as low birth weight and infant mortality, which are both significant indicators of health in children. For example, low birth weight is associated with an increased likelihood of persistent physical health, cognitive, and emotional problems; grade retention; learning disabilities; lower levels of intelligence; and decreased math and reading achievement. Furthermore, adverse birth outcomes are more likely for unmarried women, women with low educational levels, and black mothers, three populations that have high poverty rates (Brooks-Gunn & Duncan, 1997).

Early childhood interventions can be crucial in reducing the undesirable effects of poverty on the lives of children (Brooks-Gunn & Duncan, 1997). Other measures to mitigate the adverse effects of poverty in children include nutrition programs, especially those targeted toward the most undernourished; lead abatement; enhanced parental education; involvement in a home-learning environment; income policy reforms; and in-kind support programs.

Resources for Advocates

According to the Government Accounting Office (1998), approximately 60% of children in foster care belong to minority groups, and they wait twice as long to be placed in foster homes or to be adopted. The Multi-Ethnic Placement Act (1994) eliminated delaying or denying placements based on race or ethnicity; however, children under the ICWA are exempt from Multi-Ethnic Placement Act provisions because same-race placements for Native American children should be the preferred course of action when it concerns placement decisions (Pecora, 2000). However, the Multi-Ethnic Placement Act could be counterproductive as well, because minority children might not be a good fit in households or families that are not sensitive to their culture or their linguistic needs.

The DCFS in Los Angeles implemented the Permanency Partners Program (P-3) in October 2004 to find permanent homes and long-term connections for youth ages 12 to 18 placed in long-term foster care. The staff consists of retired caseworkers who review case records to find relatives or other adults who were connected to the youth. By July

2011, P-3 had served 4,635 youth, of whom 37% (1,696) have a legal permanent plan. Read about P-3 and other programs offered by DCFS in Los Angeles (DCFS, n.d.) at http://dcfs.co.la.ca.us/community/Pomona/index.html.

POLICY ADVOCACY LEARNING CHALLENGE 11.3

Connecting Micro and Macro Policy
Advocacy to Provide Culturally Sensitive Services

Anastacia is a 13-year-old Romanian girl who identifies herself as a "gypsy." She was removed from her parents on allegations that they had intentionally allowed her to be molested by an influential older man (who was a family friend) and videotaped the entire incident to financially blackmail that person. Anastacia is bilingual and conversational in both English and Romanian. The parents are, however, not very fluent in English. In addition, because they strongly identify with the gypsy culture, they believe that a girl should be homeschooled and have refused to send their daughter to a regular school. The social worker does not take the necessary steps of understanding the culture of the family and accuses the family of *educational neglect* along with the abuse charges. In addition, the social worker does not offer interpreter services to the parents and uses Anastacia to interpret for her parents.

LEARNING EXERCISE

1. How does this vignette illustrate a tendency to ignore culture in defining parental responsibilities and providing relevant services?
2. What laws could have protected this family and the child's best interests?
3. Could a social worker in this clinic have engaged in macro policy advocacy to resolve this situation?

Core Problem 4: Engaging in Advocacy to Promote Prevention—With Some Red Flag Alerts

- **Red Flag Alert 11.15.** Your agency's services are reactive and not preventive.
- **Red Flag Alert 11.16.** There is little support recourse for families struggling with poverty.
- **Red Flag Alert 11.17.** Your agency does not collaborate with other agencies to provide preventive services.

- **Red Flag Alert 11.18.** No resources are provided to families who do not meet the criteria to receive services from your agency.

Background

The lack of prevention is felt across all social sectors, and it is especially true for the child and family sector. Child welfare is a multilevel systemic problem that might have its origins in other root problems embedded in the social environment or the personal circumstances of the individual or the family. CPS is known to be a reactive agency and appears after child abuse occurs. In many cases, because of this post-incident reaction, the problem has become acute. For example, there are natural linkages between the welfare and child welfare systems. More than half the children who enter the child welfare system come from families eligible for welfare, and poverty is strongly associated with an increased risk of child maltreatment. Children in families with annual incomes less than $15,000 are 22 times more likely than children in families with annual incomes more than $30,000 to be abused or neglected (Lind, 2004).

It is essential to prevent child abuse and neglect because it has detrimental effects throughout a child's life span. Abuse and neglect have been found to negatively affect attachment style and aggression in children (Weizman, Har-Even, Shnit, Finzi, & Ram, 2001) and have negative effects on the developing brain (De Bellis et al., 1999). In a longitudinal, national study of more than 15,000 adolescents to examine the effects of childhood maltreatment on adolescent health behavior, each type of childhood maltreatment, that is, physical abuse, emotional abuse, sexual abuse, or neglect, was associated with increased smoking, alcohol use, drug use, and violent behavior during adolescence (Kotch, Chang, & Hussey, 2006).

In a well-known study that examined how early child abuse and neglect affected adult health risk behaviors and disease, referred to as adverse childhood experiences (ACE), the more ACEs that an adult experienced, the higher the likelihood that he or she would experience health risk behaviors and diseases associated with the leading causes of death in adulthood. For adults with four or more ACEs relative to adults with none, there was a fourfold to 12-fold increase in substance use, depression, and suicide attempts; a twofold to fourfold increase in smoking, self-rated poor health, number of sexual partners, and STDs; and about a 1.5-fold increase in severe obesity and physical inactivity. In addition, adults with more ACEs were more likely to have diseases such as cancer, liver disease, and chronic lung disease (Felitti et al., 1998).

Resources for Advocates

The passage of AACWA in 1980 was a direct response to discontent over the inadequate functioning of the child welfare system at that time. It amended Title IV-A and Title IV-B of the Social Security Act and created Title IV-E, thus shifting the focus from child abuse detection to prevention and permanence planning for children in out-of-home placements (Pecora, 2000). Some of the requirements that states and counties had to implement to receive federal funding consisted of the following:

1. Establish a state inventory of children in out-of-home placements, to include all children who have been in foster care during a period of six months or more.

2. Establish a statewide information system with a database whereby the sociodemographic characteristics, legal status, and goals set for a child receiving foster care services for a period of more than 12 months can be recorded and available for review if needed.

3. Implement preplacement preventive services whereby agencies document that they had offered services to a family that could have facilitated the retention of the child within the confines of his or her home.

4. Establish reunification or permanent planning services to reunify the child with his or her birth family or to find an adoptive home for the child.

5. Implement periodic case reviews with a judicial or administrative review every six months and a dispositional review by a court after 18 months of the child's being placed in the system.

6. Establish standards for care that prescribe best efforts to place children in the least restrictive settings, preferably close to their parents and their relatives.

7. Encourage participation of parents and children in the formulation of their case plans and their permanency goals as much as possible.

8. Provide adoption subsidies for children with special needs, with additional subsidies for families who adopt special needs children.

POLICY ADVOCACY LEARNING CHALLENGE 11.4

Connecting Micro, Mezzo, and Macro Policy Advocacy to Expand Preventive Services

Imagine that you are a social worker for the Los Angeles DCFS and you screen telephone calls from people calling to report suspected abuse and neglect. A grandmother calls the child protection hotline concerned that her daughter, a 19-year-old

(Continued)

(Continued)

first-time mother, is not properly caring for her one-year-old child. When asked for more details, the grandmother states that her daughter parties a lot, and that they argue about how to raise the child. After ascertaining that the young mother does not abuse her child, does not leave the child alone, and is meeting the child's medical needs, you decide that the call does not meet the criteria for abuse or neglect and determine that the family would benefit from assistance. As you speak with the grandmother further, she indicates that she and her daughter have communication problems, and she wishes her daughter would enroll in a parenting class.

As part of micro and mezzo advocacy, you consult your resource guides and provide the family with several telephone numbers to local agencies within their vicinity, including 211, a Los Angeles County–operated 24/7 telephone system. Before providing the family with a list of numbers, you call them to ensure that the family is eligible for services and that there is no wait list. You also make a follow-up telephone call to speak with the young mother and inform her of the services in her area. After listening to her discuss how she and her mother argue about how to raise her daughter, you empathize with her and discuss the many services of the close-by agencies. In addition, you provide her websites such as www.healthycity.org, where agencies can be located according to zip codes and services. You recommend that she contact the agencies for assistance with childcare, baby food, baby clothing, parenting classes, and education. She agrees to call the agency, and you follow up with her in a week to ask whether she had any trouble obtaining assistance.

Regarding mezzo and macro policy advocacy, the social worker speaks to the supervisor and administrators regarding the possibility of creating a new policy or protocol that would provide services to families who need assistance but do not meet the criteria for abuse and neglect. You also discuss the possibility of forming partnerships with other agencies for the creation of primary preventive services for families at risk for child maltreatment that come to the attention of community agencies early.

LEARNING EXERCISE

1. How does this vignette illustrate the difficulty of providing preventive services?
2. Would you describe these services as preventive or reactive services?
3. What are some disadvantages to providing services only if a family meets the criteria for child abuse and neglect?
4. Can you think of additional micro, mezzo, or macro policy advocacy that could be done in this situation?

Core Problem 5: Engaging in Advocacy to Promote Affordable and Accessible Care—With Some Red Flag Alerts

- **Red Flag Alert 11.19.** A client's recovery is impeded by lack of funding for services.
- **Red Flag Alert 11.20.** The political atmosphere does not support increased funding.
- **Red Flag Alert 11.21.** Families are reluctant to engage in services due to their immigration status.
- **Red Flag Alert 11.22.** Vulnerable families, such as immigrants, are excluded from financial benefits.

Background

Temporary Assistance for Needy Families (TANF) is a block grant created by the Personal Responsibility and Work Opportunity Reconciliation Act of 1996 as part of a federal effort to "end welfare as we know it" (Schott, 2009). The TANF block grant replaced the AFDC program, which had provided cash welfare to poor families with children since 1935 (Schott, 2009). The TANF grants are given to the states, which have the option to spend the money to promote the four basic purposes set forth by the federal government: (1) provide assistance to needy families so children may be cared for in their own homes or in the homes of relatives, (2) end the dependence of needy parents on government benefits by promoting job preparation, work, and marriage, (3) prevent and reduce the incidence of out-of-wedlock pregnancies, and (4) establish annual numerical goals for preventing and reducing the incidence of these pregnancies, encouraging the formation and maintenance of two-parent families (Schott, 2009). This act gave a lot of flexibility to states to frame their own criteria for eligibility for these services, as long as these services strove to reduce nonmarital childbearing and promote marriage (Schott, 2009). However, this act was steeped in controversy because many felt it relied too heavily on set criteria that punished people for making more money than the amount set as the eligibility limit by the act.

Approximately 700,000 children and adolescents in the United States end up in the child welfare system each year due to parental neglect, abuse, and abandonment. Although a number of these children are reunited with their families or adopted, many linger in foster care until they are kicked out of the child welfare system at age 18. According to recent estimates, roughly 20,000 18-year-olds leave foster care each year, and many of them are not prepared for the responsibilities and burdens that come with independent living (Christenson, 2009).

In California, more than 4,000 youth "age out" of the foster care system each year, and of these youth, 65% are emancipated without a place to live, less than

3% go to college, and 51% are unemployed (SSI Fact Sheet, 2009). These youth are at risk for a number of negative outcomes, including substantial periods of unemployment, homelessness, involvement with the criminal justice system, and poverty (Christenson, 2009; Needell, Cuccaro-Alamin, Brookhart, Jackman, & Shlonsky, 2002). In any given year, foster children comprise less than 0.3% of the state's population, yet 40% of persons living in homeless shelters are former foster children. A similarly disproportionate percentage of the nation's prison population is composed of former foster youth (Children Uniting Nations, n.d.).

One of the most essential building blocks for a productive and flourishing adult life for former foster youth is access to higher education. College education or some kind of vocational training is one of the best ways these youth can pull themselves out of poverty and have the means for an adequate standard of living. If child welfare agencies do not adequately prepare and support young people to enter, pay for, and complete college, the chances are good that their children, in turn, will struggle, thus resulting in a cycle of poverty (Promising Practices, 2009).

Resources for Advocates

The ASFA of 1997 introduced legislation that extended independent living services to young people whose assets did not exceed $5,000, which differed from the former $1,000 cap. According to the provisions in the act, these services should be designed to assist young people in preparing to live independently when they leave foster care (Welte, 1997). However, based on expert testimony and the realization that separate legislation is needed to allocate services and resources separately for this group of foster youth, the Foster Care Independence Act of 1999 (also named the Chafee Act after the late John H. Chafee, the senator who sponsored the bill) was passed by Congress (Graf, 2002). The main thrust of the Foster Care Independence Act was to expand the provisions for independent-living programs by doubling the allotment provided for these programs under Title IV-E, and it allowed for more flexibility in terms of providing independence-oriented services. The Chafee Act also allowed for extensions of Medicaid to youth until the age of 21 and strengthened the focus on accountability of states by allocating 1.5% of the total allotment (or $2.1 million) for the development and implementation of national evaluation and the provision of technical assistance to states in assisting youth (Graf, 2002).

In California, the Higher Education Outreach and Assistance Act for Emancipated Foster Youth (California Education Code 89340) offers more needed assistance for former foster youth by requiring California state colleges and universities to provide them with outreach services and technical assistance. It also requires California state colleges and universities to evaluate programs, improve delivery of services, track the progress of former foster youth, and engage in other activities designed to advance services and outreach for former foster youth. In addition, the McKinney–Vento Act clarified some of the educational responsibilities of child welfare agencies. According to this act, the educational goals of a foster child or youth are the shared responsibility of the child welfare agency and the schools. Thus, the McKinney–Vento Act made it clear that child welfare agencies had their share of responsibilities in supporting the educational attainment of their wards. In addition, this act mandated that child welfare agencies implement and design their own policies and practices to maximize placement stability, consider the educational consequences of any action in the child welfare case, and make sure the act is implemented efficiently and that youths derive maximum benefit from these programs (Julianelle, 2009).

There are other federal programs and resources that can also assist these youth in reaching their vocational training goals. A program called Youthbuild, operated by Housing and Urban Development (HUD), provides grants on a competitive basis to assist high-risk youth between the ages of 16 and 24 in learning housing construction job skills and completing their high school education. Program participants are able to augment their skills as they construct and/or restore affordable housing for very low income, homeless people or families. During the past seven years, HUD has released more than $300 million in grants to Youthbuild programs around the nation (NACO, 2008). Also, there are other resources for obtaining educational and vocational grants such as the Federal Pell grants (Annie E. Casey Foundation, 2001). The Pell grants authorize a maximum of more than $5,000 per student per year to support postsecondary training and education. Also, Welfare to Work and TANF programs have funding available for educational and vocational training. In addition to that, the Workforce Investment Act (WIA) has specifically allocated a part of its funding to support work experience and postsecondary vocational training for disadvantaged youth. These nontraditional funding sources can supplement the funding provided by the Foster Care Independence Act (Promising Practices, 2009).

Assembly Bill 12 (AB12) was passed in California in 2010, which allows youth to remain in foster care voluntarily until they are 21 as long as they meet one of the following conditions: completing high school or an equivalent program, enrolling in college or a vocational program, working at least 80 hours a week, participating in an employment program, or living with a medical condition that deems them unable to do any of the above (Aspiranet, n.d.). AB12 took effect in 2012 and uses Title IV-E funds to provide assistance to eligible youth involved with child welfare and probation (CDSS, n.d.a). The effects of AB12 are being felt in many areas of child welfare, including kinship care, the Kinship Guardian Assistance Program (Kin-Gap), transitional housing, and adoptions (CDSS, n.d.b).

POLICY ADVOCACY LEARNING CHALLENGE 11.5

Connecting Micro, Mezzo, and Macro Policy Advocacy

Funding Substance Abuse Services for Jose's Father

Jose is a 10-year-old Hispanic male who has been in the foster care system for a year; he was removed from his father's care because of his father's substance abuse problems. His mother's whereabouts are unknown, and Jose is receiving family reunification services. His father was court ordered to attend a residential substance abuse program; he was motivated and completed his program quickly. The father relapsed soon after, and Jose was placed back in foster care. Upon investigation, it was found that Jose's father could not access continued substance abuse and mental health services because he did not qualify for services under Medi-Cal. With no support, Jose's father returned to his drug abuse.

As a social worker assigned to this case, you try to find the resources through which Jose's father can access drug counseling or support groups. You find that Medicaid is no longer an option because of its regulations. Therefore, you look for other nonprofits in the community and find one that offers counseling and support groups for free if the client offers to volunteer for one of its services. However, you are still frustrated that there is no broad-based policy at the department level that might be able to help Jose's father. You find that Delaware used their Title IV-E funds to hire substance abuse specialists in each of their offices to take care of cases like this one (USDHHS, 2010). You present a plan to the director of the agency, detailing a similar program with data supporting the programmatic benefits and cost-effectiveness of such programs.

LEARNING EXERCISE

1. How does this vignette highlight the risks of not supporting families in recovery?
2. What are some disadvantages of having short-term case planning?
3. What type of policy advocacy needs to be done here?

Core Problem 6: Engaging in Advocacy to Promote Care for Mental Distress—With Some Red Flag Alerts

- **Red Flag Alert 11.23.** There is no communication between the child protective services agency and the agency providing therapy.
- **Red Flag Alert 11.24.** There are unaddressed mental health concerns.
- **Red Flag Alert 11.25.** The family's functioning is being severely affected by mental health problems.

- **Red Flag Alert 11.26.** A client is receiving mental health services, but they are either too little or too much.
- **Red Flag Alert 11.27.** The psychological services are not targeting the person that needs to be receiving help. For example, a family brings their child in for behavioral problems, but the child is acting out as a result of the fighting at home between the parents.

Background

The incidence of youth mental health problems in foster care is overwhelming. Anywhere from 40% to 85% of children in foster care have mental health disorders (Austin, 2004). Children in out-of-home placements not only struggle to cope with the tremendous loss of their family, but also recurrently blame themselves for being removed. Mental health services should be provided to foster youth according to their Bill of Rights, but research shows that less than one third of foster children receive mental health services (Austin, 2004). Findings from a national study that examined specialty mental health service use for children involved in child welfare across 97 U.S. counties indicated that younger children had significantly lower rates of specialty mental health service use, although they had higher levels of clinical need (Hurlburt et al., 2004). Another study, which measured emotional and behavioral outcomes for children placed in foster care by comparing children who had reunified with their families with those who had not reunified six years later, found that children who reunified with their families had worse emotional and behavioral outcomes than their nonreunified peers (Taussig, Clyman, & Landsverk, 2001). Both of these studies point to areas of need within CPS: The former highlights the unmet needs of children left in their home, and the latter indicates that some of these same problems remain even if children are detained and later reunified with their families. The provision of mental health services is further complicated by the growing needs of seriously emotionally disturbed children and the inconsistent availability of foster parent training and support, which can result in high foster parent turnover, placement disruption, inconsistent treatment, and increased trauma for the child (Austin, 2004).

Resources for Advocates

Eligibility for TANF funding for alcohol and drug treatment was expanded to include individuals at risk of involvement. In 1999, TANF significantly expanded services for family safety program clients. Fifteen million dollars (nonrecurring funds) were allocated to fund substance abuse treatment services, substance abuse prevention services, children's mental health services, and residential treatment for substance abuse clients, with priority given to family safety clients.

More recently, DHHS approved up to 10 states to waive certain requirements of Title IV-E to conduct demonstration projects to deliver and finance child welfare services through greater flexibility of the funds according to Section 1130 of the Social Security Act. The projects allow for Title IV-E foster care funds to be used to test different approaches for implementing child welfare services to improve safety, permanency, and well-being for children. California's proposal for the Title IV-E waiver was approved on March 31, 2006, and Los Angeles and Alameda were the two counties who began implementing the waiver on July 1, 2007; the end date was set for June 30, 2012 (CDSS, n.d.b).

POLICY ADVOCACY LEARNING CHALLENGE 11.6

Connecting Micro, Mezzo, and Macro Policy Advocacy

The Rodriguez Family Needs Mental Health Services

The Rodriguez family consists of 47-year-old Jennifer Rodriguez, 15-year-old Julie Rodriguez, and 12-year-old Bobby Rodriguez. The family came to the attention of the Los Angeles DCFS because of an allegation of general neglect after Julie was admitted to a psychiatric hospital for attempting to overdose on sleeping pills. As part of the allegation, it was reported that the mother was not meeting Julie's unique psychiatric needs and constantly yelled at her children.

After reading the relevant policy and identifying the mental health concerns to be addressed by the Department of Mental Health (DMH), the social worker immediately called the psychiatric hospital to find out when Julie would be released. Due to the mental health concerns and the three previous referrals for general neglect, the social worker and supervisor decided that this referral needed a team decision meeting (TDM) to best coordinate services with the family's participation. In preparation for the TDM, the social worker summarized the DCFS history and the psychiatric treatment recommendations. At the TDM, the social worker presented the information and discussed all the possible options with the family, the DMH worker, and the DCFS supervisor to come to a mutual agreement. The mother felt she could not control her daughter's behavior and was worried that her daughter would run away as soon as she got home. Because of the seriousness of Julie's mental health problems and because her mother felt as if she could not handle Julie on her own, it was agreed to open up a voluntary case and to voluntarily place Julie with a foster family while her mother received support to deal with Julie's unique mental health needs.

The social worker attempted to make Julie's transition into foster care as easy as possible by explaining the process and by having her family visit on a regular basis. Her mother was enrolled in parenting classes, and Julie began receiving therapy immediately because of the coordination with DMH. After the situation stabilized, Julie was returned to her family, and they received family preservation services to assist with the transition back home.

LEARNING EXERCISE

1. How does this vignette illustrate the importance of coordination/collaboration between various service agencies?
2. What examples of micro policy advocacy did you notice in this vignette? What other type of micro policy advocacy could the social worker have done for the family?
3. Could a social worker in this clinic have engaged in mezzo or macro policy advocacy in this scenario? Give some examples.

Core Problem 7: Engaging in Advocacy to Promote Care Linked to Communities—With Some Red Flag Alerts

- **Red Flag Alert 11.28.** Your agency cannot provide the services your client desperately needs.
- **Red Flag Alert 11.29.** Your agency competes with other agencies instead of collaborating.
- **Red Flag Alert 11.30.** There are no additional agencies that can provide the services that your client needs.
- **Red Flag Alert 11.31.** Your client fears receiving services because of their national origin.
- **Red Flag Alert 11.32.** Information between agencies involved with the same client is not shared, and there is no coordination of services.

Background

Children in the child and family sector often find themselves simultaneously involved in other public sectors such as public social services, mental health, criminal justice, immigration, education, and public social services, which are sometimes referred to as cross-sector services (Drake, Jonson-Reid, & Sapokaite, 2006). The literature reveals that from 35% to 85% of children entering foster care have significant mental health problems (Reed & Karpilow, 2002). Parental substance abuse is a factor in an estimated two thirds of cases with children in foster care. Child abuse and domestic violence most often go hand in hand, occurring in the same household and having a common perpetrator. Foster children are more likely than other children to perform poorly in school and develop conduct problems. Juvenile justice departments have also been consistently reporting a rising tide of children from foster care landing on their doorstep. Therefore, policies should be geared toward streamlining services in agencies so that people can transition from one agency to another without any bureaucratic red tape.

Resources for Advocates

Changes in TANF laws have prevented many individuals and families from receiving the financial assistance they require (Stoesz, 1999). This prevention has pushed many families beyond their limits and contributed to the growing number of child neglect cases owing to a lack of financial resources (Stoesz, 1999).

Another sector that frequently crosses over with child welfare is juvenile justice. In juvenile justice, children who are maltreated are at risk for delinquency and often end up in the juvenile justice system (Bender, 2010). It is estimated that a quarter of foster youth will serve time in jail in the first two years after high school, and nearly 70% of inmates in state penitentiaries have been in foster care (Just in Time for Foster Youth, n.d.). These youth are often referred to as crossover youth or dually involved youth, and the majority of them have problems involving school, mental health, and/or drug use (Herz et al., 2012). Furthermore, many crossover youth have witnessed domestic violence and have parents with mental health problems, substance abuse issues, and criminal justice involvement (Herz et al., 2012). National estimates indicate that children whose caregivers have been arrested have higher rates of drug use, domestic violence, and poverty (Phillips & Dettlaff, 2009).

Almost one fourth of all children in the United States have at least one parent who is an immigrant (American Humane Association, n.d.a). Although the numbers of children living with immigrant families are not certain because these statistics are usually not collected by CPS agencies, national estimates indicate that this population makes up approximately 8.6% of children reported to CPS (Dettlaff, Earner, & Phillips, 2009). Related to immigration, human trafficking has become a growing problem. With the passage of the Victims of Trafficking and Violence Protection Act in 2000, identification and treatment of victims of human trafficking has considerably improved (Fong & Berger Cardoso, 2010)—but its resources have mostly gone to adult victims rather than children. According to the Department of Justice, there were 2,515 human trafficking incidents opened for investigation between January 2008 and June 2010 (Banks & Kyckelhahn, 2011). Of these, 1,016 children were investigated for prostitution or child exploitation, accounting for more than 40% of all investigated incidents.

The following websites are relevant to the crossover between immigration and child welfare:

> American Humane Association: http://www.americanhumane.org/children/professional-resources/program-publications/child-welfare-migration/tool-kits.html
>
> Family to Family California: http://www.f2f.ca.gov/Immigrants.htm
>
> Integration: Building Inclusive Societies: http://www.unaoc.org/ibis/2011/02/21/migration-and-child-welfare-national-network/

The following websites provide services and advocacy to victims of human trafficking:

Girls Education and Mentoring Services: http://www.gems-girls.org/

Office of Refugee Resettlement: http://www.acf.hhs.gov/programs/orr/programs/anti-trafficking and http://www.acf.hhs.gov/programs/orr/resource/fact-sheet-child-victims-of-human-trafficking

SCTNow.org: http://www.sctnow.org/index.aspx?parentnavigationid=5812

Trafficking in Persons Report: http://www.state.gov/documents/organization/192587.pdf

---

POLICY ADVOCACY LEARNING CHALLENGE 11.7

Connecting Micro, Mezzo, and Macro Policy Advocacy

Finding Community Resources

Imagine that you are a social worker in the Department of Children and Family Services (DCFS) who has been assigned to 17-year-old Tommy Jones. Tommy is African American, and he walked into your office today after running away for one month. He will not say where he was and states that he returned to the office because he was tired of living on the streets. Tommy has not participated in therapy and has not taken his psychotropic medication since he went AWOL from his last group home. You look in his file and note that he was last prescribed Seroquel for psychotic disorder not otherwise specified. He also has not been in school in over six months and was on probation, although it is unclear whether it is still active.

While sitting at your desk, you notice that Tommy is staring at people and laughing for no reason at all. You ask him about drug use, and he states that he smokes tobacco and marijuana every once in a while. You ask him whether he has ever been in a psychiatric hospital, and he states that he has been hospitalized twice in the last six months (he reports that he does not remember why). You ask Tommy about whether he'll go talk to a psychiatrist to get his medication filled again, and he states that he does not want to take medication because he is Christian and God will take care of him. You further read in his file that his aunt dropped him off at a DCFS office when he was 16 because she could no longer handle his strange behavior. He still visits her once a month, but she states that she can't have him at her house for more than a few hours at a time because of his strange behavior. Aside from this aunt, his relatives' whereabouts are unknown. When you ask him what he wants, Tommy says that he just wants a place to stay.

LEARNING EXERCISE

1. How does this vignette illustrate the multiple sectors that a client can be involved with?
2. Before any type of policy advocacy can occur, what is the first step that should be taken when working with Tommy?
3. What kind of policy advocacy needs to be done with Tommy, considering he is a crossover youth?

"THINKING BIG" AS POLICY ADVOCATES IN THE CHILD AND FAMILY SECTOR

The foster youth caucus of the U.S. House of Representatives, chaired by Democratic congresswomen Karen Bass of Los Angeles, often develops legislation to assist foster children. Go to its website at http://fosteryouthcaucus-karenbass.house.gov and click on "Activities & Legislation." Select one of the pieces of legislation. Using concepts developed in Chapter 6 on policy analysis, develop some policy options that the House legislators might consider when drafting a legislative proposal with regard to one of their prioritized legislative or issue areas. Develop some criteria to be used to assess the options, such as cost and effectiveness. Decide which option appears to be meritorious.

Or examine the list of recommendations made by the Blue Ribbon Commission in Los Angeles County in the summer of 2014 to reform child welfare services. Would any of these recommendations apply to the child welfare system in your jurisdiction? Select one or several of them as possible recommendations in your jurisdiction. (You can find the Commission's recommendations at http://ceo.lacounty.gov/pdf/brc/BRCCP_Final_Report_April_18_2014.pdf.)

You may also tackle another common problem in foster care: the inability of social workers to obtain the education records of foster children from their schools on the grounds that schools do not want to breech student confidentiality. This policy, while well intended, often has bad consequences for foster children because they must often switch schools when they are shifted from one foster home to another. The lack of information about the courses these students took in other schools often leads to their repeating courses, which severely delays their schooling and jeopardizes their graduation.

Another option is to propose and seek enactment of a "children's allowance" that other industrialized nations provide to parents of children. Such a resource would be invaluable to stressed-out single parents, who often work two to three jobs just to make ends meet.

LEARNING OUTCOMES

You are now equipped to:

- Contact key advocacy groups in the child and family sector and use their Internet materials
- Critically analyze the evolution of the child welfare system in the United States
- Identify the impact of specific interest groups and organizations on child welfare policies
- Analyze how income inequality in the United States profoundly impacts the problems of children and families that require interventions by child welfare professionals
- Engage in micro, mezzo, or macro policy advocacy with respect to seven problems often experienced by children and families in the child and family sector
- Apply the eight challenges in the multilevel policy empowerment framework to the child and family sector

REFERENCES

American Humane Association. (n.d.a). *Child welfare and migration.* Retrieved from http://www .americanhumane.org/children/programs/child-welfare-migration/

American Humane Association. (n.d.b). *Disparities in child welfare.* Retrieved from http://www .americanhumane.org/children/programs/disparities-in-child-welfare.html

Anderson, P. G. (1989). The origin, emergence, and professional recognition of child protection. *Social Service Review, 63*(2), 222–244. doi: 10.1086/603695

Annie E. Casey Foundation. (2001). *Promising practices: School to career and postsecondary education for foster care youth: A guide for policymakers and practitioners.* Retrieved from: http://collegeforamerica.org/reports/promisingpractices2.pdf

Areen, J. (1975). Intervention between parent and child: A reappraisal of the state's role in child neglect and abuse cases. *Georgetown Law Journal, 63*(4), 887–937.

Arkansas Advocates. (2005). *The Arkansas child welfare system.* Retrieved from http://www .aradvocates.org/_images/pdfs/ArkChildWelfareSystem.pdf

Aspiranet: Transition Age Youth Services. (n.d.). *Building the bridge between foster care and independence.* Retrieved from http://www.aspiranetthpplus.org/ab12-benefits-aging-out-of -foster-care/

Austin, L. (2004). *Mental health needs of youth in foster care: Challenges and strategies.* Retrieved from http://www.casanet.org/library/foster-care/mental-health-%5Bconnection -04%5D.pdf

Banks, D., & Kyckelhahn, T. (2011). *Characteristics of suspected human trafficking incidents, 2008–2010.* U.S. Department of Justice, Office of Justice Programs, Bureau of Justice Statistics. Retrieved from http://bjs.ojp.usdoj.gov/index.cfm?ty=tp&tid=40#data_collections

Bardach, E. (1996). The eight-step path of policy analysis. In *Best practices.* Berkeley, CA: Berkeley Academic Press. Retrieved from http://www.newwaystowork.org/initiatives/ytat/ practices.html

Bender, K. (2010). Why do some maltreated youth become juvenile offenders? A call for further investigation and adaptation of youth services. *Children and Youth Services Review*, *32*(3), 466–473. doi: 10.1016/j.childyouth.2009.10.022

Bluecommissionla.com. (n.d.). *The road to safety for our children*. Retrieved from http://ceo.lacounty.gov/pdf/brc/BRCCP_Final_Report_April_18_2014.pdf

Brittain, C., & Hunt, D. E. (2004). *Helping in child protective services: A competency-based casework handbook*. Cambridge, UK: Oxford University Press.

Brooks-Gunn, J., & Duncan, G. J. (1997). The effects of poverty on children. *Future of Children*, *7*(2), 55–71.

California Department of Social Services. (n.d.a). *Assembly Bill 12*. Retrieved from http://www.childsworld.ca.gov/PG2902.htm

California Department of Social Services. (n.d.b). *Title IV-E Child Welfare Waiver Demonstration Capped Allocation Project (CAP)*. Retrieved from http://www.dss.cahwnet.gov/cfsweb/PG1333.htm

Child protective services. (n.d.). *Wikipedia*. Retrieved May 28, 2014, from http://en.wikipedia.org/wiki/Child_Protective_Services#Child_Protective_Services_Recidivism_in_the_United_States

Child Welfare Information Gateway. (n.d.a). *Clients' rights*. Retrieved from http://www.childwelfare.gov/management/ethical/client_rights.cfm

Child Welfare Information Gateway. (n.d.b). *Evidence-based practice in child welfare*. Retrieved from http://www.childwelfare.gov/management/practice_improvement/evidence/ebp.cfm

Child Welfare Information Gateway. (2009). *Adoption assistance for children adopted from foster care*. Retrieved from http://www.childwelfare.gov/can/defining/federal.cfm

Child Welfare Information Gateway. (2011). *Adoption assistance for children adopted from foster care*. Retrieved from https://www.childwelfare.gov/pubs/f_subsid.pdf#page=1&view=Introduction

Child Welfare League of America. (n.d.). *Summary of the Adoption and Safe Families Act of 1997 (P.L. 105-89)*. Retrieved from http://www.cwla.org/advocacy/asfapl105-89summary.htm

Children Uniting Nations. (n.d.). *Foster care statistics*. Retrieved June 27, 2014, from http://www.childrenunitingnations.org/who-we-are/foster-care-statistics/

Christenson, B. L. (2009). *Youth exiting foster care: Efficacy of foster care in the state of Idaho*. Retrieved from http://www.jimcaseyyouth.org/docs/exitingfoster.pdf

Costin, L. B., Karger, H. J., & Stoesz, D. (1996). *The politics of child abuse in America*. New York, NY: Oxford University Press.

De Bellis, M. D., Keshavan, M. S., Clark, D. B., Casey, B. J., Giedd, J. N., Boring, A. M., & Ryan, N. D. (1999). Developmental traumatology: Part II. Brain development. *Biological Psychiatry, 45,* 1271–1284.

Department of Children and Family Services. (n.d.). *DCFS office outreach: Pomona*. Retrieved from http://dcfs.co.la.ca.us/community/Pomona/index.html

Department of Children and Family Services. (2014). *Community response services, alternative response services and up-front assessments 0070-548.00*. Retrieved from http://policy.dcfs.lacounty.gov/default.htm#POE_ARS_Communit.htm#Topic1

Dettlaff, A. J., Earner, I., & Phillips, S. D. (2009). Latino children of immigrants in the child welfare system: Prevalence, characteristics, and risk. *Children and Youth Services Review, 31*(7), 775–783.

Doherty, S. (2005). *Rights of children in foster care.* Retrieved from http://www.hunter.cuny.edu/socwork/nrcfcpp/downloads/rights-children-foster-care.pdf

Drake, B., Jonson-Reid, M., & Sapokaite, L. (2006). Rereporting of child maltreatment: Does participation in other public sector services moderate the likelihood of a second maltreatment report? *Child Abuse and Neglect, 30*(11), 1201–1226. doi: 10.1016/j.chiabu.2006.05.008

Fearnotlaw.com. (n.d.). *In re A.J..* Retrieved from http://www.fearnotlaw.com/articles/article28570.html

Felitti, V. J., Anda, R. F., Nordenberg, D., Williamson, D. F., Spitz, A. M., Edwards, V., & Marks, J. S. (1998). Relationship of childhood abuse and household dysfunction to many of the leading causes of death in adults. *American Journal of Preventive Medicine, 14*(4), 245–258. doi: 10.1016/S0749-3797(98)00017-8

Fogarty, J. (2008). Some aspects of the early history of child protection in Australia. *Family Matters, 78,* 52–59.

Fong, R., & Berger Cardoso, J. (2010). Child human trafficking victims: Challenges for the child welfare system. *Evaluation and Program Planning, 33*(3), 311–316.

Fryer, R. G., Jr., & Levitt, S. D. (2004). Understanding the black–white test score gap in the first two years of school. *Review of Economics and Statistics, 86*(2), 447–464.

Gelles, R. J. (2001). Family preservation and reunification: How effective a social policy? In *Handbook of youth and justice* (pp. 367–376). New York, NY: Kluwer Academic/Plenum.

Glisson, C. (2009). Organizational climate and culture and performance in the human services. In R. Patti (Ed.), *The handbook of social welfare management* (pp. 119–141). Thousand Oaks, CA: SAGE.

Government Accounting Office, Report to the Chairman, Subcommittee on Human Resources, Committee on Ways and Means, House of Representatives. (1998). *Foster care implementation of the multiethnic placement act poses difficult challenges.* Retrieved from http://www.gao.gov/archive/1998/he98204.pdf

Graf, B. (2002). *Foster Care Independence Act.* Retrieved from http://www.hunter.cuny.edu/socwork/nrcfcpp/downloads/information_packets/foster_care_independence_act-pkt.pdf

Harding, D. J. (2003). Counterfactual models of neighborhood effects: The effect of neighborhood poverty on dropping out and teenage pregnancy. *American Journal of Sociology, 109*(3), 676–719.

Herz, D., Lee, P., Lutz, L., Stewart, M., Tuell, J., & Wiig, J. (2012). *Addressing the needs of multi-system youth: Strengthening the connection between child welfare and juvenile justice.* Washington, DC: Georgetown University Center for Juvenile Justice Reform / Boston: RFK Children's Action Corps. Retrieved from http://cjjr.georgetown.edu/pdfs/msy/AddressingtheNeedsofMultiSystemYouth.pdf

Hill, B. (2006). *Synthesis of research on disproportionality in child welfare: An update.* Retrieved from http://www.racemattersconsortium.org/docs/BobHillPaper_FINAL.pdf

Hurlburt, M., Leslie, L. K., Landsverk, J., Barth, R. P., Burns, B. J., Gibbons, R. D., . . . Zhang, J. (2004). Contextual predictors of mental health service use among children open to child welfare. *Archives of General Psychiatry, 61*(12), 1217–1224. doi: 10.1001/archpsyc.61.12.1217

Jackson, K. (2009). Building cultural competence: A systematic evaluation of the effectiveness of culturally sensitive interventions with ethnic minority youth. *Children and Youth Services Review, 31*(11), 1192–1198.

Julianelle, P. (2009). *The McKinney-Vento Act and children and youth awaiting foster care placement.* Retrieved from National Association for the Education of Homeless Children and Youth: http://www.naehcy.org/dl/mv_afcp.pdf

Just in Time for Foster Youth. (n.d.). *Outcomes.* Retrieved June 21, 2014, from http://jitfosteryouth.org/outcomes/

Kotch, J. B., Chang, J. J., & Hussey, J. M. (2006). Child maltreatment in the United States: Prevalence, risk factors, and adolescent health consequences. *Pediatrics, 118*(3), 933–942. doi: 10.1542/peds.2005-2452

Lee, J. (2002). Racial and ethnic achievement gap trends: Reversing the progress toward equity. *Educational Researcher, 31*(1), 3–12.

Lehmann, B., & Guyer, J. (2012). *Child welfare and the Affordable Care Act: Key provisions for foster care children and youth.* Washington, DC: Center for Children and Families. Retrieved from Georgetown University: http://ccf.georgetown.edu/wp-content/uploads/2012/07/Child-Welfare-and-the-ACA.pdf

Lind, C. (2004). *Developing and supporting a continuum of child welfare services.* Retrieved from http://www.financeproject.org/publications/developingandsupportingIN.pdf

Menchik, P. L. (1993). Economic status as a determinant of mortality among black and white older men: Does poverty kill? *Population Studies, 47*(3), 427–436.

Morales, A., Sheafor, B. W., & Scott, M. E. (2011). *Social work: A profession of many faces.* Boston, MA: Allyn & Bacon.

Murray, K., & Gesiriech, S. (2005). *A brief legislative history of the child welfare system.* Retrieved from http://pewfostercare.org/research/docs/Legislative.pdf

Myers, J. E. B. (2008). Short history of child protection in America. *Family Law Quarterly, 449,* 449–463.

NACO. (2008). *Youth aging out of foster care: Strategies and best practices.* Retrieved from http://www.naco.org/Content/ContentGroups/Issue_Briefs/IB-YouthAgingoutof Foster-2008.pdf

Needell, B., Cuccaro-Alamin, S., Brookhart, A., Jackman, W., & Shlonsky, A. (2002). Youth emancipating from foster care in California: Findings using linked administrative data. Berkeley, CA: Center for Social Services Research.

Patton, C. V., & Sawicki, D. S. (1993). *Basic methods of policy analysis & planning* (2nd ed.). Englewood Cliffs, NJ: Prentice Hall.

Pecora, P. J. (2000). *The child welfare challenge: Policy, practice and research.* New York, NY: Aldine Gruyter.

Penn State. (n.d.). In *Wikipedia.* Retrieved July 31, 2014, from http://en.wikipedia.org/wiki/Penn_State_child_sex_abuse_scandal

Phillips, S. D., & Dettlaff, A. J. (2009). More than parents in prison: The broader overlap between the criminal justice and child welfare systems. *Journal of Public Child Welfare, 3*(1), 3–22.

Promising Practices. (2009). *School to career and post-secondary education for foster youth.* Retrieved August 3, 2014, from http://www.workforcestrategy.org/publications/promisingpractices2.pdf

Reed, F. D., & Karpilow, K. (2002). *Understanding the child welfare system in California: A primer for service providers and policymakers.* Retrieved from http://www.ccrwf .org/pdf/ChildWelfarePrimer.pdf

Sampson, R. J., & Wilson, W. J. (1995). Toward a theory of race, crime, and urban inequality. In *Race, crime, and justice: A reader* (pp. 177–190). Retrieved from http://faculty .washington.edu/matsueda/courses/371/Readings/Sampson%20Wilson.pdf

Schene, P. A. (1998). Past, present, and future roles of child protective services. *Future of Children, 8*(1), 23–38.

Schene, P. (2005). The emergence of differential response. *Protecting Children, 20*(2–3), 4–7. Retrieved from http://www.americanhumane.org/assets/pdfs/children/protecting -children-journal/pc-20-2-3.pdf#page=5

Schott, L. (2009). *Policy basics: An introduction to TANF.* Retrieved from http://www .cbpp.org/cms/?fa=view&id=93

Sedlak, A. J., Mettenburg, J., Basena, M., Petta, I., McPherson, K., Greene, A., & Li, S. (2010). *Fourth National Incidence Study of Child Abuse and Neglect (NIS–4): Report to Congress.* Washington, DC: U.S. Department of Health and Human Services, Administration for Children and Families.

SSI Fact Sheet. (2009). *SSI fact sheet for foster youth.* Retrieved from http://www.ssitransitions .org/pdfs/AB%201331%20Information%20Sheet.pdf

Stoesz, D. (1999). Unraveling welfare reform. *Society, 36*(4), 53–61.

Stoltzfus, E. (2011). *Child welfare: The Child and Family Services Improvement and Innovation Act (P.L. 112-34).* Congressional Research Service, Library of Congress. Retrieved from http://greenbook.waysandmeans.house.gov/sites/greenbook.waysand means.house.gov/files/2011/images/R42027_gb.pdf

Taussig, H. N., Clyman, R. B., & Landsverk, J. (2001). Children who return home from foster care: A 6-year prospective study of behavioral health outcomes in adolescence. *Pediatrics, 208,* E10. Retrieved from http://pediatrics.aappublications.org/cgi/ content/full/108/1/e10#otherarticle

Therolf, G. (2013, May 31). Boy's death prompts outrage, red flags of child abuse "ignored." *Los Angeles Times.* Retrieved from http://articles.latimes.com/2013 /may/31/local/la-me-ln-boy-killed-20130531

Trattner, W. I. (1999). *From poor law to welfare state.* New York, NY: Free Press.

Twiname, J. (1975). *Using Title XX to serve children and youth.* Retrieved from http://www .eric.ed.gov/ERICDocs/data/ericdocs2sql/content_storage_01/0000019b/80/31/5b/a7.pdf

U.S. Department of Health and Human Services, Substance Abuse and Mental Health Services Administration, Administration for Children and Families. (2010). *Substance abuse specialists in child welfare agencies and dependency courts considerations for program designers and evaluators.* Retrieved from https://www.ncsacw.samhsa.gov /files/SubstanceAbuseSpecialists.pdf

U.S. Department of Health and Human Services, Administration for Children and Families, Administration on Children, Youth and Families, Children's Bureau. (2013). *Child maltreatment 2012.* Retrieved from http://www.acf.hhs.gov/programs/cb /research-data-technology/statistics-research/child-maltreatment

Wang, C. T., & Holton, J. (2007). *Total estimated cost of child abuse and neglect in the United States.* Chicago, IL: Prevent Child Abuse America.

Weizman, A., Har-Even, D., Shnit, D., Finzi, R., & Ram, A. (2001). Attachment styles and aggression in physically abused and neglected children. *Journal of Youth and Adolescence, 30*(6), 769–786. doi: 10.1023/A:1012237813771

Welte, C. (1997). *Detailed summary of the Adoption and Safe Families Act.* Retrieved from http://www.casanet.org/reference/asfa-summary.htm

Wilkins, A. (2004). *The Indian Child Welfare Act and the states.* Retrieved from http://www.ncsl.org/IssuesResearch/StateTribal/TheIndianChildWelfareActandthe States/tabid/13275/Default.aspx

Wulczyn, F. (2009). Epidemiological perspectives on maltreatment prevention. *Future of Children, 19*(2), 39–66.

Chapter 12

BECOMING POLICY ADVOCATES IN THE EDUCATION SECTOR

Bruce S. Jansson, Elaine Sanchez Wilson, and Vivien Villaverde

---

LEARNING OBJECTIVES

In this chapter, you will learn how to:

1. Analyze how the American educational system has evolved

2. Identify educational problems caused by economic inequality

3. Analyze the education sector's current political economy, including powerful players and interests as well as key advocacy groups

4. Identify problematic issues that impact students' educational and personal outcomes

5. Discuss advocacy strategies social workers can utilize as they encounter seven major problems

---

Students must navigate not only the often overcrowded hallways of their schools but also a bevy of institutional hurdles. They face increasing pressure to demonstrate proficiency in math and reading without a mastery of the subjects' foundations. They often lack a sufficient support system at home to help them with their studies or cultivate their learning. They often have overworked teachers who are not attentive to their personal issues. They often must contend with bullies. Many of them have serious undiagnosed or poorly treated mental conditions like autism, attention deficit disorder, anxiety, and depression. Substance abuse is widespread among students. Some go to their beds hungry, while others may not have their own beds at all.

Educational institutions lie at the heart of the American dream of upward mobility and personal success. Social workers assume a critical role in helping students in these institutions. They can provide micro, mezzo, and macro policy advocacy that draw upon their unique empowerment perspectives.

ANALYZING THE EVOLUTION OF THE AMERICAN EDUCATION SYSTEM

VIDEO LINK 12.1
Placing Social
Work Units in
Schools

This timeline represents the historical forces that influenced the current processes and policies of the U.S. educational system, particularly for primary and secondary education:

- The Massachusetts Act of 1642 mandated colonial-era parents and masters to teach their children and apprentices about moral character as well as their new homeland's laws. Children received lessons in reading, writing, math, and prayers. Those in lower socioeconomic groups became apprentices to specialize in particular trades.
- The United States implemented its first national system of public schools, beginning with primary and elementary grades, in the middle part of the 19th century, and enacted compulsory high school education in the latter part of the 19th century and early part of the 20th century.
- Despite making civil rights gains in the aftermath of the Civil War, African Americans endured a major blow at the hands of the Supreme Court, which validated the "separate but equal" doctrine in its 1896 *Plessy v. Ferguson* decision. States had the right to separate facilities by race as long as they provided equal counterparts. This ruling led to the legitimization of separate educational institutions that were largely inferior in the case of minorities.
- Compulsory education laws, first seen in Massachusetts during the colonial period, were adopted nationwide by 1918.
- Goals shifted during the 1930s (Allen-Meares, 2007). Tight budgets reduced or cut visiting teachers' programs (Areson, 1923). Instead of serving as liaisons between school and home, school social workers focused on improving children's mental health and providing emotional support (Hall, 1936).
- In the famous court case *Brown v. Board of Education*, the U.S. Supreme Court overturned *Plessy v. Ferguson* by ruling that separate educational institutions were inherently unequal.
- First applied in the labor setting, the term "affirmative action" was introduced by President John F. Kennedy in a 1961 executive order that required government contractors to "take affirmative action to ensure that all applicants are

employed, and that employees are treated during employment, without regard to their race, creed, color, or national origin" (Executive Order No. 10925). The policy was extended to include women in 1967.

- The Bilingual Education Act of 1968, later amended in 1974 and 1988, granted funding to school districts to set up their own bilingual educational programs, teacher training, and materials.
- The NASW Council on Social Work in Schools held its first meeting in 1973, where it discussed the issues that field workers encountered. Among these were embattled parent–child relationships involving emotionally disturbed students from low-income areas (two thirds of whom were white), overwhelming caseloads, excessive referrals, and unclear job descriptions.
- Passing Congress in 2001 with widespread bipartisan support, No Child Left Behind is the latest version of the omnibus 1965 Elementary and Secondary Education Act. The legislation, proposed and signed into law by President George W. Bush, aimed to improve student achievement, especially among disadvantaged students, through an expanded federal role in education.
- President Barack Obama developed a revised version of Bush's legislation called "Race to the Top." It gave states greater latitude to develop their educational systems, allowing states to develop their own methods of evaluating the quality of students' education as long as they include students' test scores in their evaluations of teachers and principals.

RECOGNIZING EDUCATIONAL PROBLEMS CREATED BY AN INEGALITARIAN NATION

President George W. Bush famously implored Americans to "attack the soft bigotry of low expectations" and work to narrow the achievement gap between black and white students when he enacted No Child Left Behind. The gap to which the president was referring has been widening since the late 1980s. The average black or Hispanic student at 17 years old is performing worse on standardized tests than at least 80% of his or her white classmates (Thernstrom & Thernstrom, 2003). While the academic divide is present in suburban and urban districts, students from "distressed neighborhoods" are at greatest risk of lacking the minimum skills and knowledge they need to prosper as adults (Thernstrom & Thernstrom, 2003).

Other theorists go even farther in analyzing the causes of educational disparities. Low-income children, they note, receive substantially less preparation for school during their early years. They hear far fewer words than middle- and upper-income children from their parents and peers. Minus considerable reinforcement of their education by preschools and by Head Start, they are often destined to perform at lower levels than their more affluent counterparts. Many experts want even greater funding of preschool programs, including Head Start.

School choice laws of the 1980s drew support from free-market proponents such as President Ronald Reagan. Traditionally, low-income, largely minority, parents who were unable to relocate to better school districts or to afford private school had no choice but to send their children to underfinanced neighborhood schools (Sawhill & Smith, 2000). With the passage of public school choice laws, students would be able to transfer from their schools to others in the same district or outside their home district. Public school alternatives include public and private voucher programs, homeschooling, and charter schools, or privately run public schools that are free from many state and district regulations.

ANALYZING THE POLITICAL ECONOMY OF THE EDUCATION SECTOR

The dynamics among educational stakeholders, including school board members, superintendents, teachers, parents, and students, are often wrought with tension.

For example, one key roadblock to much-needed educational reform is teacher quality, which research shows has a significant impact on student learning (Thernstrom & Thernstrom, 2003). School administrators have not held back their harsh criticisms against their fellow educators. Iowa Department of Education director Jason Glass said quality, not seniority, should be the determining criteria in layoffs. Michelle Rhee, former Washington, DC, chancellor of schools, drew fire for her plan to terminate ineffective teachers at will. The Educational Trust shone a spotlight on the glaring difference between schools in poor districts and schools that serve students of higher income levels, noting "a pervasive, almost chilling difference in the quality of their teachers."

Teachers' unions, on the other hand, say the blame is too quickly placed on its members. Many teachers work well past school hours, crafting lessons and grading assignments into the night. Salaries are modest, classrooms are overcrowded, and with today's tight budgets, many teachers face job insecurity. As a result, some educators call for parents to meet them halfway. Schools cannot do all the work; rather, families must put in the effort to work with their children at home and impose higher expectations. President Obama summed up this sentiment in a fiery 2009 speech to the NAACP, during which he told parents,

> We can't tell our kids to do well in school and then fail to support them when they get home. For our kids to excel, we have to accept our responsibility to help them learn . . . We've got to say to our children . . . your destiny is in your hands . . . No excuses. (Sweet, 2009)

Advocacy groups are increasingly influencing education policy through lobbying and aggressive campaigning, especially at the state level. (See Table 12.1.)

Table 12.1 Selected Advocacy Groups for Educational Reforms

Education Reform Now seeks educational reforms for low-income students in 14 states. **www.edreform.org**

The **Education Trust** engages in advocacy for low-income students at all levels of education. **www.edtrust.org**

Stand for Children advocates public education. **www.stand.org**

Democrats for Education Reform advocates accountable public schools. **www.dfer.org**

The **National Indian Education Association** seeks to improve schools for American Indians. **www.niea.org**

The **National School Boards Association** provides training for board members and disseminates research on critical issues. **www.nsba.org**

Parents for Public Schools seeks to improve public schools by mobilizing parents. **www.parents4publicschools.org**

The **Mexican American Legal Defense and Educational Fund (MALDEF)** seeks to improve schools for Latino children. **www.maldef.org**

ANALYZING SEVEN CORE PROBLEMS IN THE AMERICAN EDUCATION SYSTEM

Core Problem 1: Engaging in Advocacy to Promote Ethical Rights, Human Rights, and Economic Justice—With Some Red Flag Alerts

Ethics can take on different forms in the education sector, and it is essential for social workers to identify potential issues at the student level or, even more broadly, at the school or district level. These concerns lead social workers to assess whether students in their schools are receiving their right to an education and challenge administration to engage in addressing these questions.

- **Red Flag Alert 12.1.** A school refuses to honor a parent's request for her child's academic record.
- **Red Flag Alert 12.2.** Students are suspended for personal views, such as wearing a shirt in support of the death penalty.
- **Red Flag Alert 12.3.** A student is forced to sit in the corner in time-out for refusing to recite the Pledge of Allegiance.

- **Red Flag Alert 12.4.** A student receives a slap on the wrist for classroom disruption.
- **Red Flag Alert 12.5.** A student is expelled without a hearing.
- **Red Flag Alert 12.6.** School personnel search student lockers without providing a reason.
- **Red Flag Alert 12.7.** School administrators prevent a school newspaper from publishing an editorial about teen pregnancy.
- **Red Flag Alert 12.8.** A group of students are prohibited from assembling a gay–straight alliance.
- **Red Flag Alert 12.9.** Juvenile bullying is a frequent occurrence.
- **Red Flag Alert 12.10.** Schools discriminate against lesbian and gay students.

Background

Most elementary, middle, and—arguably—high school students are simply not aware of their personal rights, and as a result, they represent a vulnerable population. Although some pupils may be equipped with this knowledge, the teacher–student dynamic makes it challenging for youngsters to assert and defend these rights. They may feel intimidated or fear punishment from school administration or parents.

Certain minority groups are possibly at greater risk of experiencing a violation of their rights. Non-English-speaking parents may not understand the entire situation affecting their children. Some Asian American families find it difficult to deviate from their cultural norm of not questioning persons in authority.

Resources for Advocates

As students, parents, teachers, and school administrators encounter and struggle with these ethical and educational rights issues, education advocates can use the different education policies, statutes and constitutional rights, state and federal regulations, and court rulings to guide their advocacy.

Statutes and the Constitution. Article 26 of the Universal Declaration of Human Rights states that every person is entitled to an education. It endorses a free public elementary and secondary education. "Education shall be directed to the full development of the human personality and to the strengthening of respect for human rights and fundamental freedoms," it proclaims, adding that parents have the right to select the type of education their children receive. Nevertheless, school choice is not always available to families. Some low-income students are not offered an alternative to their dilapidated classrooms, noncredentialed faculty, and lack of educational resources. Their schooling does not lift them up to their full academic potential, and as a result, many will struggle with employment later in life.

The Family Educational Rights and Privacy Act, enacted in 1974, protects the privacy of student records (20 U.S.C. 1232g; 34 CFR Part 99). Schools that receive any Department of Education funds are subject to the policy; therefore, private and parochial schools are not legally bound to comply. Parents, or eligible students 18 years of age or older, have the right to review students' academic records and request changes if they believe the document is inaccurate or misleading. If a school does not grant the change, parents can ask for a formal hearing. If the review panel also denies the request, parents have the right to include a written statement about the contested information in their child's record. Schools are prohibited from sharing information from a student's education record except in a few cases, such as academic institutions to which the student may be transferring or officials within a juvenile justice system.

The Equal Access Act, ratified in 1984, provides that secondary schools that utilize federal funds must grant their students equal access to extracurricular activities. If the institution already possesses a "limited open forum," or in other words already permits one student-led club to meet outside class time, it must allow additional clubs to organize and be given equal access to meeting spaces and publications.

Court Rulings. A number of court cases have also shaped the ethical standards that are upheld in schools. For example, in the 1943 *West Virginia State Board of Education v. Barnette* trial, the Supreme Court ruled that students could not be forced to salute the American flag or recite the Pledge of Allegiance in school. The 1969 *Tinker v. Des Moines Independent Community School District* decision produced what is today known as the Tinker test, which courts apply in assessing whether academic disciplinary decisions violate students' First Amendment right of free speech. In this particular case, students Mary Beth Tinker, John Tinker, and Christopher Eckhardt wore black armbands to school in protest of the Vietnam War and were subsequently suspended. In its majority opinion, the Court concluded, "It can hardly be argued that either teachers or students shed their constitutional rights to free speech or expression at the schoolhouse gate" (393 U.S. 503). Exceptions to this policy include speech that infringes on the rights of others; interferes with school operations; is obscene, lewd, or offensive; or is school-sponsored. Students' freedom of expression did not fare so well in the 1988 ruling, *Hazelwood School District et al. v. Kuhlmeier et al.*, when it was ruled for the first time that school administration can censor content in school-sponsored student publications.

POLICY ADVOCACY LEARNING CHALLENGE 12.1

**Connecting Micro, Mezzo, and
Macro Policy Advocacy to Protect a Student's Ethical Rights**

Alison came from a loving household with parents who supported her. As a result of the trust she developed with them, she came out as a lesbian and introduced them to her girlfriend Caroline. Both seniors in high school, the two girls were excited to attend the upcoming homecoming ball, and they naturally wanted to go together. Although Alison's parents were proud that their daughter had found happiness and was brave enough to share it with the world, they worried about the fallout she might experience in her school. Despite her parents' warnings, Alison decided to list Caroline as her date when she RSVP'd for the event.

A week later, the student homecoming coordinator, a classmate of Alison and Caroline's, approached the girls in the cafeteria. She proclaimed that she did not agree with their "chosen lifestyle" and that students were allowed only to bring dates of the other sex. The pair refused to comply and said they would not change their plans to arrive to ball together. The next day, Alison and Caroline wore matching gay pride T-shirts to school. After the homecoming coordinator noticed this act of defiance, she informed the school's principal about the girls' intentions. He immediately called Alison and Caroline into his office. Not only were they prohibited from going together to prom, but they were also suspended from school for violating the dress code. During periods of suspension, students are not allowed to participate in any school-sponsored events or activities. As a result, Alison and Caroline missed their homecoming ball.

LEARNING EXERCISE

1. How could a case advocate have assisted with Alison and Caroline's situation?
2. What are some of the challenges an advocate might encounter in addressing this controversial issue?
3. What were some of the federal policies the school administration neglected to follow?
4. How can a school social worker initiate policy advocacy at the district level, or beyond?

Core Problem 2: Engaging in Advocacy to Promote Quality Education—With Some Red Flag Alerts

Although more than five decades have passed since the Supreme Court's *Brown v. Board* decision declared that separate schools are inherently unequal, children across the country still receive very separate and very unequal educations. An achievement gap exists, as divergent test scores and college attendance rates between black and white Americans suggest (Fox, Connolly, & Snyder, 2005).

- **Red Flag Alert 12.11.** A student who is failing in math lives in a one-parent household in a distressed neighborhood.
- **Red Flag Alert 12.12.** A student is habitually absent from science class.
- **Red Flag Alert 12.13.** A school uses decades-old textbooks in poor condition.
- **Red Flag Alert 12.14.** A school is not equipped with more advanced technology, such as computer stations.
- **Red Flag Alert 12.15.** A student is reading at a grade level well below that of others her age.
- **Red Flag Alert 12.16.** A student is prevented from enrolling because he is without documentation.
- **Red Flag Alert 12.17.** A high school dropout wishes to enroll back in school to earn his diploma.
- **Red Flag Alert 12.18.** A parent has expressed a desire for her child to attend a local charter school, but is not assisted in exploring this option by local school officials.
- **Red Flag Alert 12.19.** A teacher frequently arrives late to class and is known to call in sick for work.

Background

While the government must ensure that children have access to an education, it does not enforce access to a quality one. That is, many children and adolescents are bound to their neighborhood schools, which may be equipped with inept personnel, outdated learning materials, inadequate funds, and unsafe atmospheres. Young students face various risks on their journeys to adulthood, including but not limited to poverty, racial discrimination and injustice, limited opportunities for education and employment, child abuse, parental conflict, and biomedical problems (Kirby & Fraser, 1997). Furthermore, affluent persons are more likely to exercise school choice (Orfield & Eaton, 1996), as low-income, minority parents tend not to have the requisite social capital (Smrekar & Goldring, 1999).

Resources for Advocates

With the adoption of the Fourteenth Amendment to the United States Constitution in 1868, all persons in every state were granted equal protection under the law. After the *Brown v. Board* decision, Title VI of the Civil Rights Act of 1964 made its way through Congress and forbade discrimination based on race, color, creed, or national origin in federally sponsored programs. These pieces of legislation paved the way for the Equal Educational Opportunities Act, which declares that all public school attendees are entitled to "equal educational opportunity" without regard to race, color, sex, or national origin. It directed local educational agencies to restructure dual school systems, which had historically separated students. Furthermore, it acknowledged that "excessive transportation" disrupted the educational process, noting that the assignment of a student to a school "nearest his place of residence which provides the appropriate grade level and type of education for such student is not a denial of equal educational opportunity" unless the intention is to segregate students deliberately (20 USC Sec. 1705). Essentially, the legislation admits that government cannot help the fact that students are bound to their local schools, even if those academic institutions are not of the highest quality, as long as there is no proof of racial motivation. Yet the truth remains that these schools are often subpar even if they are easy to access.

Undocumented youth were often precluded from attending schools—a policy overridden in 1982 when the U.S. Supreme Court ruled in *Plyler v. Doe* that a Texas law that denied enrollment to illegal immigrant children was unconstitutional. The court's ruling maintained that access to a quality education for undocumented youth would likely lead to "the creation and perpetuation of a subclass of illiterates within our boundaries, surely adding to the problems and costs of unemployment, welfare, and crime." This policy has been restricted to primary and secondary schooling, however, so many states do not allow undocumented students to enter state colleges and universities or to receive in-state tuition and financial aid. President Obama was prevented from enacting the so-called DREAM Act to provide federal subsidies for these students by Republican opposition in the Senate in 2011, but he signed an executive order in 2012 to stop their deportation. Some states, such as California, have enacted their own DREAM Acts.

Considerable research demonstrates that individuals with relatively high levels of education are far less likely to become unemployed than individuals with lower levels—and to earn higher salaries or wages (Kleinbard, 2014, pp. 289–298). This connection was weakened, however, during and after the Great Recession of 2007 into 2009 as unemployment rates soared for people with college degrees and community college degrees. President Obama has proposed the launch of a "Bridge to Work" program that matches employees with businesses for on-the-job training while they are still receiving unemployment benefits. He also supports a tax credit of up to $4,000 for businesses that hire the long-term unemployed, or people who have been out of work for more than six months (White House, 2011a). The U.S. Department of Labor reveals that number to be 6 million people (U.S. Department of Labor, 2012).

POLICY ADVOCACY LEARNING CHALLENGE 12.2

Connecting Micro, Mezzo, and Macro Policy Advocacy to Promote Quality Education

Ms. Lopez is a school social worker working with a 10th-grade student named John. His mother comes to school asking for help in transferring her son to a new charter school in the neighborhood. John's mother expresses that she is concerned that John is falling through the cracks and not getting the attention he needs in school in order to perform at grade level. John is very shy and tends to disappear in a big class size. John has had minor behavior problems and is a C-average student. The mother expresses that when they lived in another district with a smaller class size, his grades were better. The mother is scared that John is starting to regress and isolate. He is now at risk of failing.

The mother has attempted to enroll her son at the new charter school and has been told that her son does not meet the qualifications for acceptance. She is confused because it was said that there are still openings at the school and they are accepting new students. The school social worker agreed to contact the charter school and follow up. Ms. Lopez was informed of the same information. John does not meet the grade requirement and his behavior and attendance history do not make him a good candidate. The school social worker tried to advocate for the student, but to no avail; she was concerned about this, so she did a little bit of a research. She found that the charter school has the right to set the requirement and criteria for acceptance in her school district and state. The California Department of Education (2011) states that in general, charter schools are not mandated to follow most district, state, or federal guidelines. Further research showed that this particular charter school has a reputation for targeting and accepting students who are high performers and college bound. In fact, there was a transfer of the school's high-performing students to the charter school when it first opened recently. Ms. Lopez informs the mother of this. The mother is outraged, but she has no choice but to keep John at the same school. The mother has limited income and cannot afford to send John to a school outside the neighborhood.

LEARNING EXERCISE

1. What could the school do to prevent losing their high-performing students to a charter school?
2. How could John's mother advocate for him? How can Ms. Lopez and the school help advocate for John?

(Continued)

(Continued)

3. What impact would the student/family's ethnicity have on the advocacy efforts?
4. Is it legal for the charter school to exclude certain students from their school?
5. What can local schools and districts do to prevent losing their high-performing students to charter schools from a policy perspective? How can they increase inclusion?
6. What is the responsibility of the state/federal government in this process? How can it be more equitable?

Core Problem 3: Engaging in Advocacy to Promote Culturally Competent Education—With Some Red Flag Alerts

- **Red Flag Alert 12.20.** A school's faculty are mostly white.
- **Red Flag Alert 12.21.** Parents with limited English skills attend their child's disciplinary hearing without the presence of a translator.
- **Red Flag Alert 12.22.** Schools send home announcements that are written only in English.
- **Red Flag Alert 12.23.** A Hispanic child acts as translator for her parents during parent–teacher conferences.
- **Red Flag Alert 12.24.** An Asian American child or a girl is hesitant to participate in class.
- **Red Flag Alert 12.25.** Black students are frequently referred to the principal's office.
- **Red Flag Alert 12.26.** An immigrant student consistently shows up to school without completed homework.
- **Red Flag Alert 12.27.** A bilingual student is recommended for a general-track program.

Background

Not every child learns the same way, and when one throws race and ethnicity into the mix, the notion of what constitutes effective and appropriate teaching methods becomes even more complicated. Take Asian Americans, for example. As a group, they are seen as the model minority and perceived as enjoying the higher ground in the academic achievement gap and performing well in standardized testing. Yet, a closer look into the effects of their cultural experience reveals a much grimmer depiction of their educational paths.

Immigration stress for children manifests as behavioral disorders in the classroom (Aronowitz, 1984). Immigrant students indicate that school and communication are two of the biggest areas of cultural adjustment difficulties (Yeh &

Inose, 2003). Parental involvement, or rather the lack thereof, is a reality for many Asian American students. In one study, Chinese American children commonly felt they lacked the necessary support from parents, who routinely work long shifts (Chan & Leong, 1994). Some immigrant parents do not give their children adequate attention, especially during early resettlement, because they themselves are dealing with demands that require time and emotional energy (Moon & Lee, 2009). The long work hours of working-class parents, who also have limited educational attainment, prevent them from assisting their children with homework (Louie, 2001). On the other hand, for Asian American parents who exhibit a desire to engage in their child's education, their inability to navigate American educational institutions greatly restricts their level of participation (Ngo, 2006). Because of their parents' lack of knowledge, students commonly manage the daunting college admissions process on their own or with the help of friends and older siblings (Ngo, 2006).

People from many other ethnic and racial groups, including Latino/as, African Americans, and Native Americans, also experience problems in schools, where teachers and other school personnel are often insensitive to their cultures. School personnel can be inattentive to the needs of girls as well, such as by allowing boys to dominate classroom discussions.

Social workers, guidance counselors, teachers, and administration should be aware of the unique challenges of immigrants' upbringing. They should be trained to adapt their practices to better serve a growing diverse student population.

Resources for Advocates

Teacher Recruitment. Many college-educated African Americans worked as teachers before the passage of civil rights legislation (Cole, 1986). However, after the Civil Rights Act of 1964, 38,000 out of the total black teaching force of 82,000 lost their jobs. Schools hired white teachers to handle the influx of desegregated school populations, while blacks were either demoted or dismissed. According to the Urban Institute, reasons for the underrepresentation of minority teachers today include inadequate academic preparation, the attraction of other careers, unsupportive working conditions, the lack of cultural and support groups, increased standards and competency testing, and financial considerations, among others. The absence of teachers of color may have a negative effect on minority students, as research has suggested that having a teacher of the same race may result in positive gains in student performance (Dee, 2005).

Bilingual Education. The first state to pass a law permitting bilingual education was Ohio, which allowed instruction in German upon parental request in 1868.

Louisiana soon followed, giving the green light to French–English instruction, and in the following decade New Mexico said yes to Spanish–English instruction. Nevertheless, a number of laws passed in U.S. history took on a more nationalistic zeal. Native American children were required to be taught in English rather than their own languages; later, they would be taken off reservations and brought into boarding schools that promoted assimilation. The influx of immigrants at the turn of the 19th century alarmed the federal government into issuing the 1906 Nationality Act, which mandated that all immigrants speak English as a requirement for citizenship. Thirty-four states had English-only instruction laws in place by the 1920s.

Since then, the government has stepped forward to recognize the needs of immigrant students. The 1965 Elementary and Secondary Education Act set aside federal funds for bilingual education, paving the way for the Bilingual Education Act of 1968. The act specifically aimed to promote experiential educational programs for non-English native speakers entering the American school system. The grant-in-aid program provided school districts funds to foster native language instructional models and, later, English-only programs. Today, there are an estimated 5 million students with limited English skills that impact their learning (Payan & Nettles, n.d.).

Bilingual education advocates suffered a setback in 1998, when California passed Proposition 227, and again in 2000, when Arizona enacted Proposition 203. As part of the "English for the Children" campaign, the initiatives sought to eliminate bilingual education in the United States. The California proposition is written in language that allows for flexibility, and the state has affirmed parents' right to choose bilingual education for their children. According to a court ruling, the law "was designed to wrest from school boards and administrators decision-making authority for selecting between LEP [limited English proficiency] educational options, and repose this power exclusively in parents of LEP students." The Arizona proposition contains much stricter language, by contrast, essentially mandating English-only instruction by severely constraining parental choice (Wright, 2005).

References to "bilingualism" as an education goal were eliminated in the No Child Left Behind program, and the Bilingual Education Act was renamed the English Language Acquisition, Language Enhancement, and Academic Achievement Act. States are required to demonstrate marked progress in the academic achievement of LEP students. The legislation also set up the Office of English Language Acquisition (OELA), charged with identifying the needs of English language learners (ELL students; those who study English as a second language) and assisting school districts with issues such as academic standards, accountability, professional training, and parental involvement. Specifically, the office distributes funding for language programs designed for LEP students. Supporting the OELA is the National Clearinghouse for English Language Acquisition, which collects and analyzes data about LEP instructional programs.

Translation Services. Per the requirements of Title IV of the 1964 Civil Rights Act and the Equal Educational Opportunity Act of 1974, school districts must adequately notify LEP parents about school-related activities that it reports to other parents. In other words, administration must provide written or oral translation of school announcements and notices. If the U.S. Department of Justice discovers noncompliance, it may call on the offending district to implement specific practices, such as:

- Securing adequate interpreter and translation resources within the district and outside it, when needed, to meet the language needs of LEP parents
- Ensuring that district staff have access to these resources in a timely manner
- Developing district procedures for the timely and competent provision of translation and interpreter services, and training district staff regarding these procedures
- Providing notice to parents about the availability of translation and interpreter services and how to request them
- Requiring translations of documents containing essential information
- Prior to conducting an individualized education program meeting, notifying parents of the availability of interpreters and providing interpreters on request, with reasonable notice
- Prohibiting the use of students as translators or interpreters except in the event of an emergency

In 2000, President Bill Clinton issued an executive order for federal agencies to "develop and implement a system by which limited-English-proficient (LEP) persons can meaningfully access the agency's services" (Executive Order No. 13166). Following the announcement, many state departments of education issued guidelines that directed public schools on how to provide adequate translation and interpretation services. In California, for example, schools are instructed not to use children as intermediaries in parent–teacher communications. "Some discussions with families involve discipline, medical or mental issues, or academic performance and may make the child uncomfortable and produce biased results" (California Department of Education, 2012). Still, individuals and groups who work on language-access issues say districts are not adhering to protocols (Zehr, 2011).

POLICY ADVOCACY LEARNING CHALLENGE 12.3

Connecting Micro, Mezzo, and Macro Policy Advocacy to Provide Culturally Sensitive Education and Services

Linda was a social worker assigned to a public high school in the heart of Chinatown. This was no ordinary academic institution; rather, it was designed as a transfer program for non–native English speakers who were either recent immigrants or had failed out of traditional schools. Because of its location, the majority of students were of Chinese descent. Many felt a special connection to Linda, as she was the only social worker who shared their nationality. When parents were not showing up to parent–teacher conferences, Linda prodded the school to schedule these meetings later in the evening in order to accommodate the busy schedules of mostly restaurant workers. When a teacher reported that a student had disrespected him in class, Linda explained that the student's evasion of eye contact was actually a sign of respect in China. When a student brought up her interest in nursing, Linda linked her with a volunteer candy-striping program at a nearby hospital and paired her with a supervising mentor at the facility.

Lately, Linda has been feeling overworked and underappreciated. She is frequently called upon to serve as a translator during meetings, although her fluency is in Mandarin, not Cantonese and other dialects. Her office is always packed with students who need her help with various school-related issues, such as scheduling, classroom conflict, and college preparation. Furthermore, students have turned to her for counsel in out-of-school matters, such as disagreements with parents, relationship advice, and career aspirations. When Linda told her supervisor about her overwhelming caseload, her boss responded sympathetically but reminded her that "everyone is in the same boat." Linda loves her students, but she is not sure whether she is physically and mentally able to keep up with all her duties.

LEARNING EXERCISE

1. How is Linda an example of an effective case advocate? Is there anything she should be doing differently to manage her caseload?
2. What are some ways that Linda can engage in policy advocacy to improve the situation at her school?

Core Problem 4: Engaging in Advocacy to Promote Prevention—With Some Red Flag Alerts

- **Red Flag Alert 12.28.** A parent asks for support for her son, who she thinks is being bullied. She is asked to report it every time it happens, but no services are provided.
- **Red Flag Alert 12.29.** A parent is not responding to the school's effort to link a student to services in school.
- **Red Flag Alert 12.30.** A parent refuses to sign the consent form for an anger management group to which his son has been referred.
- **Red Flag Alert 12.31.** All year, a teacher has been referring a student who is at risk of failing the sixth grade, but she has been told repeatedly to give it time. The school year ends and the teacher is told that middle school will deal with it.
- **Red Flag Alert 12.32.** Two counselors at a middle school try to develop an at-risk student group but have problems getting it going because they keep losing counseling staff and have to take on their caseload.
- **Red Flag Alert 12.33.** A mother of a third-grade student requests that her son participate in the after-school reading enhancement program. She is given the application, and upon submitting it she is told there is a four-month waiting period. The mother complains to the school, but the school is unable to do anything due to limited funding.
- **Red Flag Alert 12.34.** An elementary principal proposed a change in instruction as recommended by her district. She decided to add a social skills curriculum that would be done in the morning for 45 minutes twice a week. The teachers were trained and given the materials. Upon unannounced class visits, the principal finds that half the teachers are not following this directive.
- **Red Flag Alert 12.35.** Several parents from a local middle school go to the school with their concern regarding an increase in crime in the neighborhood and the safety of their children as they walk to and from school.

Background

An estimated one third of all school-aged children, or around 13 million students, are bullied each year (White House, 2011b). According to a national survey in 2010, daily marijuana use is up among 8th-, 10th-, and 12th-graders and, by some measures, has even surpassed cigarette smoking (National Institute on Drug Abuse, 2012). Suicide remains the third leading cause of death among 15- to 24-year-olds.

Even more startling, the Centers for Disease Control and Prevention reported in 2007 that the rate in American teenagers had jumped by 8% in 2003 to 2004, the largest increase observed in 15 years. Risk factors include biomedical predisposition, depression, substance abuse, sexual orientation–related factors, poor coping and interpersonal skills, stressful life events, and suicide in one's family history (Peebles-Wilkins, 2006).

Schools across the country frequently implement prevention programs designed to mitigate the many dangers and risks that youngsters face in the classroom, on the playground, and beyond. Services can include mental health hotlines, drug and substance abuse awareness programs, anti-bullying initiatives, remedial tutoring, and sex education, among others. Schools can also adopt in-service training programs on behavior management, conflict resolution, and anger control. According to Whitted and Dupper (2005), "school-level interventions should aim at clarifying and communicating behavioral norms—that is, developing classroom and school-wide rules that prohibit bullying and promote adult modeling of respectful and nonviolent behavior."

Resources for Advocates

Initiatives/Recommendations. Many early intervention and prevention initiatives are being developed at the local, state, and federal levels. All aim to address disparity at an early stage. Education advocates should keep abreast of these initiatives and utilize them to decrease and prevent gaps in services.

Under No Child Left Behind, school safety was identified as a top priority in terms of educational goals. As part of the Unsafe School Choice option, each state must establish a definition of what constitutes a "persistently dangerous" school, and students who attend that school can transfer to a safer school in the same district.

In March 2011, President Obama and First Lady Michelle held a White House Conference on Bullying Prevention to raise awareness of bullying in schools and recommend ways to make schoolchildren feel safer in their learning environments. To combat this harmful practice, six federal agencies, consisting of the Departments of Education, Health and Human Services, Justice, Defense, Agriculture, and the Interior, collaborated to form the Federal Partners in Bullying Prevention Steering Committee, which launched StopBullying.gov. Many states, such as New Jersey, have their own anti-bullying laws.

Schools should adopt evidence-based practices, such as the Screening for Mental Health program called Signs of Suicide. This particular program has demonstrated effectiveness in reducing suicidal behavior and improving student outcomes, attitudes, and awareness (Aseltine & DeMartino, 2004).

POLICY ADVOCACY LEARNING CHALLENGE 12.4

**Connecting Micro, Mezzo,
and Macro Policy Advocacy to Promote Prevention**

Averting Truancy

A school social worker (Mr. Jones) is working with a ninth-grade student (David) who is truant and at risk of failing. He's had multiple absences since the seventh grade but has not been flagged until now. He is failing multiple classes and now on the list to be processed for the Student Attendance Review Board (SARB). As defined by the California Department of Education (2012), SARB comprises members from different organizations providing services to families and youths. It focuses on helping truant students by determining the cause of the truancy and addressing needs through available school and community resources.

A pre-SARB meeting is held to discuss the student, his history, and possible supports. Mr. Jones attends the meeting to support David and his father. The meeting reveals that David's problems started in fifth grade when his mother died. His grades and his attendance started deteriorating. He started complaining of being sick and asked to stay home. The paternal grandmother watched David and his two younger siblings while the father worked two jobs to make ends meet. He attended a few parent–teacher meetings but missed most of them. The grandmother was not able to attend either because of her age and some mobility issues. David had to stay home from school to help when his grandmother was sick. Both the father and the grandmother have shared some of the information with a teacher in the past. The grandmother's health has deteriorated over the past two years and David has had to stay home more to help out. The family has very limited resources and is trying to cope with the situation.

The SARB team was not aware of this information. Mr. Jones had been asked to meet with the family for a thorough assessment and to coordinate with the team for possible resources.

LEARNING EXERCISE

1. Are teachers trained on how to respond to community and family issues students bring into the classroom? What support could the school offer the family? What can administration do to respond early to such issues?
2. Who could the school partner with to support David's family?
3. What impact does the student/family's ethnicity, race, SES, and so forth have on identifying a student in need of services? How about access to resources?
4. What policy changes can the local school or the district engage in for early identification of student support service needs?

Core Problem 5: Engaging in Advocacy to Promote Affordable and Accessible Education—With Some Red Flag Alerts

- **Red Flag Alert 12.36.** A parent asks for a special education assessment but is told it is too late in the year to do so.
- **Red Flag Alert 12.37.** A parent is not able to attend an individualized education program (IEP) meeting due to work constraints.
- **Red Flag Alert 12.38.** A school's IEP team decides on a program for the student without parent participation.
- **Red Flag Alert 12.39.** Letters and pamphlets are sent to students' homes in English only.
- **Red Flag Alert 12.40.** A foster child tries to enroll in a school without school records or with fragmented ones.
- **Red Flag Alert 12.41.** A foster child in the process of moving for the third time in a year wants to stay in the same school.
- **Red Flag Alert 12.42.** A student is suspended for the third time, resulting in a possible opportunity transfer or expulsion without support linkages or due process.
- **Red Flag Alert 12.43.** A parent does not respond to any school communication or attempts to meet.
- **Red Flag Alert 12.44.** Some teachers do not attend staff meetings or understand programs and policy changes at their school.
- **Red Flag Alert 12.45.** Some schools do not implement district mandates.

Background

The Condition of Education reports in 2007–2008 indicated that 16,122 schools were ranked as high-poverty schools (U.S. Department of Education, 2010). The majority of the students in these schools qualify for free or reduced-price meals. The report also states that there has been a 17% increase in high-poverty schools, identifying 20% of elementary schools and 9% of secondary schools as high poverty (Aud et al., 2010). Most of these schools are located in urban settings and have, on average, 68% graduation rates, compared with 91% graduation rates for low-poverty schools. They are Title I schools that need more services for their at-risk students: Twelve percent to 15% of their students need individualized education plans (Aud et al., 2010). These high-poverty schools are faced with the heavy burden of responding to multiple needs. They are disadvantaged in accessing available resources in order to respond to the needs. They are faced with the tough choice of picking only those programs that they can finance to help decrease these achievement gaps, forcing them to decide which support services will best reduce the gaps.

Families with limited resources also encounter multiple challenges when trying to engage in and support the education of their children. They face financial constraints, which hinder them from taking advantage of some of the options and programs available to them. Many of them cannot use school voucher and charter school programs due to transportation and childcare issues. Many are intimidated from going to schools outside their communities due to perceived lifestyle issues. Extracurricular activities and school supplies are not included in the voucher programs, placing additional financial pressure on these low-income families. Data from the Children's Defense Fund's 2004 survey shows the following key facts (Allen-Meares, 2007, p. 223):

- Two in five eligible children do not participate in Head Start
- One in three is behind a year or more in school
- One in three is born to unmarried parents
- One in four lives with only one parent
- One in five is poor now
- One in eight lives in a family receiving food stamps
- One in eight has no health insurance
- One in 12 has a disability
- One in 14 lives at less than half the poverty level
- One in five is born to a mother who did not graduate from high school
- One in seven never graduates from high school

Parents' lack of information or knowledge about school programs, policies, and processes and procedures is a significant impediment in receiving equal educational opportunities. Parents are often unaware of what support/program to ask for, the timeline involved, and to what services students are entitled, including special education, truancy prevention, enrollment, and school transfer programs. Some schools may not advertise programs due to the financial cost of advertising. There may also be language barriers that keep parents from knowing about specific services. Many parents of low-income children are too intimidated to inquire about specific options.

Resources for Advocates

There are multiple statutes and constitutional rights, state and federal regulations, court rulings, and private and public initiatives supporting at-risk students who are from low-income families.

Head Start Program (1965). Head Start is a comprehensive child development program designed to support the cognitive and socioemotional development of low-income children. Initially established in 1965, it has been reauthorized and expanded, serving close to 30 million children. It seeks to prepare at-risk children to enter school. Allen-Meares points out that two in five Head Start–qualified children do not participate (2007, p. 223). President Obama proposed a Preschool for All Initiative in 2013 through a cost-sharing agreement with states, but Congress has failed to take the necessary action.

McKinney-Vento Act (2001). This legislation requires all states to address the educational needs of homeless children by creating equal access and opportunities (Allen-Meares, 2007).

Title I, Part A of the Elementary and Secondary Education Act (ESEA; 1965). This legislation provides financial assistance to states and school districts to meet the needs of educationally at-risk students. It aims to provide extra instructional services and support services to students at risk of failing or already failing.

California Assembly Bill 490 (2003). This is a California law establishing the rights and regulations of foster care children regarding enrollment, school transfer, access to records, and many other issues. Its goal is to provide educational access, opportunities, and stability for foster care children (Youth Law Center/Children's Law Center of Los Angeles, 2003).

Charter School Laws/Voucher Programs. Charter schools are publicly funded institutions but not fully regulated by state or local laws. According to Sipple (2007), about 40 states had passed a law allowing the formation of charter schools by 2005. On the other hand, the voucher program provides a fixed amount that could be used to pay the tuition to the parent's school of choice. This was found constitutional by the U.S. Supreme Court in 2002 in *Zelman v. Simmons-Harris* (Sipple, 2007), opening the doors for states and local districts to establish such a program if they choose.

POLICY ADVOCACY LEARNING CHALLENGE 12.5

Connecting Micro, Mezzo, and Macro
Policy Advocacy to Promote Affordable and Accessible Education

Foster Children and Schools

Joe is a 14-year-old foster child who has been moved to a different foster home four times in the last year. The last two moves were emergency moves and the new foster parent does not have his school records. The foster mother tried to enroll him in a Southern California school but was told he could not be enrolled because the school records were missing. She was told to come back when she had all his records. She went home and tried to ask Joe about his school history. Joe remembered the last two schools but was unclear about the others. Joe lived in different cities and even went to a school in another state at one point. The foster mother finally contacted child services and asked for his records. The social worker told her that she was still gathering his records but that he should be allowed to enroll because of the AB 490 law. The foster mother did not know what this was, and so the social worker met both Joe and the foster mother at the school to assist with enrollment. The school registrar was not aware of this law either and had to check with the principal and the district office to proceed. Joe was finally enrolled after a week, even though the records were still not available.

LEARNING EXERCISE

1. Should Joe have been enrolled in school the first time he went?
2. What should administration do to improve knowledge regarding existing and new policies?
3. What can child protective services agencies and schools do to respond better to foster children's needs?
4. What responsibility did the foster mother have in advocating for Joe?
5. What is the responsibility of school staff regarding knowing and understanding school policy? How are they made accountable?

Core Problem 6: Engaging in Advocacy to Promote Care for Students' Mental Distress—With Some Red Flag Alerts

- **Red Flag Alert 12.46.** A student needs mental health services, but her parent refuses to sign the consent for services.
- **Red Flag Alert 12.47.** A student is disengaged and isolated but does not exhibit behavior problems.
- **Red Flag Alert 12.48.** A group of middle-school students are rumored to engage in "cutting behavior."
- **Red Flag Alert 12.49.** An elementary student cries every day in school.
- **Red Flag Alert 12.50.** A teacher complains that a ninth-grader who is being pulled out from her class once a week for counseling will fall behind other students.
- **Red Flag Alert 12.51.** A student who often exhibits serious behavior issues is at risk of expulsion.

VIDEO LINK 12.2
Children With Mental Illness and Trauma

- **Red Flag Alert 12.52.** A teacher walks away despite hearing a student inform another student that he is suicidal.
- **Red Flag Alert 12.53.** A school has just lost its assigned designated instruction service (DIS) counselor and has difficulty identifying a new one. The school has two students with an individualized education plan (IEP) requiring weekly behavior support and DIS counseling.
- **Red Flag Alert 12.54.** A parent asks the school to let a community social worker/mental health worker access the student at school with parental consent. The school has no clear policy regarding this.
- **Red Flag Alert 12.55.** The district leaves it up to the school to decide what support services to purchase each year.

Background

"Education Takes a Beating Nationwide: More Layoffs, Bigger Classes, Fewer Programs . . ." was the title of an article in the July 31, 2011, issue of the *Los Angeles Times* (Ceasar & Watanabe, 2011). The article talks about recent budget cuts impacting schools nationwide. The cuts have led to reduced school days; noninstructional employee layoffs (of school social workers, counselors, psychologist, and nurses); and the reduction or elimination of support services programs, including but not limited to tutoring, summer school, after-school programs, prevention programs, and other health and human services programs (Ceasar & Watanabe, 2011). The impact of the budget cuts was felt all around, but the brunt of it was felt by those who were the most vulnerable populations in schools: lower-income and minority students.

Although the budget cuts in schools are a nationwide trend, the effects are not felt equally. One of the vulnerable populations that are directly affected is school-aged children and adolescents needing mental health services. About 10 million or more youths are in need of mental health services (Franklin, Harris, & Allen-Mears, 2007). Franklin and Harris also highlight an existing discrepancy between the 70% of youths who expect to access mental health services in schools and the actual number who receive them.

Unaddressed mental health problems of students negatively impact schools, parents, teachers, and, of course, the students themselves. Schools have to deal with disruptions of their classes and poor student performance when they are under increasing pressure to produce academically proficient students. Parents often have to leave their jobs to care for children who do not receive care. Teachers are burdened with students with unaddressed mental health conditions. They are being asked to devote extra time for these students and at the same time teach their classes.

The mental health needs of children in specific schools vary significantly and are shaped by their demographics, their culture, and their available resources. Developing and delivering the appropriate mental health services within the school system is an enormous undertaking. Schools recognize the need to respond to this growing issue by having a wide variety of support services available to students. Current mental health services within schools take many forms, from preventive to intensive wraparound care programs. The American Academy of Pediatrics (AAP, 2004) released a policy statement stating that one way to categorize a school's mental health program is by using the three-tiered model. The three-tiered system categorizes the severity of mental health needs and the intensity of the services provided. The first tier is the preventive tier, increasing resilience and school connectedness. It offers many programs targeting all types of students in an attempt to decrease risk factors and increase achievement (AAP, 2004). The second tier provides more specific services to students who have more identifiable mental health issues but are still able to function in school (AAP, 2004). Students in this tier might receive multiple services to help them reach their education goals. The third tier is the most intensive of the three. It is geared toward providing services to a small population comprising the most seriously affected and at-risk students. These students will receive multiple intensive services from multiple professionals (AAP, 2004). This categorization helps create a framework for a continuum of care that is in line with the current model of Response-to-Intervention (RTI; Fuchs & Fuchs, 2006) used by educators for early identification and support of students with learning difficulties.

Resources for Advocates

A recent American Academy of Pediatrics (AAP) policy statement (2004) states that families do not address their mental health needs for multiple reasons. Some barriers include inadequate insurance coverage, lack of transportation, financial constraints, a shortage of adequately trained mental health professionals, and the stigma attached to mental health problems (AAP, 2004). Schools encounter multiple barriers as they attempt to respond to the mental health needs of students. Limited resources force many schools to limit or cut plans for supportive services. Even when schools do set aside resources, administrators are unsure if those funds will be available the following year. Resource shortages make it even more difficult to determine priorities, such as whether to focus on preventive or curative mental health programs and whether to contract these services to external agencies or provide them internally.

Statutes and the Constitution. The Individuals with Disabilities and Education Improvement Act (IDEA) was reauthorized by Congress in 2004. Originally known as Public Law 92-142 (the Education for All Handicapped Children Act), it was passed by Congress in 1975 and has been amended and expanded several times to become what is now known as IDEA 2004. This legislation established a "bill of rights" for children with disabilities within the education system (Atkins-Burnett, 2007, p. 187). IDEA, as it stands today, authorizes funds and sets the guidelines for meeting the needs of children with disabilities within the education system. It specifies the different categories that qualify as disability, including autism, learning disability, and emotional disturbance. It requires identification, assessment, and service provision to these children and adolescents. A more recent expansion of the mental health service provision is incorporated in the Affordable Care Act (ACA) of 2010. This legislation calls for expansion of insurance coverage of mental health issues as well as an increase in the scope of coverage. Schools are in a position to explore ways to promote improved mental health in light of this recent policy change, especially in a time where there is a strong push for the creation of school-based health services and wellness center programs within school campuses.

Policy Brief/Recommendations. The 2012 Condition of Education report states that about 6.5 million students received special education services from 2009 to 2010 (Aud et al., 2012). A 1999 report from the surgeon general states, "One in five children and adolescents have emotional or behavioral problems sufficient to warrant a mental health diagnosis" (as cited in Brener, Weist, Adelman, Taylor, & Vernon-Smiley, 2007). The Robert Wood Johnson Foundation (2009) also emphasizes the need for early childhood intervention programs to promote life-long success and well-being.

Not having clear policy mandates (except for IDEA) results in great variation in mental health service provision among school districts and states. Varying policy briefs, recommendations, and initiatives reveal a need to address the mental health needs of school-aged children. Education advocates will have to keep abreast of pertinent information and changes in available funding streams to engage in the discourse and access available resources as they advocate funding and services. These circumstances and challenges make it even more important to know and be aware of the changing local, state, and federal policies and initiatives.

POLICY ADVOCACY LEARNING CHALLENGE 12.6

Connecting Micro, Mezzo, and Macro
Policy Advocacy to Promote Care for Students' Mental Distress

Daryl is a ninth-grader who has been referred to the dean of discipline multiple times due to classroom disruption, verbal altercations with the teacher and peers, refusing to do his work, not turning in his homework, not being in uniform, sleeping in class, shoving classroom furniture, and many other infractions. The teacher has stated that he seems angry all the time and has a short fuse. The dean has suspended him from class, as well as from school, several times, but the behavior continues. The teacher is frustrated and has started complaining about the lack of support and how the other students are affected by his constant disruption. The teacher talks to the dean almost every day to complain about Daryl and the situation and has started talking to the school counselor about him; she has mentioned wanting him out of her class and transferred to another teacher. The counselor has done a little investigation and alerted the school social worker, Ms. Silva, about the student.

Ms. Silva asked the teacher to send Daryl to her the next time he was in class or before she sent him back to the dean. It took several days, but Ms. Silva finally met with Daryl. Daryl refused to talk to her and asked if he was in trouble. Ms. Silva told him he was not in trouble and explained her role in the school and the services she offers. Daryl continued to be suspicious of the social worker and asked if he could go back to class. Ms. Silva agreed and asked if she could talk to him briefly once a week. She also gave him a business card and asked him to make sure to ask for her next time he got in trouble. Daryl responded by saying, "Whatever; it makes no difference who I see. I'm on my way out anyways."

Ms. Silva decided to find out more about Daryl, so she sought out the dean and the counselor. She found out that Daryl had a history of barely passing his classes and had several fails. He also had multiple absences. His records showed that his elementary school grades had been significantly better and that the decline started in sixth grade. When Ms. Silva asked if the counselor knew anything about his personal life, the counselor stated, "Not really. This is his first year at this school, and I don't really know him. I have a lot of students assigned to me and I'm still trying to get to know all of them, especially the ninth-graders."

Ms. Silva then decided to meet with the dean to discuss Daryl. The dean recognized Ms. Silva but had not had many interactions with her. This was Ms. Silva's second year at the school and she had tried to familiarize all the staff with her role and responsibilities, but it had been very challenging. Ms. Silva had been assigned to coordinate and provide mental health services at the school. She saw students individually and in groups and linked them to additional services. She had attended several staff meetings and sent memos explaining the services, but she had been inundated with a heavy caseload, so it had been difficult to connect with all the school staff.

After reminding the dean of her role, Ms. Silva proceeded to ask about Daryl. The dean explained the nature of her contacts with Daryl as well as his mother. She told Ms. Silva of the behavior problems and the multiple suspensions. She also stated that Daryl's records showed problems from the previous middle school and that she knew from the first referral that Daryl might become a frequent referral. The dean shared that it was difficult to schedule a meeting with Daryl's mother and that she seemed to want to help Daryl but was frustrated with all the problems he was causing. The dean had never met the father—and Daryl refused to talk about him. All the dean knew was that

(Continued)

(Continued)

Daryl had two young siblings and spent a lot of time with them. She also shared that she was looking into an opportunity transfer for Daryl if the behavior continued.

Ms. Silva asked if the dean would be willing to try out a few interventions before going that route. She asked the dean to let her know the next time Daryl was referred to her for a behavior problem. Ms. Silva offered to collaborate in exploring ways to work with Daryl and turn the situation around. She also informed the dean that she had met Daryl and offered him her services but that he had been wary of accepting them. The dean agreed to talk to Daryl's mother to get her consent for Daryl to avail himself of the services.

Ms. Silva left the dean's office with a plan of saying hi to Daryl in the halls and meeting with him weekly just to check in. She also wanted to make sure that the teacher was aware that she was available for support and that she would let her know when Daryl was referred to the dean again. Ms. Silva wanted to make sure to be present at the next meeting with the dean to help advocate for services rather than having Daryl transferred to another school.

LEARNING EXERCISE

1. How could Ms. Silva advocate for Daryl? Other students with discipline issues? Ninth-graders transitioning from middle school?
2. Do the student/family's race or ethnicity, socioeconomic status, or other demographic factors impact the tolerance level and response to discipline issues?
3. How could the school social worker improve the identification of students with mental health needs and make sure they receive the services they need? What policy advocacy work is needed to make sure that this becomes an automatic process?
4. Are any federal, state, or local policies being violated by any school staff?
5. What policy/program advocacy can Ms. Silva engage in to increase the mental health services at the school?

Core Problem 7: Engaging in Advocacy to Promote Education Linked to Students' Communities—With Some Red Flag Alerts

- **Red Flag Alert 12.56.** A social worker needs to meet with a student at school but lacks a private space to meet.
- **Red Flag Alert 12.57.** A teacher inquires about the progress of a student he has referred for counseling services.

- **Red Flag Alert 12.58.** A teacher refuses to release a student from class to meet with a service provider.
- **Red Flag Alert 12.59.** A community agency provider asks to meet with a student during second period two times weekly.
- **Red Flag Alert 12.60.** A community agency leaves health or mental health-related messages about students for the school social worker or coordinator with the front office worker.
- **Red Flag Alert 12.61.** An administrator keeps tabling the school social worker/coordinator's presentation at the faculty meeting.
- **Red Flag Alert 12.62.** Teachers refer all problems in the classroom to the school social worker/coordinator.
- **Red Flag Alert 12.63.** An administrator fails to attend key collaborative meetings.
- **Red Flag Alert 12.64.** A student receives services from three different agencies at the school, revealing the need for collaboration and coordination.

Background

The U.S. Department of Justice (2009) reports that in 2008, about 2.11 million individuals under the age of 18 were arrested for various reasons. The same bulletin states, "Juveniles accounted for 16% of violent crime arrests and 26% of all property crime arrests in 2008" (p. 1). According to Furlong, Paige, and Osher (2003), "In 2000, suicide and homicide were the third and fourth leading causes of death for children ages 10–14, and among individuals ages 15–19, homicide and suicide were the second and third leading causes of death." These data clearly demonstrate the issues students bring in to school campuses and ultimately to the classroom. Many schools realize they have limited resources to deal with all the problems originating in students' families and communities, so they are increasingly partnering with community-based agencies and governmental agencies to create school-based services, wellness centers, community resource partnerships, and many more.

Resources for Advocates

Although collaboration and community partnerships are advantageous to schools, they can also strain an already thinly stretched system. They require countless hours of work, and for the most part they entail many additional duties (Dryfoos, 2005). Collaborators must be vested in the work, have specialized training, and fully understand all systems and stakeholders. It is often difficult to establish partnerships because of differing policies, operating procedures, ethical and legal mandates, and goals. Schools follow the regulations set forth by the Family Educational Rights and Privacy Act (FERPA) of 1974 when it comes to school-related information, while community agencies follow the policies set forth by the Health Insurance Portability and Accountability Act (HIPAA) of 1996. All partners must learn to navigate these intricacies to protect students' rights as they engage in collaboration to increase support services to students.

Federal agencies are also taking initiatives to link schools with community agencies. Safe Schools/Healthy Students (SSHS), for example, is a collaboration between the federal Departments of Education, Justice, and Health and Human Services to promote and provide resources for school–community preventive services, healthy child development, health services, safe-school services, intensive mental health services, and use of evidence-based practices (Furlong et al., 2003). SSHS is only one of the many initiatives currently in existence. As another example, the Children's Health Program Act (CHIP) was created in 1997 and reauthorized in 2009 to help states insure low-income children who are ineligible for Medicaid but cannot afford private insurance. Schools collaborate and team with this program to help identify students who qualify for CHIP and to educate parents about how to access it and use its benefits. Many schools are also partnering with community organizations for after-school programming. These are a few ways schools are taking the initiative to create partnerships and collaboration to increase resources and services.

POLICY ADVOCACY LEARNING CHALLENGE 12.7

Connecting Micro, Mezzo, and Macro Policy Advocacy

Opening Schools to Surrounding Communities

It is the first day of a new school year. Ms. Valdez, a school social worker, has been assigned to implement a grant received by a local school cluster to simultaneously provide services to students and create a wellness center in a local high school. Administrators and a few community agencies that already provide services in the school have planned the program. A new principal has now replaced the principal who helped to write the grant.

The summer prior to the school year, a space at the high school was identified, and it was to be cleared so that it would be ready for the new program for the fall. Summer passed and school started. The space was still full of supplies and furniture the previous program had left behind. Ms. Valdez was introduced to the new principal and the six assistant principals who jointly manage the school. Ms. Valdez was given the task of creating a program following the mandates of the initiative but was not given any instructions on how to do so. She also had to deal with suspicions from school staff who did not know who she was and what her role was going to be. Ms. Valdez had been assigned from the district office and had not been chosen by the school administrator. The teachers had not been fully involved in the planning and did not fully understand the grant.

Ms. Valdez was at a loss as to where to start. She decided to work on the physical space and at the same time get to know the school. Ms. Valdez and her interns worked on clearing the room of unwanted items and salvaging furniture to furnish the office. She did this with the help of the MSW interns assigned to her. At the same time, Ms. Valdez started meeting with as many school staff as she could on an individual basis. Her goal was to get to know them and their understanding of the program. She also wanted the staff to become familiar with her and learn her role in the school. She did the same with all the different community agencies that provided services on campus, whether they were part of the initiative or not. She eventually set up a structure that encouraged outside agencies to check in at the wellness center and work with her when providing services to the students.

Ms. Valdez learned about the school and the community culture when she decided to do this. She learned of different facts and issues unique to the school as she got to know the school and the staff:

- The school and the community are a closed system.
- Faith-based organizations play a key role in this community.
- There have been several administrator turnovers over the years.
- There have been many programs that have come and gone over the years.
- The school had very limited participation in the actual program development and implementation, although it took part in the planning.
- The school has its own vision of how to develop and implement the program that differs from that of the district.

Ms. Valdez was now faced with three major tasks:

1. Deal with the above issues to pave the way for the program
2. Align herself with multiple stakeholders to get buy-in and support for the program
3. Create an infrastructure to foster strong collaboration, start the delivery of services, and streamline access to the services

The three tasks were the focus of the work for the first academic year. Ms. Valdez and the interns worked on building their relationship with the students, the school staff, and the community agencies. By the end of the school year, students were receiving services at school or linked services in the community. The students were either referred by the teacher or by other staff or self-referred. Unfortunately, parent participation was still at a minimum when school ended. Things were by no means where they should be, but at this point most of the school staff and the majority of the community agencies were familiar with who Ms. Valdez was. The wellness center had become a functioning resource center.

LEARNING EXERCISE

1. Who should have been involved in planning, program development, and implementation?
2. How can Ms. Valdez work on aligning the school staff's vision and the district's vision for the initiative?
3. What could Ms. Valdez do to increase parent participation?
4. How can Ms. Valdez generate stakeholder participation and buy-in at this point in the implementation?
5. Is there any policy-related work that needs to be done or incorporated in the implementation to promote sustainability?

"THINKING BIG" AS ADVOCATES IN THE EDUCATION SECTOR

President Obama was determined to improve the nation's schools. Despite the enactment in 2001 of No Child Left Behind (NCLB), students had lower scores on standardized Math and English tests than many of their counterparts in Europe, Canada, and Asia. President Obama devoted $80 billion of the stimulus bill to education; this was geared mostly toward avoiding laying off teachers during the recession. NCLB had set 2014 as the year when every child, including persons of color, disabled students, and low-income students, could read and do math at grade level,. Many states, too, had embraced the establishment of charter schools to give parents a choice of private schools, usually nonprofit ones, that would establish their own curriculum and policies and whose teachers weren't usually members of teacher unions. But results of all this effort proved elusive.

President Obama and Arne Duncan, his secretary of education, proposed to replace No Child Left Behind with an initiative known as Race to the Top, which would give states producing plans that met goals established by the U.S. Department of Education grants from a pool of $4.3 billion. It was a clever strategy to avoid the political problem that had dogged educational reforms since the 1950s whenever school reformers proposed initiatives that appeared to allow federal officials to "interfere" with secondary education, which was widely viewed as "belonging" to states. By asking states to compete for funds based on innovations they had developed, President Obama and Duncan avoided this problem.

A basic problem remained, however. Secondary education often remained behind the times. Rather than helping students grapple with ideas and math at a conceptual level, it often had a cookbook quality. Between 2008 and 2014, however, a remarkable development took place: Most states had accepted the concept of a "Common Core Curriculum." This movement began in 2008 when Bill Gates was persuaded by two educational reformers to endorse the Common Core: an approach to education that emphasized problem-solving in reading and math. In the ensuing five years, the Gates Foundation dispersed tens of millions of dollars to school districts and public officials across the United States to support efforts to write and use curriculum based on common core precepts. In turn, the Obama administration made it known to school districts and states that they stood a better chance of obtaining grants from Race to the Top if they included the adoption of the Common Core Curriculum in their proposals.

Adoption of the Common Core was widely accepted by liberals and conservatives—until 2014, when critics appeared. Some conservatives even named the Common Core "Obamacore." Some liberals doubted that evidence existed to show that changes in curriculum standards lead to better educational achievement.

If Gates and President Obama emphasized curriculum reforms, a national movement to provide supportive assistance to students, particularly those with learning and behavior problems, was absent, even though evidence-based reforms demonstrated that teams of social workers, teachers, and other personnel had remarkable success in decreasing truancy, school dropout, and low achievement. Once they saw warning signs in specific youth that they were falling behind or were becoming truant, they immersed these youth in supportive services. They visited their homes. They kept track of their truancy, finding them in their communities and shepherding them back to school. They involved their parents.

Stories fill the Internet about the cost to individuals, families, and American society of high dropout rates by low-income students, minority students, and others. Many evidence-based projects to cut truancy have been effective.

So why don't social workers take the lead in developing a national program that works to decrease dropout, truancy, and poor performance by addressing students' mental health, economic, and social needs? Why shouldn't social workers take a leading role?

Discussion Tasks

1. Develop a national program for cutting truancy and underachievement where social workers have a leading role.

2. Estimate the likely cost of this program if it is applied to thousands of school districts with a large percentage of low-income children.

3. Give the program a name.

4. Send copies of the program to representatives and senators from your state.

5. Send copies of the program to the national director of NASW and ask that person to assume a leadership role on Capitol Hill in pushing the program.

LEARNING OUTCOMES

You are now equipped to:

- Identify key policies that shape the American educational system, with special emphasis on those that promote special services to students, collaborations between schools and community agencies, and honoring of students' ethical rights
- Identify important eras in the development of the American educational system
- Identify seven core problems experienced by students, parents, and schools
- Identify specific Red Flag Alerts that inform social workers when they might need to provide micro or macro policy interventions
- Develop connected micro, mezzo, and macro policy interventions

REFERENCES

Allen-Meares, P. (2007). *Social work services in schools* (5th ed.). New York, NY: Pearson.

American Academy of Pediatrics, Committee on School Health. (2004). School-based mental health services. *Pediatrics, 113*(6), 1839–1845. Retrieved from http://pediatrics.aappublica tions.org/content/113/6/1839.full

Areson, C. W. (1923). Status of children's work in the United States. *Proceedings of the National Conference of Social Work.* Chicago, IL: University of Chicago Press.

Aronowitz, M. (1984). The social and emotional adjustment of immigrant children: A review of the literature. *International Migration Review, 237*–257.

Aseltine, R. H., Jr., & DeMartino, R. (2004). An outcome evaluation of the SOS suicide prevention program. *American Journal of Public Health, 94*(3), 446.

Atkins-Burnett, S. (2007). Children with disabilities. In P. Allen-Meares (Ed.), *Social work services in schools* (pp.182–221). New York, NY: Pearson.

Aud, S., Hussar, W., Planty, M., Snyder, T., Bianco, K., Fox, M. A., . . . Hannes, G. (2010). *The condition of education: Closer look 2010 (High-poverty schools).* Retrieved from: http://nces .ed.gov/programs/coe/analysis/2010-index.asp

Aud, S., Hussar, W., Johnson, F., Kena, G., Roth, E., Manning, E., . . . Yohn, C. (2012). *The conditions of education 2012: Children and youth with disabilities (Indicator 9).* Retrieved from http://nces.ed.gov/pubs2012/2012045.pdf

Brener, N. D., Weist, M., Adelman, H., Taylor, L, & Vernon-Smiley, M. (2007). Mental health and social services: Results from the School Health Policies and Programs Study 2006. *Journal of School Health, 77*(8), 486–499.

California Department of Education. (2011, November 3). *Charter Schools CalEdFacts.* Retrieved from http://www.cde.ca.gov/sp/cs/re/cefcharterschools.asp

California Department of Education. (2012, September 17). *School attendance review boards.* Retrieved from http://www.cde.ca.gov/ls/ai/sb/

Ceasar, S., & Watanabe, T. (2011, July 31). Education takes a beating nationwide: More layoffs, bigger classes, fewer programs and higher tuition are nothing new to U.S. educators, but analysts say this year stands out. *Los Angeles Times.* Retrieved from http://articles.latimes.com/2011/jul/31/nation/la-na-education-budget-cuts-20110731

Chan, S., & Leong, C. W. (1994). Chinese families in transition: Cultural conflicts and adjustment problems. *Journal of Social Distress and the Homeless, 3*(3), 263–281.

Cole, B. P. (1986). The Black educator: An endangered species. *Journal of Negro Education, 55*(3), 326–334.

Dee, T. S. (2005). A teacher like me: Does race, ethnicity, or gender matter? *American Economic Review, 95*(2), 158-165.

Dryfoos, J. (2005). Full-service community schools: A strategy—not a program. *New Directions for Youth Development, 2005*(107), 7–14. doi: 10.1002/yd.124

Fox, M. A., Connolly, B. A., & Snyder, T. D. (2005). *Youth indicators, 2005: Trends in the well-being of American Youth* (NCES 2005-050). U.S. Department of Education.

Franklin, C., Harris, M., & Allen-Mears, P. (2007). *The school services sourcebook: A guide for school-based professionals.* New York, NY: Oxford University Press.

Fuchs, D., & Fuchs, L. (2006). Introduction to response to intervention: What, why, and how valid is it? *Reading Research Quarterly, 41*(1), 93–99. doi: 10.1598/RRQ.41.1.4

Furlong, M., Paige, L. Z., & Osher, D. (2003). The Safe Schools/Healthy Students (SS/HS) initiative: Lessons learned from implementing comprehensive youth development programs. *Psychology in the Schools, 40*(5), 447–456. doi: 10.1002/pits.10102

Hall, G. E. (1936). Changing concepts in visiting teacher work. *Visiting Teachers Bulletin*, p. 12.

Kirby, L. D., & Fraser, M. W. (1997). Risk and resilience in childhood. In M. W. Fraser, *Risk and resilience in childhood: An ecological perspective* (pp. 10–33). Washington, DC: NASW Press.

Kleinbard, E. (2014). *We are better than this: How government should spend your money.* Oxford, UK: Oxford University Press.

Louie, V. (2005). Immigrant newcomer populations, ESEA, and the pipeline to college: Current considerations and future lines of inquiry. *Review of Research in Education, 29,* 69–105.

Moon, S. S., & Lee, J. (2009). Multiple predictors of Asian American children's school achievement. *Early Education and Development, 20*(1), 129–147.

National Institute on Drug Abuse. (2012). *DrugFacts: High school and youth trends.* Washington, DC: National Institutes of Health. Retrieved November 11, 2011, from http://www.nida.nih.gov/infofacts/hsyouthtrends.html

Ngo, B. (2006). Learning from the margins: The education of Southeast and South Asian Americans in context. *Race, Ethnicity and Education, 9*(1), 51–65.

Orfield, G., & Eaton, S. (1996). *Dismantling desegregation: The quiet reversal of* Brown v. Board of Education. New York, NY: New Press.

Payan, R. M., & Nettles, M. T. (n.d.). *Current state of English-language learners in the US K–12 student population.* Retrieved November 2, 2012, from http://www.ets.org/Media/Conferences_and_Events/pdf/ELLsympsium/ELL_factsheet.pdf

Peebles-Wilkins, W. (2006). Evidence-based suicide prevention. *Children and Schools, 28*(4), 195–196.

Robert Woods Johnson Foundation. (2009). *Beyond health care: New directions to a healthier America.* Retrieved from www.commissionhealth.org

Sawhill, I. V., & Smith, S. L. (2000). Vouchers for elementary and secondary education. In C. Steuerle, V. Ooms, G. Peterson, & R. Reischauer (Eds.), *Vouchers and the provision of public services* (pp. 251–292). Washington DC: Brookings Institution Press.

Sipple, J. W., (2007). Major issues in American schools. In P. Allen-Meares (Ed.), *Social work services in schools* (pp.1–25). New York, NY: Pearson.

Smrekar, C., & Goldring, E. (1999). *School choice in urban America: Magnet schools and the pursuit of equity.* Critical Issues in Educational Leadership Series. Williston, VT: Teachers College Press.

Sweet, L. (2009). Obama's NAACP speech, July 16, 2009: Transcript. *Chicago Sun-Times.* Retrieved November 1, 2011, from http://blogs.suntimes.com/sweet/2009/07/obamas_naacp _speech.html

Thernstrom, A., & Thernstrom, S. (2003). *No excuses: Closing the racial gap in learning.* New York, NY: Simon & Schuster.

U.S. Department of Education, National Center for Education Statistics. (2010). *2010 spotlight: High-poverty public schools.* Retrieved January 8, 2014, from http://www.nces.ed.gov

U.S. Department of Labor, Bureau of Labor Statistics. (2012, November 2). *Economic news release.* Retrieved November 2, 2012, from http://www.bls.gov/news.release/empsit.t12.htm

White House, Office of the Press Secretary. (2011a, September 8). *Fact sheet: The American Jobs Act.* Retrieved November 3, 2011, from http://www.whitehouse.gov/the-press-office/ 2011/09/08/fact-sheet-american-jobs-act

White House, Office of the Press Secretary. (2011b). *President and First Lady call for a united effort to address bullying.* Retrieved November 11, 2011, from ww.whitehouse .gov/the-press-office/2011/03/10/president-and-first-lady-call-united-effort-address-bullying

Whitted, K. S., & Dupper, D. R. (2005). Best practices for preventing or reducing bullying in schools. *Children and Schools, 27*(3), 167–175.

Wright, W. E. (2005). The political spectacle of Arizona's Proposition 203. *Educational Policy, 19*(5), 662–700.

Yeh, C. J., & Inose, M. (2003). International students' reported English fluency, social support satisfaction, and social connectedness as predictors of acculturative stress. *Counselling Psychology Quarterly, 16*(1), 15–28.

Youth Law Center/Children's Law Center of Los Angeles. (2003, December). Ensuring educational rights and stability for foster youth: AB 490 summary. Retrieved http://www.youthlaw.org/filead min/ncyl/youthlaw/events_trainings/ab490/AB490_Summary.pdf

Zehr, M. A. (2011, March 3). Advocacy groups push for better translation services. *Education Week.* Retrieved November 2, 2012, from http://blogs.edweek.org/edweek/learning-the language/2011/03/advocacy_groups_push_for_bette.html

Chapter 13

BECOMING POLICY ADVOCATES IN THE IMMIGRATION SECTOR

LEARNING OBJECTIVES

In this chapter, you will learn:

1. Why many social problems are shaped by global events, including the plight of many migrants across national borders

2. How American foreign policy, international institutions, and American immigration policies evolved during the seven eras of American history

3. The causes of migration across national borders

4. How problems of immigrants are linked to inequality in the United States

5. How to identify powerful players and interests, as well as unrepresented populations and interests, in the global economy

6. How to identify seven problems that immigrants experience and that impact American immigration policies; statutes, regulations, and policies that are germane to each of them; and Red-Flag Alerts that point toward micro and macro policy interventions

7. How to apply the eight challenges in the multilevel policy advocacy framework to the immigration sector

The United States has had waves of immigration throughout its history. Social workers often need to be advocates for immigrants no matter the policy sector where they work.

ANALYZING THE EVOLUTION OF AMERICA'S IMMIGRATION POLICIES

VIDEO LINK 13.1
Undocumented
Youth in Detention
Centers

From the inception of the Republic, colonial authorities, specific states, and the federal government have enacted immigration policies, as this brief overview demonstrates:

- In the early Republic, Congress allowed immigrants to enter the United States with a minimal health test, no literacy test, no annual limits, and no limits on specific nations.
- The American Constitution vested power over immigration with the federal government, not individual states, when it was enacted in 1789.
- Congress enacted legislation in 1790 that restricted citizenship to Caucasians, leading to noncitizenship for persons of African descent, Native Americans, and (later) persons of Asian descent.
- Immigrants flooded into the United States as it industrialized from 1860 to 1920.
- Many immigrants experienced considerable discrimination in the 19th and early 20th centuries, including people from Ireland, China, Japan, Italy, Mexico, and Eastern Europe along with emancipated slaves, African Americans, Jews and Catholics. Not technically immigrants because they were indigenous, Native Americans were cruelly attacked and exploited as they were pushed off land as white Americans moved westward, as were persons of Mexican and Spanish descent.
- Harsh legislation was enacted against immigrants from China and Japan in 1907.
- The Immigration Act of 1924 cut immigration from Eastern and Southern Europe as well as Asia while increasing immigration from Northern Europe in an effort to decrease nonwhite immigrants as well as Catholic immigrants and Jewish immigrants.
- The Bracero program was initiated in 1942. It allowed a specific number of Mexicans to enter the U.S. to meet labor shortages on farms and ranches. It was accompanied by supposed protections for them, such as guaranteeing them a suitable wage and preserving their civil rights, but these were mostly ignored by American employers such as ranchers. The program ended in 1964.
- The Immigration Act of 1965, the Indochina Migration and Refugee Assistance Act of 1975, and the 1980 Immigration Act abolished quotas for specific nations and regions—and led to a huge upswing in immigration from Asia, as well as Central America, the Caribbean, the Middle East, Russia, and Eastern Europe.
- The Immigration Act of 1986 provided amnesty to 3 million undocumented immigrants, mostly from Mexico and Central America, if they could prove they had lived in the U.S. for four years.

- Proposition 187 was enacted in California in 1994. It declared immigrants to be ineligible for medical, social, and educational services—but was not implemented due to court challenges. The Personal Responsibility and Work Opportunity Reconciliation Act of 1996 banned access by undocumented immigrants to many medical, safety-net, and social services.
- Due to bipartisan agreement between leaders of both parties, Congress appeared ready to enact sweeping immigration reforms in 2007 that would have legalized as many as 12 million undocumented persons, but could not surmount partisan gridlock.
- President Barack Obama promised to secure sweeping immigration reforms during both his first and second terms, but could not succeed due to intense opposition from conservatives. Conservatives spearheaded anti-immigrant policies in many states, including Arizona, North Carolina, Alabama, and Georgia, such as those that allowed police to check the citizenship of anyone who "looked like" an undocumented person. The U.S. Supreme Court overturned many of these policies when it ruled that the U.S. Constitution vested power over immigration with the federal government rather than with the states.
- In 2014, thousands of children and youth came over the border between Mexico and the United States—many from Central American nations like Guatemala—seeking to reunite themselves with their parents and relatives. They were housed in makeshift settings in the United States as Congress refused to pass a request for more than $3 billion by President Obama to meet their housing and medical needs. The president promised to decide by the end of the summer of 2014 whether to allow them entry or to deport them to their nations of origin while accusing Republicans of blocking major immigration reforms.

ANALYZING THE MOVEMENT OF PEOPLE ACROSS NATIONAL BOUNDARIES

We cannot understand American immigrants without placing them in a global context. Persons move between many nations, as documented by the fact that roughly 214 million people—or 3.1% of the world's population—lived outside their nations of birth worldwide in 2011 (International Organization for Migration, 2011). These migrants are evenly split between males and females. They send payments (often called remittances) to family members that total $440 billion per year.

The United States has attracted the greatest number of immigrants relative to other countries, with 38.5 million foreign-born persons (12.5% of its total population), including many from Mexico (29.9%), the Philippines (4.5%), India (4.3%), China (3.7%), Vietnam (3%), El Salvador (3%), Korea (2.6%), Cuba (2.6%), Canada (2.1%), and the Dominican Republic (2.1%) (Migration Policy Institute,

2011). About half of these immigrants are people with limited English proficiency (LEPs) who report on surveys that they speak English "not at all" or "not well" as compared to "well." The immigrants speak many languages, although 62% of them speak Spanish. These immigrants are evenly split by gender. About one fourth of the immigrants have a bachelor's degree or higher, while about one third lack a high school diploma. Roughly two in five of them are naturalized U.S. citizens, and the remaining immigrants are split between legal permanent residents, unauthorized (or undocumented) immigrants, and legal residents on temporary visas as students or workers (Migration Policy Institute, 2011). Immigrants from Mexico are concentrated in California (37.5%), Texas (20.9%), Illinois (6%), Arizona (5.2%), and Georgia (2.4%). Immigrants constitute roughly 16% of the American workforce (Migration Policy Institute, 2011).

Households that have one or more of their heads born in other nations vary widely in their economic status. Roughly one fourth of the 26 million households are middle class, with a total annual income between $47,000 and $79,000. These immigrant adults tend to have a high school education and some postsecondary credential short of a bachelor's degree (International Organization for Migration, 2011). Many immigrants fall beneath federal poverty standards. Immigrants cross the age spectrum, including about 16.9 million children at or under age 17 (Migration Policy Institute, 2011).

Over 1 million persons become new lawful permanent residents each year, roughly one half as immediate relatives of U.S. citizens, one fifth through a family-sponsored preference, one-tenth through employment-based preference, 16% from refugee or asylum status, and 4% as diversity-lottery winners who win annual lotteries established by the federal government to increase entry from nations with low rates of immigration to the U.S. (Migration Policy Institute, 2011).

Roughly 11.2 million unauthorized immigrants lived in the U.S. in 2010—or 28% of the nation's foreign-born population and 5% of the nation's workers (Pew Hispanic Center, 2012). Immigration of unauthorized persons ebbs and flows with economic conditions, falling from 850,000 per year from March 2000 to March 2005, for example, to only 300,000 per year during the economic downturn in March 2007 to March 2009 (Pew Hispanic Center, 2012). The economic well-being of unauthorized immigrants in the U.S. markedly declined during the Great Recession, with the downturn in agriculture, tourism, and industry leading some of them to return to Mexico and other nations. Their economic duress was experienced as well by broader Hispanic, African American, and white households, whose wealth respectively declined by 66%, 53%, and 16% from 2005 through 2009 (Pew Hispanic Center, 2011). Immigration of Latino/as to the U.S. from Mexico had *reversed* by 2012 as more of them exited than entered the U.S. (Pew Hispanic Center, 2012).

Immigrants are both "pulled" and "pushed" across national boundaries. They are *pulled* by economic factors when they seek improved economic conditions in another nation. Immigrants constitute about 6% of the populations in rich nations as opposed to just 1% in poor countries. A considerable proportion of immigrants send "remittances" to family members who remain in their native lands in order to provide them with needed capital. India received the largest volume of remittances ($21.7 billion) in 2004), followed by China ($21.3 billion) and Mexico ($18.1 billion).

Many immigrants are *pushed* by intolerable economic and social conditions in their native lands, including violations of human rights, wars between nations, civil wars, genocide, tribal or sectarian conflict, and famine. We can distinguish between *refugees, asylum seekers, and internally displaced person* (IDPs). Refugees are persons who are pushed away from their homes and can document that they have been persecuted for reasons of race, religion, nationality, membership in a particular social group, or political opinion. Some LGBTQQ persons seek refugee status due to discrimination and physical attacks in their native lands. Refugees include persons displaced by wars or disturbances of public order; many persons emigrated to the U.S. during civil wars in Nicaragua, El Salvador, Cuba, Afghanistan, and Iraq, while many others came to the U.S. in the wake of the Vietnam War. Asylum seekers are individuals whose claim to be refugees has not yet been documented. IDPs are persons who must migrate due to natural disasters, tribal warfare, or internal discord. The United Nations High Commissioner for Refugees (UNHCR; n.d.), which coordinates refugee protection, estimated that 10.5 million refugees existed in 2010. Most refugees flee to neighboring nations, but many seek refuge in distant lands, such as Vietnamese persons who came to the U.S. in the wake of the Vietnam War in the 1970s and later.

Many immigrant women come to the U.S. due to human trafficking, including sex trafficking and use of people for labor or services through force, fraud, or coercion (ACLU, n.d.). Some parents insist that their oldest child migrate to provide them with needed resources. Droughts, floods, tsunamis, and earthquakes have often led to the destruction of food and housing in many nations—leading many people to flee to other nations or to refugee camps funded by nongovernmental organizations, the UN, or specific governments.

ANALYZING THE LEGAL STATUS OF IMMIGRANTS IN THE UNITED STATES

Migrants to other nations are a heterogeneous group with respect to their legal status. Many of them are "undocumented" and cross borders without the approval of host nations. They often exist in a state of limbo. Employers frequently exploit them. They often do not report burglaries and physical attacks because they fear deportation. They often work and even pay taxes, but find it difficult to access social programs and education—whether because host nations deny them these benefits or because they fear deportation if they claim benefits. Undocumented persons have some rights, however, as we discuss subsequently.

People need visas to legalize temporary stays, obtained through petitions filed with the U.S. Citizenship and Immigration Services, or USCIS (VisaPro Immigration Attorneys, n.d.). *Family visas* include those for people with close relations with a U.S. citizen, such as fiancés, spouses, and children, as well as visas for persons with more distant family relationships with a U.S citizen. *Green cards* grant lawful permanent residency, including permission to live and work in the U.S. Holders must maintain permanent resident status and can be removed from the U.S. if certain conditions of this status are not met. Roughly 140,000 *work visas* are issued each year, such as those for business visitors, registered nurses, and people of extraordinary ability in the arts, athletics, business, education, science, or agriculture. Some work visas are given only to temporary immigrants sponsored for a specified period by an American employer (U.S. Department of State, n.d.). A system of priorities exists. First priority is given to persons with extraordinary ability, researchers, professors, and multinational managers or executives. Second priority goes to professionals holding advanced degrees. Third priority is given to skilled workers, professionals, and unskilled workers. Fourth preference goes to certain special immigrants, including Iraqi and Afghan interpreters and translators and persons recruited to the U.S. armed forces outside the nation. Fifth priority goes to immigrant investors and entrepreneurs.

Student visas are given to academic or language students, exchange visitors, or vocational or nonacademic students. *Other visas* include those for people seeking asylum from persecution by governments in other nations as well as those for people who have come to the U.S. via human trafficking. Some persons have uncertain immigration status, such as persons who wait for extended periods in the U.S. as they seek citizenship—waits that can last months or years. American citizens who wish to adopt children from other nations petition United States Citizenship and Immigration Services (USCIS).

Family members and some employers file petitions to help people emigrate to the U.S., often becoming their financial "sponsors" by filing an "affidavit of support" where they promise to support the immigrant and even to repay certain benefits that the immigrant uses, as required by the 1996 welfare law (National Immigration Law Center, 2005). Under the 1996 legislation, sponsors' income is sometimes added to immigrants' income to determine their eligibility for specific public benefit programs, even for 10 or more years after immigrants enter the nation. (Exceptions include survivors of domestic violence and immigrants who would become hungry or homeless without assistance.)

People who criticize undocumented immigrants, or even those with work visas, fail to understand benefits that they bring to the United States. Immigrants often take jobs that naturalized Americans do not want, particularly low-paying and undesirable jobs in agriculture, tourism, healthcare, and industry. These jobs often expose immigrants to health and other risks. These immigrants pay sales taxes and social security taxes. Many researchers conclude that immigrants contribute more resources to the American economy than they take from it because they make relatively little use of American safety-net programs, whether because they are ineligible to use them or because they fear deportation if they *do* use them. Americans will increasingly need labor from immigrants due to the aging of the American population.

The United States pursues conflicting policies. On the one hand, it invites the inflow of undocumented persons through its immigration policies. By not providing sufficient work visas to fill existing jobs that are not claimed by American citizens, the U.S. creates an employment vacuum that is filled by undocumented persons who want and need employment. Needing their labor, employers often do not check workers' documents to ascertain if they have entered the U.S. legally—and pressure immigration authorities *not* to conduct raids on their workforces. Having enticed them to enter the United States, Americans often harass undocumented workers. Public agencies raid places of work and even the homes of undocumented persons. They deport undocumented persons. They allow employers to defraud immigrants by not paying them minimum wages—or not paying them at all. They forbid immigrants to use many of the nation's health and social service programs.

Sweeping immigration reform is needed that legalizes immigrants sufficiently to meet the nation's economic needs and preserve immigrants' dignity and human rights. It should provide amnesty to millions of immigrants who have "paid their dues" by working in the U.S. for extended periods. It should give temporary work visas to immigrants needed for the nation's economy.

Many groups have provided micro, mezzo, and macro policy advocacy for immigrants throughout American history by seeking to improve their legal status (see Table 13.1 for some contemporary advocacy groups).

RECOGNIZING PROBLEMS FOR IMMIGRANTS CREATED BY AN INEGALITARIAN NATION

Immigrants work disproportionately in low-income, unskilled or semiskilled positions in American society, including janitorial work, the tourist industry, agriculture, construction, restaurants, and the health system. They receive even lower wages than their counterparts in Canada and Europe, where economic inequality is not as marked as in the United States. Their economic marginalization is often accentuated by widespread prejudice against undocumented persons—even as most Americans agree that immigrants' labor is indispensable to the American economy. Undocumented immigrants are often stereotyped as using social programs excessively, committing crimes, and having babies to obtain citizenship for them, even when considerable research indicates these stereotypes are false (ACLU, 2008).

Table 13.1   Some Advocacy Groups for Immigrants

The **American Civil Liberties Union** (ACLU) has fought for the rights of immigrants in courts, legislatures, and regulatory bodies. **www.aclu.org**

The **American Friends Service Committee** (AFSC) operates advocacy programs for immigrants along the Mexican border. **www.afsc.org**

The **Asian American Justice Center** (AAJC), founded in 1991 as the National Asian Pacific American Legal Consortium, works to "advance the human and civil rights of Asian Americans through advocacy, public policy, public education, and litigation." **www.advancingequality.org**

The **Center for Immigration Studies** (CIS), founded in 1985, is an independent, nonpartisan, nonprofit research organization devoted to research and policy analysis dealing with the economic, social, demographic, fiscal, and other implications of immigration for the United States. **www.cis.org**

The **Centro Humanitario para los Trabajadores** provides work opportunities and safe working conditions for immigrants. **www.centrohumanitario.org**

The **International Organization for Migration** (IOM) is the world's primary intergovernmental organization focusing on the issue of migration, with 116 member states. **www.iom.int**

The **Mexican American Legal Defense and Educational Fund** (MALDEF) is a leading advocate for Latino/as. **www.maldef.org**

The **Migrants Rights International (**MRI) is a membership organization of migration and human rights experts and practitioners. **www.migrantwatch.org**

The **Migration Policy Institute** (MPI), founded in 2001, conducts research on the movement of people worldwide and provides analysis for local, national, and international migration and refugee policies. **www.migrationpolicy.org** and **www.migrationinformation.org**

The **National Council of La Raza** (NCLR) is a national Hispanic civil rights advocacy organization in the United States. **www.nclr.org**

The **National Immigration Forum** (NIF) advocates public policies for immigrants and refugees. **www.immigrationforum.org**

The **National Immigration Law Center** (NILC) is a leading expert on immigration, public benefits, and employment laws affecting immigrants and refugees. **www.nilc.org**

The **National Network for Immigrant and Refugee Rights** (NNIRR) develops and coordinates plans of action on important immigrant and refugee issues. **www.nnirr.org**

The **Office of the United Nations High Commissioner for Refugees** (UNHCR) has helped approximately 50 million refugees looking to restart their lives. **www.unhcr.org**

The **Pew Hispanic Center** conducts research on migration flows from Mexico, Central America, and South America. **www.pewhispanic.org**

The **Population Reference Bureau** (PRB) works to "inform people around the world about population, health, and the environment." **www.prb.org**

The sheer level of poverty and marginal economic status for many American citizens stimulates hostility toward immigrants by American citizens. Many persons "on the edge" fear that immigrants take away their employment, since they often cluster in low-wage jobs in tourism, nonunionized industrial jobs, agriculture, construction, and other areas—even when many indigenous citizens are unwilling to work in many of these positions. Leaders of American trade unions have often been hostile to immigrants, since they observe how immigrants are often used by employers to "bust" unions.

UNDERSTANDING THE POLITICAL ECONOMY OF THE IMMIGRATION SECTOR

Controversy swirls around immigrants in the United States. Suspicion of immigrants was triggered by the bombings of the Twin Towers on September 11, 2001, which brought heightened fear of terrorists. The Great Recession of 2007–2009 was followed by continuing high unemployment, which sustained distrust of immigrants, who were widely seen as taking jobs from American citizens. The rise of the Tea Party in 2009, with the election of many Tea Party members and sympathizers to Congress and other legislatures, sustained animus toward immigrants.

Many conservatives insist that immigrants should be allowed to reside in the U.S. only if they have legal status. Many of them support raids on their homes and places of work as a prelude to incarceration and deportation. Many of them favor construction of a wall from Tijuana to Texas, as well as use of drones, sensors, and military personnel to restrict entry by undocumented persons. They lament that federal immigration authorities often do not enforce federal penalties against employers for hiring undocumented persons. Many liberals contend that the U.S. hypocritically uses the labor from undocumented immigrants for its agricultural, tourism, janitorial, restaurant, and other enterprises—but exploits them by providing them with low wages, harsh working conditions, and harassment by police. They argue that immigrants take jobs that most Americans would not accept. Some immigrant advocates, led by rabbis and ministers in the Sanctuary Movement, have given safe havens to undocumented immigrants in churches and temples in defiance of harsh laws. Supporters of programs and legislation that provide education, job training, and other amenities to immigrants contend, too, that they benefit the nation. For example, calculations by the nonpartisan Congressional Budget Office (CBO) indicate that the proposed federal DREAM Act, which would have subsidized the education of certain undocumented students, would have increased government tax revenues by $2.3 billion from the enhanced income they would earn over the next 10 years (CBO, 2010).

An upsurge of voting by Latino/as in local, state, and federal elections has markedly changed the political dynamics of immigration. More than 70% of Latino/as voted for President Barack Obama in 2012, as well as Democratic candidates at all levels of government. Latino/as have increasingly demanded immigration from members of both political parties, as well as developing widely publicized marches and demonstrations. Some leaders of the Republican Party fear that their party will suffer major political defeats if it does not support federal immigration reforms—and if its members continue to propose anti-immigration legislation in many states. Growing numbers of Latino/as are voting in a population that will rise to 20% of the American population in 2020.

ANALYZING SEVEN CORE PROBLEMS IN THE IMMIGRATION SECTOR

Core Problem 1: Engaging in Advocacy to Promote Ethical Rights, Human Rights, and Economic Justice—With Some Red Flag Alerts

Immigrants often confront situations where their rights are violated, as the following Red Flag Alerts indicate. They will often need legal assistance, as revealed by cases handled by volunteer attorneys and law students at the Stanford University law clinic (see www.law.stanford.edu/program/clinics/immigrantsrights/).

- **Red Flag Alert 13.1.** Specific immigrants are victimized by employers, realtors, moneylenders, or the police and need assistance in finding remedies from immigration attorneys or public officials.
- **Red Flag Alert 13.2.** Specific immigrants are detained in centers that do not meet standards of decency and need assistance in finding remedies from immigration attorneys or public officials.
- **Red Flag Alert 13.3.** Specific immigrants experience threats to their privacy through illegal searches and seizures or surveillance by Homeland Security and need assistance in finding remedies from immigration attorneys or public officials.
- **Red Flag Alert 13.4.** Specific immigrants are wrongly denied specific benefits or services and need assistance in finding remedies from immigration attorneys, legal aid, or public officials.
- **Red Flag Alert 13.5.** Staff in agencies that disperse public benefits wrongly act as immigration enforcers by demanding documents, asking unnecessary questions, and issuing unnecessary warnings to specific immigrants—and these immigrants need help in finding remedies from immigration attorneys, legal aid, or public officials.
- **Red Flag Alert 13.6.** Specific refugees fail to receive visas or eventual naturalization, so they need help from immigration attorneys, legal aid, or public officials.

- **Red Flag Alert 13.7.** Specific immigrants are wrongly placed in the "unqualified" category established by the welfare legislation of 1996 and wrongly deemed to be ineligible for specific federal public benefit programs, so they need help from immigration attorneys, legal aid, public officials, or advocacy groups.
- **Red Flag Alert 13.8.** Specific immigrants placed in the "unqualified" category established by the 1996 welfare legislation are wrongly declared to be ineligible for protection of their lives and the safety imparted by work safety regulations, so they need help from immigration attorneys, legal aid, or public officials.
- **Red Flag Alert 13.9.** Specific immigrants placed in the "unqualified" category established by the 1996 welfare legislation are wrongly deemed to be ineligible for Meals on Wheels, shelters for homeless persons, summer food programs, medical care from public systems of care, public education, and services from specific nonprofit agencies.
- **Red Flag Alert 13.10.** Specific immigrants fail to ask for a reliable immigration attorney if Immigration and Customs Enforcement arrests them.
- **Red Flag Alert 13.11.** Specific immigrants are deported without a hearing before a judge, so they need legal counsel (roughly 160,000 immigrants are annually deported under these conditions).
- **Red Flag Alert 13.12.** Specific immigrants are subjected to racial profiling, including searches and seizures without sufficient cause or denial of benefits without sufficient cause.
- **Red Flag Alert 13.13.** Specific immigrants or immigrant communities are subjected to intrusive police actions, such as searches without probable cause, including knocking on doors in the middle of the night to catch "fugitive aliens" (Weiland & Sylvester, 2008).
- **Red Flag Alert 13.14.** Specific immigrants are not granted asylum when they face genuine threats of detention, injury, and death if they return home.
- **Red Flag Alert 13.15.** Victims of human trafficking are often lured to the U.S. through false promises of better income and lives, but are prevented from returning to their homelands or leaving prostitution by coercion from their captors (ACLU, 2011b).
- **Red Flag Alert 13.16.** Immigrants lack legal representation when they are threatened with deportation due to minor or old drug offenses.
- **Red Flag Alert 13.17.** Immigrants do not realize that they may qualify for a U Visa that protects victims of crime even if they are undocumented.
- **Red Flag Alert 13.18.** Roughly 5.5 million children have undocumented immigrant parents—and about 75% of these children are U.S. citizens, since they were born in the U.S. Over 100,000 parents with citizen children have been deported from the U.S. since 1999 (U.S. Department of Homeland Security, 2009). These citizen children are subject to hardships and trauma that

often negatively impact them, such as fear of deportation and possible separation from deported parents (Chaudry et al., 2009). A gap in immigration law means that the interests of these citizen children are not considered in many deportation proceedings, despite that fact that nations such as Spain, as well as the United Nations, have or favor regulations not to separate family members through deportation (Finno, 2010). Social workers should become advocates for children.

Background

In the wake of the attack on the World Trade Center on September 11, 2001, surveillance at the nation's borders, particularly the border with Mexico, was tightened with National Guard troops, sensors, cameras, and aircraft. Immigrants often died as they crossed more remote deserts. They paid higher fees to so-called coyotes that escorted them across the border. These innovations condemned increasing numbers of immigrants to deaths and injuries (ACLU, 2009). The Department of Homeland Security (DHS) instituted the National Security Entry–Exit Registration System (NSEERS) in the wake of 9/11, requiring men and boys from Arab- and Muslim-majority nations to register with DHS. NSEERS led to the deportation of thousands of Muslims for civil immigration violations and "brought an abrupt end to their productive jobs, property ownership and community ties including to U.S. citizen family members" (ACLU, 2011b). Some legislators demanded a national ID to identify undocumented persons, that is, a national biometric system of required Social Security cards that would serve as an employment verification system but could also serve for travel, voting, financial transactions, student identification, and other areas (ACLU, 2010) Would this innovation, some persons wondered, intrude on the privacy of American citizens while not preventing hiring of undocumented immigrants through false documents and corrupt employers? Other threats to privacy arose, including unauthorized use of credit cards, social networking, travel, and mobile phone surveillance by Homeland Security.

It is sometimes difficult to determine what rights immigrants possess due to ambiguities and flux in existing laws (Leicher, 2004). When immigrants seek a change in their immigration status, for example, such as obtaining permanent residency through a green card, immigration officials sometimes deny their requests because they might become "public charges." It is often unclear, however, *how* they decide that someone *will* become a charge—and someone may be denied a green card due even to relatively brief use of food stamps. In fact, few government agencies have sought reimbursement for immigrants' use of public benefits (National Immigration Law Center, 2005).

Immigrants often discover that specific protections available to American citizens do not exist for them in federal legislation (such as minimum wage protections) or in state laws that provide lesser protections. Federal and state authorities do not enforce many protections, however, against sexual harassment, employer negligence that leads to injuries, and workers' right to workmen's compensation (ACLU, 2006). It is not surprising that undocumented immigrants, who live in a state of legal and social limbo, are often victimized, because the perpetrators realize that law enforcement and government officials often will not come to their defense or enforce their rights *because* they are a marginalized population—and because immigrants often do not assert their rights for fear of deportation. Immigrants are abused by many employers, who pay them even less than the minimum wage and expose them to dangerous work conditions, poor housing, and lack of basic services in this legal limbo. They are subject to hate crimes. They are victims of harsh legislation, as reflected by welfare and immigration legislation by Congress in 1996 and harsh policies recently enacted by legislatures in Arizona, Georgia, Alabama, and South Carolina.

Resources for Advocates

Principles in the U.S. Constitution, state constitutions, and legal precedents are often used to block implementation of harsh provisions against immigrants, including unlawful search and seizure, invasion of privacy, and racial profiling—as well as the constitutional provision that gives the federal government rather than states the sole authority over immigration matters. As the executive director of the ACLU of South Carolina argued, "By requiring local law enforcement officials to act as immigration agents, this law invites discrimination against anyone who looks or sounds 'foreign,' including American citizens and legal residents" (ACLU, 2011a).

Numerous ethical issues arise with respect to immigrants. Employers, realtors, moneylenders, and the police often victimize them. They often have their privacy invaded through searches and seizures at variance with current laws. Their families are often divided in deportation proceedings. They are often detained for extended periods in centers that do not meet standards of decency. They fear deportation even from using services and programs to which they are entitled.

An informal "contract" existed in the United States prior to 2000. While border patrols made it difficult for undocumented immigrants to enter the U.S., those who made it to the U.S. could usually stay if they worked hard—and millions of them received amnesty in 1986 if they could prove residency of four years or more. In the 21st century, however, the U.S. government made immigration far more difficult when it installed or used fences, patrols, aircraft, and sensors at borders, leading to higher rates of injury and death as more immigrants used hazardous routes across deserts— and had to pay large sums to so-called coyotes to escort them. Raids on employers have increased, as well, in recent years—leading to increasing numbers of deportations. Many experts contend that immigrants' ethical rights can only be protected by enacting sweeping immigration reforms that allow many persons to migrate to the U.S. for time-limited employment as legal immigrants under a regulated system that protects their rights and gives them access to programs needed for their safety and well-being.

The term "legal permanent residents" (LPR) describes persons who have been granted the right to reside permanently in the U.S., such as persons with green cards.

Both qualified and unqualified immigrants are eligible for many programs that do not require income eligibility, but are required to protect people's lives and safety. They are eligible, for example, for federal and state safeguards of workers' safety on their jobs, Meals on Wheels, and shelters for homeless persons.

Considerable variation exists between states regarding immigrants' eligibility for specific programs. While the 1996 welfare legislation excludes many immigrants from "federal public benefits," for example, many federal agencies have not specified which specific programs are covered by it—so state and local agencies are not required to verify immigration status for some programs. The welfare legislation also exempts nonprofit charitable organizations from obtaining proof of eligibility for such benefits (Los Angeles Coalition to End Hunger and Homelessness, 2010).

States often have considerable latitude in their treatment of immigrants. They can decide whether to grant benefits to immigrants excluded from federal benefits by funding them with state funds. They can decide not to require verification of immigration status in those programs not specifically identified as needing it by federal agencies.

Immigrants' advocates must remember that, despite harsh American laws, *all* immigrants, including undocumented ones, may qualify for prenatal care, emergency and minor consent Medicaid, immunizations for children, WIC, school breakfast and lunch, summer food, medical care from the public system of care, public education, help from shelters, and services from many nonprofit agencies (Los Angeles Coalition to End Hunger and Homelessness, 2010).

Immigrants who are arrested by the Immigration and Customs Enforcement (ICE) should remain silent, ask to speak to a reliable immigration attorney, know their alien registration number if they have one and place it where family members can find it, prepare a form or document that authorizes another adult to care for their minor children, and tell family members who do not want to be questioned by the ICE to stay away from the place where they are detained (Los Angeles Coalition to End Hunger and Homelessness, 2010).

The Illegal Immigration Reform and Immigrant Responsibility Act of 1996 allowed immediate deportation of legal permanent residents even for minor offenses such as shoplifting, as opposed to prior regulations that required offenses that could lead to five or more years in jail. It restricted the use of waivers that had allowed many convicted immigrants to remain in the U.S. on grounds of their close family relations or the length of time they had been in the U.S. (Morawetz, 2000). It removed the ability of immigration judges to *not* deport parents because they have children who are U.S.-born citizens—and immigration judges have usually ruled that citizen children should accompany their deported parents because they lack the ability to make decisions about where to live (Demleitner, 2003). It allowed deportees to be kept in jails for months and even up to two years. It allowed the secretary of homeland security to permit designated state and local law enforcement officers to perform immigration law enforcement functions rather than relying only on federal officials. The deportation of undocumented persons and other persons who do not have green cards is even more likely than deportation of LPRs, whether because they have committed crimes or because they lack visas. They must show that they or their citizen children or spouses would suffer "exceptional and extremely unusual hardship" if they were deported (Demleitner, 2003).

The plight of citizen children of undocumented persons received considerable publicity during raids of worksites by the ICE from 1996 to 2008 because many of their parents had been in the U.S. for long periods and had not committed crimes. Their families were immediately disrupted. Children of arrested parents often did not even have childcare after their arrest. They lacked income with the arrest of the breadwinners. They often left the U.S. abruptly, because many arrested parents chose to immediately leave the U.S. to avoid court hearings and sentences that would make them ineligible to reenter the U.S. at a later point in time (Capps, Casteneda, Chaudry, & Santos, 2007). Many immigrants feared even to request legal assistance for fear of retaliation by the ICE. Families that chose not to leave the U.S. at once suffered considerable turmoil. While local agencies and schools often offered them assistance, parents were often detained for months as family and community members took care of their children.

Partly due to public outcry, worksite raids were greatly decreased in 2008 as more emphasis was given to fining employers who did not check applicants' documents. But they increased again during the Obama administration, until it decided in 2012 to focus the efforts of the ICE on finding and deporting immigrants who had committed crimes.

POLICY ADVOCACY LEARNING CHALLENGE 13.1

Connecting Micro, Mezzo, and Macro Policy Advocacy

Advocacy for Immigrant Children

Children and parents are often separated during deportation proceedings. While ICE officials are mandated to identify and locate parents' children, they sometimes do not. Advocates should insist that children not be separated from their parents, such as by

(Continued)

(Continued)

allowing parents to remain in the community with electronic monitoring and asking that children be allowed to stay with parents in deportation centers. To the extent that children *are* separated from their parents, advocates should seek to have the children live with family members pending deportation outcomes. Child welfare social workers should be informed of deportation cases that involve children so that they can be advocates for them.

Micro policy advocacy can be linked with macro policy advocacy to change state or federal law to make clearer that ICE and child welfare officials should work together to keep families intact, including allowing undocumented parents with citizen children to remain in the U.S. legally. If citizen children often choose to live in the United States when they become adults, why not enhance their well-being by minimizing dislocation and trauma caused by deportation?

Advocacy for immigrant children became a national issue in 2014 as President Obama and the Congress faced thousands of children from Central America who crossed the U.S. border at Mexico seeking asylum as refugees—often without their parents. The children often secured attorneys, who sought asylum for them under U.S. law that allows refugee status for persons who are victims of natural disasters or wars. Yet the immigration system was "stacked" against these children because they often did not meet these two conditions, and the U.S. law established a ceiling of 5,000 asylum grants. The system also presumes that an asylum seeker does not qualify for asylum—a presumption of guilt—unlike in U.S. criminal law, where persons have a presumption of innocence. President Obama said he would come up with a solution by the end of the summer of 2014. If he had the political will, he could invoke the Immigration Act of 1990 that allows temporary protected status for persons who seek refugee status.

Blocked by Congress from enacting a DREAM Act to grant children who had been brought to the United States by their parents illegally the right to remain in the U.S. as they finished their education and held employment for several years, President Obama established his own program using his executive authority. It granted these persons two years of work before any deportation proceedings could be held if they paid a fee, had no criminal offenses, and were self-supporting. Only about half of the eligible population applied by 2014 because they could not afford the fee or feared that the application process would give information to the ICE that would get them deported.

Core Problem 2: Engaging in Advocacy to Promote Quality Programs for Immigrants—With Some Red Flag Alerts

Research that establishes evidence-based practices and policies for immigrants is "evolving," so we often do not know what services work well for them, such as best practices with newcomer youth (Delgado, Jones, & Rohani, 2005). Service providers are sometimes prejudiced against them, such as by assigning them to low-achieving classrooms in schools, not offering them translation services, or refusing to serve them. Advocates should insist that immigrants receive services comparable to those given other persons whenever possible.

- **Red Flag Alert 13.19.** Immigrants are assigned to lower-quality services than others due to prejudice by service providers against them (Fores, 2005).
- **Red Flag Alert 13.20.** Immigrants are not given evidence-based services.

Core Problem 3: Engaging in Advocacy to Promote Culturally Competent Services for Immigrants—With Some Red Flag Alerts

- **Red Flag Alert 13.21.** LEP immigrants fail to receive translation services in specific social service settings.
- **Red Flag Alert 13.22.** People do not obtain services that are sensitive to their specific culture in specific settings.
- **Red Flag Alert 13.23.** Staff are not diversified in specific service settings.

Background

The United States is possibly the most culturally diverse society in human history, when we include first-generation immigrants and their second-generation descendants—or roughly, for example, 16.9 million children with at least one immigrant parent and 14.6 million second-generation children. Two challenges confront social workers and other professionals: They need to be able to converse with immigrants, and they need to be culturally competent. Conversing with immigrants is difficult when roughly 52% of the 38.3 foreign-born persons over the age of five have limited English proficiency (LEP), self-reporting that they speak English "not at all" or "not well." For example, at least 224 languages have been identified in Los Angeles County, not including differing dialects, while only 92 of them have been identified among students in the Los Angeles Unified School District (Los Angeles Almanac, 2011).

Conversing with people in foreign languages presents daunting challenges. Professionals need to recognize specific words *and* understand immigrants' questions and assertions at a deeper level, including shades of meaning, subtle expressions, and hidden emotions. Conversations that lack deeper levels of understanding are often superficial ones, particularly when persons discuss important topics like whether to have a life-threatening surgery, to relinquish custody of a child, or resolve marital conflict. Most of us can sustain conversations at these deeper levels only in a single language—or possibly another language at most. A shortage of professionals who can converse at high levels of proficiency often exists in specific settings, such as in mental health clinics. Agencies and programs often lack resources to hire staff who are proficient in specific languages— or to fund translation services over the telephone, such as those provided by the American Telephone and Telegraph Company (AT&T).

It is difficult to recruit people from different ethnic backgrounds even into the profession of social work to significantly decrease shortages of culturally competent staff. People from some ethnic groups do not know about social work—and often gravitate toward higher-paying fields. The need is particularly acute with respect to recruitment of Spanish-speaking staff in light of the sheer number of Spanish-speaking first- and second-generation immigrants in the U.S.

In the case of mental health services, for example, "undocumented persons have the least access and many times the highest need for mental health services" (Vega, Kolody, Aguilar-Gaxiola, & Catalona, 1999). Many immigrant cultures lack understanding of mental health problems even when many of their members possess them.

Resources for Advocates

Title VI of the 1964 Civil Rights Act *requires* that no persons be excluded from federally funded programs because they cannot understand English—and this Act has been reinforced by presidential executive orders, court rulings, and policy guidance (Kao & Jansson, 2011). A mélange of state and local laws also exist. California, for example, has more than 150 laws germane to language access, as compared to some states that have less than 10 of them. The Department of Health and Human Services issued guidance in 2003 that required health providers to give language assistance services by using four factors, including the number of LEP persons served, the frequency that specific LEP persons interact with their programs, the nature or importance of those programs, and available resources. Federal laws and laws in various states generally state that agencies should provide translation services to those populations that constitute 5% or more of their client base. It is widely accepted that minor children should never be used as translators— and that relatives should rarely assume this role and only with the concurrence of immigrant clients.

Hospitals and some health clinics make extensive use of phone-based translation services partly because of statutes and court rulings that require them to obtain patients' informed consent before providing them with medical care. These clinics and hospitals can lose their accreditation and their Medicare and Medicaid funding—and face litigation from patients—if they do not obtain informed consent from their patients. Phone-based translation services are often helpful, but they have limitations. They are cumbersome because patients and health personnel converse with a bilingual speaker who is not in their presence and who cannot see the patients' body language or other cues.

Core Problem 4: Engaging in Advocacy to Promote Preventive Services for Immigrants—With Some Red Flag Alerts

- **Red Flag Alert 13.24.** Immigrants are wrongly informed that they are not eligible for specific programs that may prevent poverty.
- **Red Flag Alert 13.25.** Immigrants are wrongly informed that they will suffer possible deportation if their children use educational, preschool, and other programs for which they qualify.
- **Red Flag Alert 13.26.** Immigrants needlessly jeopardize their eligibility for specific programs by inadvertently providing unnecessary information.

Resources for Advocates

Many Americans have been so preoccupied with the alleged law breaking of adult immigrants that they fail to realize that they often are parents with young children who are citizens because they were born in the U.S. (Four million children of immigrants attended schools in 2010—or nearly one student in every public classroom in the U.S.) When Americans restrict the access of immigrant adults to safety-net programs, they are *also* restricting the access of children to these programs— consigning many of them to live in grinding poverty (Yoshikawa, 2011).

Researchers have shown that immigrant children have lower cognitive skills and poorer development when their parents are undocumented, partly because their parents are preoccupied with surviving, often holding multiple and onerous jobs, often suffer from anxiety and depression stemming from their poverty and undocumented status, and fear deportation that might even lead to separation from their citizen children. It is likely that children would benefit from two immigration reforms: giving parents temporary and legal work visas and providing them with a path to eventual citizenship (Yoshikawa, 2011). With legal status, parents would be more likely to use safety-net programs and search for preschool and center-based childcare programs. They would be more likely to search for better and higher-paying jobs for themselves. They would be less likely to be victimized by employers if they had legal status, including receiving at least the minimum wage. Exclusion of adult undocumented immigrants from GED examinations, as well as from publicly funded education and job training, precludes them from improving their work skills and finding better jobs.

Immigrants and their children often do not realize that they qualify for specific programs in the United States—or fear they may be deported if they step forward to use them. Citizen children of undocumented parents are eligible for more programs than undocumented children of undocumented parents. Eligibility for specific programs sometimes hinges on specific visas. Eligibility sometimes hinges, too, on whether specific programs, such as Head Start, have available slots due to funding shortages for them. Undocumented adults are eligible for specific health benefits, but sometimes don't claim them because they are *not* eligible for other health benefits. Confusion often stems, too, from variations between states. Some states (but not most states) have enacted programs that enable undocumented youth to attend colleges modeled on the DREAM Act (Development, Relief, and Education for Alien Minors) introduced in the U.S. Senate in 2001 and reintroduced on May 11, 2011, but defeated by congressional conservatives—and then considered and enacted by such states as California in 2011 to be effective in 2013 (McGreevy & York, 2011). The California legislation gives undocumented students who graduate from high school access to state scholarships and provides loans for low-income students who attend junior colleges and four-year colleges and universities.

The steadfast opposition of many conservatives to policies to enhance preventive programs for immigrants has blocked many reforms. Liberals counter that children, often brought to the U.S. at an early age by undocumented parents, should not be punished for acts beyond their control. They argue that preventive programs could help millions of citizen children of undocumented parents who will remain in the U.S. to be more productive.

Some federal regulations deter prevention of immigrants' health problems, such as the five-year ban on immigrants' eligibility for Medicaid and CHIP from the point they receive green cards. Policies that deter immigrants who are victims of domestic violence from obtaining safety-net benefits, such as the five-year ban or liability of sponsors, make it more difficult for them to leave abusive relationships (National Immigration Law Center, 2005).

All immigrants are eligible for an array of preventive programs linked to their immigration status. Many programs do not have immigration requirements, so undocumented persons often qualify. These include prenatal care; emergency Medicaid and Medicaid for minors; immunizations for children; the Special Supplemental Nutrition Program for Women, Infants, and Children (WIC); school breakfast and lunch; summer food; county healthcare; public education; food pantries; shelters; and services from many nonprofit agencies.

The Los Angeles Coalition to End Hunger and Homelessness (2010) advises undocumented persons as follows:

> These programs don't have immigration requirements . . . If anyone asks you about your immigration status, be careful. You do not need to tell anyone that you or anyone else who lives with you are undocumented. Your workers do not need to ask about your immigration status if you are not getting benefits for yourself. If they do ask you, simply tell them that you are a "not qualified" immigrant ("not qualified" is not the same as undocumented). That is all they need to know.

The LA Coalition (2010) also advises immigrants to write "none" on forms, or leave blanks where schools or child centers request social security numbers—and states they may not give the form or information to a government agency. It also advises immigrants, who often do not get correct information or become discouraged, to "be strong . . . insist on talking to a supervisor, and seek out the help of someone who will advocate for you. Insist on speaking to someone who is fluent in your language or call Legal Aid."

Persons who have limited English proficiency (LEP) are entitled to interpreters free of charge, whether from the departments of public social services and health services or the Social Security Administration. These include bilingual workers or telephone interpreter services, as well as possible translation or explanations of documents written in English.

Children born in the United States automatically become American citizens. Citizen children of undocumented immigrants number roughly 4 million, constituting about one third of all immigrants' children and roughly one student in each classroom of every American elementary school (Yoshikawa, 2011). These children are entitled to participate in programs available to children of American citizens subject to the availability of funding for them in specific jurisdictions. These programs include Head Start; publicly subsidized childcare; kindergarten, primary, and secondary education; and SNAP. These children are eligible for health benefits from Medicaid, the Children's Health Insurance Program (CHIP), and family health benefits provided by employers of their parents.

The cognitive development of these children is strongly linked to the extent that they and their families take advantage of early-child programs, as indicated by national studies after adjusting for social class, parental education, and family structure (Yoshikawa, 2011). Conflicting data exist about the behavioral development of children of undocumented parents, but a major California study suggests that these children are at risk of delayed development because their parent or parents confront formidable obstacles as undocumented persons. They must often work long hours in two jobs. They experience psychological distress from their marginal legal position. They are sometimes isolated with weak support systems. They often experience extreme poverty and food insecurity due to low wages and poor working conditions that are exacerbated by the lack of enforcement of wage and workplace regulations, as well as accumulated debt. They often live in crowded apartments shared by several families. Their parents are often unaware that they are eligible for programs like Head Start, government-subsidized infant childcare, and income-enhancing programs (Yoshikawa, 2011). Undocumented parents and their children are less likely to have a usual source of healthcare or to use healthcare at the levels of children of documented parents. Their parents are not eligible for public housing or Section 8 subsidized housing.

The children of undocumented immigrants who were born in their nation of origin, but who migrate to the U.S., are not entitled to citizenship. They have been allowed to attend public schools—and schools have not divulged their undocumented status to immigration authorities. Recent legislation by some states, such as Alabama, requires school administrators to identify students and parents who are undocumented and to report them to federal immigration authorities—although these laws are subject to legal challenge in the courts.

Clinics and hospitals are required to offer medical treatment to *anyone* who possesses life-threatening health conditions or who is in child labor under the Emergency Medical Treatment and Active Labor Act (EMTALA) of 1986, as well as laws in many states. These patients cannot be transferred to other health institutions or their communities until they are medically stabilized. Treatment cannot be made conditional upon income or citizenship. EMTALA guidelines are available from the Centers for Medicare and Medicaid Services (CMS) at http://www.cms .hhs.gov/manuals/Downloads/som107ap_v_emerg.pdf. Undocumented adults are also eligible for some public health programs offered by specific states or local units of government, such as prevention programs for TB and HIV/AIDS.

The Fair Labor Standards Act (FLSA) of 1938, which established the federal minimum wage, maximum hours, and overtime pay standards, covers all American workers, including undocumented ones, except volunteers and independent contractors. Yet more than one third of undocumented workers in New York City work below the federal minimum wage, work more than 40 hours per work, and do not receive overtime pay, which is required by the FLSA to be at least 1.5 times normal pay (Yoshikawa, 2011). (The work hours of these undocumented parents routinely exceed 54 hours a week.) Undocumented workers are usually employed, as well, in jobs with low job autonomy—and both low wages and low job autonomy are linked to low child cognitive ability at 36 months (Yoshikawa, 2011). These poor work conditions and pay are caused by poor enforcement of the FLSA, because the number of federal inspectors decreased by 31% between 1980 and 2007 (Yoshikawa, 2011).

The work conditions of undocumented persons would likely improve if more of them become unionized, as has occurred with undocumented janitors in Los Angeles since the late 1990s in the wake of registration of many Latino/a voters and an increase in pro-Latino/a political leaders. But this will occur only if immigrants are organized politically and if community organizations are developed that advocate their needs.

Immigrants often prefer non-welfare programs like WIC that give them non-cash resources such as food and nutritional counseling that help their children, as well as obstetrics and childbirth medical services and primary care health clinics. They often prefer to receive these services from immigrant-friendly organizations in their communities, such as those in the Chinatowns of New York and Los Angeles. They prefer programs that do not require extensive paperwork and complex applications. These programs need to be expanded to include parenting and child development programs (Yoshikawa, 2011).

> ## POLICY ADVOCACY LEARNING CHALLENGE 13.2
>
> **Connecting Micro, Mezzo, and Macro Policy Interventions**
>
> Improving the Cognitive Skills of Immigrants' Children
>
> Research demonstrates that immigrant children benefit cognitively from participating in preschool and educational programs. Advocates can use micro policy advocacy to obtain their enrollments in these programs while also working against the enactment of policies that require administrators of these programs to ask parents where they are documented.
>
> We have discussed how participation in preschool and center-based childcare enhances the cognitive levels of children of undocumented parents. Advocates can engage in micro policy advocacy to link specific immigrant families to these services. They can also work to form community organizations in communities with high concentrations of immigrant families that can provide micro policy advocacy and develop outreach to immigrants to inform them of benefits of participating in these programs and help increase their access to them (Yoshikawa, 2011).

Core Problem 5: Engaging in Advocacy to Promote Affordable and Accessible Services and Programs for Immigrants—With Some Red Flag Alerts

- **Red Flag Alert 13.27.** Immigrants are wrongly informed that they do not qualify for safety-net programs.
- **Red Flag Alert 13.28.** Undocumented parents, who may not qualify for specific safety-net programs, are not informed that their citizen children *do* qualify for benefits.
- **Red Flag Alert 13.29.** Many immigrants do not know they are eligible for specific programs. In California, for example, macro policy advocates developed and distributed a brochure informing them of their right in California to resources from the state's California Cash Assistance Program for Immigrants (CAPI) that provides monthly financial assistance to certain elderly, blind, or disabled noncitizens not eligible for SSI due to their immigration status (Stanford Law School, n.d.).
- **Red Flag Alert 13.30.** Immigrants encounter adverse financial impacts due to specific federal policies, like the five-year ban on the use of CHIP and Medicaid by green card holders and time limits placed on the use of SSI by some refugees. While these time limits were temporarily extended in 2008 by the Bush administration, they have now expired so that almost 50,000 time-limited noncitizen SSI recipients lost their SSI benefits after August 2011— with half of them being on SSI due to disabilities and half due to extreme age, including "Kurdish victims of Saddam Hussein, Jews who were persecuted in

Russia, Hmong tribesmen who fought for the U.S in Vietnam, and victims of sex trafficking" (National Immigration Law Center, 2011).

Resources for Advocates

Widespread confusion often exists about the eligibility of immigrants for specific programs due to "the complex interaction of immigration and welfare laws, differences in eligibility criteria for various state and federal programs, and lack of adequate training on the rules by agency personnel" (National Immigration Law Center, 2005). Many eligible immigrants are mistakenly denied services or benefits. Immigrants often need expert advocacy from immigration attorneys or from staff of organizations that specialize in assisting immigrants in specific jurisdictions.

A distinction was established in 1996 between "qualified" and "unqualified" immigrants. "Qualified" immigrants include persons with green cards, refugees, asylees, persons granted withholding of deportation or removal, Cuban and Haitian entrants, persons paroled into the U.S. for at least one year, conditional entrants, and certain spouses and children who are victims of domestic violence (Los Angeles Coalition to End Hunger and Homelessness, 2010). The term "legal permanent residents" (LPRs) describes persons who have been granted the right to reside permanently in the U.S., such as persons with green cards. The federal welfare law does not define "federal public benefits" precisely, but the U.S. Department of Health and Human Services (DHHS) included Medicaid, CHIP, Medicare, TANF, foster care, adoption assistance, the Child Care and Development Fund, and the Low-Income Home Energy Assistance Program in 1998. It must be noted, however, that Congress imposed restrictions on the use of TANF, Medicaid, and CHIP by distinguishing between those who entered the U.S. before, on, or after August 22, 1996, when the welfare legislation was enacted. The welfare law barred most qualified immigrants from receiving SSI, SNAP, nonemergency Medicaid, TANF, and CHIP during the five years *after* they secured "qualified" status—while exempting refugees, victims of trafficking, veterans, Cuban/Haitian entrants, and Amerasian immigrants from this requirement (National Immigration Law Center, 2005). (About 20 states use state funds to give some of these benefits to immigrants subject to the five-year ban.)

"Unqualified" immigrants include undocumented immigrants, immigrants with temporary protected status (TPS); immigrants who are permanently residing under color of law (PRUCOL), whom immigration authorities know to be in the U.S. but do not plan to deport; persons in the U.S. on a temporary nonimmigrant visa; applicants for U Visa/interim relief; and victims of trafficking. Unqualified immigrants are not eligible for most federal public benefit programs. When a federal agency does designate a program as a federal public benefit for which "not qualified" immigrants are ineligible, federal law requires that state or local agencies verify *all* immigrants' immigration and citizenship status.

The Affordable Care Act was not kind to immigrants. Roughly one third of immigrants lacked private or public insurance in 2009 before its enactment in 2010. (Roughly half of these 13.4 million uninsured immigrants were undocumented ones, while roughly one third of them were lawful permanent residents and another fifth were naturalized citizens.) Rather than expanding coverage to include them, the ACA did not grant undocumented immigrants health coverage, so they are largely restricted to care for emergency conditions, obstetrics, and some public health preventive programs such as for tuberculosis. Their lack of health insurance often disqualifies these immigrants, moreover, from mental health services unless they develop emergency mental health conditions that qualify them for care in ERs.

Even when immigrants *are* eligible for specific services and resources, they often avoid them for fear that providers will report them to the (ICE). Immigrants often need micro policy advocacy to help them navigate the complex rules that the American welfare state has established—and to help them dispel false fears of deportation when they are eligible for benefits and services.

Many agencies that provide public benefits mistakenly believe that their personnel are supposed to act as immigration enforcers, such as by demanding immigration documents and social security numbers (SSNs), asking unnecessary questions on application forms, and issuing unnecessary warnings on the walls of waiting rooms (National Immigration Law Center, 2005). A series of federal guidance to federal benefit providers has narrowed the questions that agency personnel can ask immigrants and their family members. When agency personnel exceed these limits, they not only violate immigrants' privacy, but they frighten them from using services and benefits to which they are entitled.

POLICY ADVOCACY LEARNING CHALLENGE 13.3

Connecting Micro, Mezzo, and Macro Policy Interventions

Expanding Benefits to Immigrants

Micro policy advocates help green card holders to meet their survival needs when they face five-year bans on the use of Medicaid and CHIP, such as by informing them that they can use public systems of healthcare as well as emergency medical services. Macro policy advocates work to eliminate these five-year bans from federal law, following the lead of the National Immigration Law Center. Macro policy advocates can fight for other policies, such as the Immigrant Children's Health Improvement Act (ICHIA) to allow states to provide Medicaid and CHIP to lawfully present children and pregnant women regardless of entry into the U.S. They can seek to overturn specific provisions in restrictive immigration legislation enacted in 1996 and 1997.

Core Problem 6: Engaging in Advocacy to Promote Care for Immigrants' Mental Distress—With Some Red Flag Alerts

- **Red Flag Alert 13.31.** Immigrants and refugees who have been subjected to traumatic events in their homelands have not been diagnosed or treated for posttraumatic stress disorder (Marshall, 2005).
- **Red Flag Alert 13.32.** Some hospital emergency rooms may not medically stabilize immigrants who come to them with mental health problems that endanger their lives or the lives of other persons.
- **Red Flag Alert 13.33.** Specific immigrants lack supports from immigrants from their nation of origin, such as membership in churches, social groups, or community groups. This isolation may cause mental distress (Yoshikawa, 2011).
- **Red Flag Alert 13.34.** Specific immigrants are wrongly denied mental health services from specific mental health agencies, whether nonprofit or public ones.
- **Red Flag Alert 13.35.** Some hospital emergency rooms may not provide quality services to immigrant women who have been sexually or physically abused (Stanford Law School, n.d.).
- **Red Flag Alert 13.36.** Specific immigrants are given inferior mental health services due to the prejudice of service providers.
- **Red Flag Alert 13.37.** Some immigrants do not obtain mental health services because they cannot afford the fees charged by nonprofit and public agencies at a time when many of them have a budget shortfall. Or they may encounter long waits due to staff cuts caused by these budget shortfalls.
- **Red Flag Alert 13.38.** Immigrants do not receive services for substance abuse from public and nonprofit counseling agencies due to long waits caused by funding cuts or failure of their staff to prioritize them.
- **Red Flag Alert 13.39.** Immigrants lack legal representation when they are threatened with deportation for a minor drug offense that requires no jail time (Stanford Law School, n.d.).

Resources for Advocates

The marginalized status of immigrants, as well as their poverty, causes or exacerbates mental problems for a significant number of them. Unauthorized immigrants have the poorest access and the greatest need for mental health services, even though many of them experience anxiety, depression, and other mental health disorders due to their poverty, marginal status, and fears of deportation (Vega et al., 1999). Many immigrants and refugees have been subjected to trauma in their native lands, including rape, murder, and civil wars—often causing PTSD and other mental conditions (Marshall, 2005).

Translation services are unavailable in many nonprofit agencies because they are not subject to government regulations when they receive no federal or state funds and because budget shortfalls make it difficult to purchase telephone trans-lation services.

Some barriers to services derive from immigrants' culture. Many Asian and Asian American persons, as well as immigrants from many other nations, do not like to admit to or talk about mental health problems with family members or with mental health professionals. They often do not even visit mental health clinics. They often rely upon herbs and other natural substances. Mental health condi-tions may be most likely among immigrants who lack strong supports from other immigrants from their nations of origin (Yoshikawa, 2011).

All immigrants qualify for in-kind programs that protect their lives and safety, including child and adult protective services. All immigrants qualify for mental health services for life-threatening mental health conditions, such as psychosis, depression, and anxiety that make it likely that they have attempted suicide or are at risk of attempting it. Some immigrants qualify for mental health services funded by Medicaid. Immigrants qualify for mental health services provided by many nonprofit agencies. Some immigrants qualify for mental health services funded by states and local units of government. Some immigrants cannot afford fees that are charged by mental health clinics that have become more onerous with cuts in government funding as well as donations to nonprofit agencies.

POLICY ADVOCACY LEARNING CHALLENGE 13.4

Connecting Micro, Mezzo, and Macro Policy Advocacy

Improving Translation Services in Mental Health Agencies

Assume that you work for a nonprofit mental health counseling agency and have engaged in *micro policy advocacy* to secure translation services for immigrants by referring them to other agencies due to the paucity of in-house translation services. You decide that you want to develop a plan for increasing translation services in your agency. How might you engage in *mezzo policy advocacy* to achieve approval of this plan by the executive direc-tor? How might you advance to *macro policy advocacy* to change citywide or statewide regulations related to translation services for immigrants in mental health settings?

Core Problem 7: Engaging in Advocacy to Link Services for Immigrants to Their Communities—With a Red Flag Alert

- **Red Flag Alert 13.40.** Immigrants receive services and benefits from profes-sionals who do not know where they live, their living conditions, or the nature of their work. Lack of knowledge of these realities makes it difficult for professionals to be micro, mezzo, or macro policy advocates.

Barriers

Many professionals possess limited knowledge of the geographic location of immigrants, even in their immediate areas. A list of the 20 American cities with the most immigrants as a percentage of their populations illustrates the sheer number of immigrants ("20 U.S. Cities"), as seen in Table 13.2. An advocate working in these cities would want to identify specific ethnic enclaves within them to better understand their needs and resources.

Table 13.2 American Metro Areas With the Highest Proportion of Immigrants

City	Percentage	Number
1. Miami–Fort Lauderdale–Pompano Beach, FL	36.90%	1.995 mil
2. San Jose–Sunnyvale–Santa Clara, CA	36.31%	.650 mil
3. Los Angeles–Long Beach–Santa Ana, CA	34.28%	4.394 mil
4. San Francisco–Oakland–Fremont, CA	29.50%	1.246 mil
5. New York–Northern New Jersey–Long Island, NY–NJ–PA	28.10%	5.300 mil
6. Chicago–Naperville–Joliet, IL	17.64%	1.676 mil
7. Dallas–Fort Worth–Arlington, TX	17.73%	1.090 mil
8. Washington–Arlington–Alexandria, DC–VA	20.23%	1.074 mil
9. Houston–Sugar Land–Baytown, TX	21.39%	1.120 mil
10. Los Vegas–Paradise, NV	21.81%	1.471 mil
11. Riverside–San Bernardino–Ontario, CA	22.04%	.894 mil
12. San Diego–Carlsbad–San Marcos, CA	22.64%	.672 mil
13. Sacramento–Arden–Arcade–Roseville, CA	17.21%	.358 mil
14. Phoenix–Mesa–Scottsdale, AZ	16.63%	.692 mil
15. Boston–Cambridge–Quincy, MA	15.94%	.716 mil
16. Orlando–Kissmee, FL	15.85%	.321 mil
17. Seattle–Tacoma–Bellevue, WA	15.57%	.514 mil
18. Austin–Round Rock, TX	14.63%	.228 mil
19. Atlanta–Sandy Springs–Marietta, GA	12.84%	.674 mil
20. Denver–Aurora, CO	12.60%	.309 mil

Urban enclaves of immigrants exist in every metropolitan area in every state, as well as in smaller towns and rural areas in light of the spread of Latino/as and other immigrants throughout the United States. Immigrant farmworkers and ranch workers, disproportionately from Mexico and Central America, have proven indispensable to American growers and ranchers for more than a century. Some immigrants are migrants who relocate frequently, such as farmworkers who move to new locations as crops are planted, cultivated, and harvested.

Staff in agencies and programs that help these populations need to use the information throughout this chapter to provide advocacy services for immigrants that are linked to the communities and enclaves where they reside. Too often, immigrants are invisible persons who come to and from their jobs, but are otherwise anonymous individuals who make relatively little use of organized services.

POLICY ADVOCACY LEARNING CHALLENGE 13.5

Connecting Micro, Mezzo, and Macro Advocacy

Invisible Persons

Ramiro Gomez, a Latino folk artist, makes life-sized cardboard cutouts of immigrant laborers who serve as nannies, gardeners, valet workers, and housekeepers in wealthy areas of Los Angeles. He uses acrylic paint to depict these persons, giving them names. He places them at various points in these wealthy areas, such as near George Clooney's home just prior to a fundraiser attended by President Barack Obama. Gomez contends, "We see the beautiful homes. The hedges are trimmed, the gardens are perfect, the children are cared for. We've come to expect it to be this way. But who maintains all this? Who looks after it? And do we treat the workers with the dignity they deserve? Do we stop and notice them?" Sometimes the police, hotel staff, or property owners remove this folk art, which is attached to trees or propped against hedges. The Secret Service asked it to be removed from Clooney's neighborhood. Most pieces only make it a day or two.

LEARNING EXERCISE

1. Are immigrants sometimes "invisible," as well, among professionals who serve them or see them?
2. Can professionals effectively link their services to the communities of immigrants if they do not know where immigrant enclaves exist?

"THINKING BIG" AS POLICY ADVOCATES IN THE IMMIGRATION SECTOR

Immigration policy issues are frequently associated with political conflict. When President Obama, along with a bipartisan group of senators, crafted immigration legislation in early 2013, he knew they would be tested in the coming months as Republicans, Democrats, trade unions, agricultural interests, tourism companies, construction companies, persons living in states and communities bordering Mexico, Latino leaders, African American leaders, the Mexican government, and other groups entered the fray. Unfortunately, immigration reform fell victim to political gridlock, so no progress had been made by the congressional elections of 2014.

Leading politicians were acutely aware of the politics of immigration in 2007. The Comprehensive Immigration Reform Act of 2007 (also known as the Secure Borders, Economic Opportunity and Immigration Reform Act of 2007) that failed to pass Congress provides one example of large-scale reform. It proposed to provide amnesty to more than 10 million immigrant residents by creating a "Z visa" to allow everyone in the U.S. without a valid visa on January 1, 2008, to have the legal right to remain in the U.S. for the rest of his or her life, as well as a Social Security number. Holders of this visa would be eligible for a green card once they had paid a $2,000 fine and back taxes for some of the period in which they worked. Like other green card holders, they could begin the process of becoming a U.S. citizen five years later. The bill strengthened border enforcement, funding 20,000 border patrol agents, 105 camera and radar towers, and 300 miles of vehicle barriers. It replaced the employer-sponsored facet of the immigration system with a point-based merit system based on a combination of education, job skills, family connections, and English proficiency. The legislation had bipartisan support, including (for the Democrats) Majority Leader Harry Reid and Senator Ted Kennedy, and (for the Republicans) Senator John McCain, Senator Jon Kyl, and President George W. Bush.

Several points of contention proved fatal to its passage. Some conservatives argued it needed even more focus on border enforcement and sanctions against employers hiring "illegals" as well as more stringent standards for obtaining a Z visa. Some liberals argued that it gave excessive concessions to highly skilled immigrants, failed to sufficiently support family reunification of immigrants to allow relatives from outside the U.S. to obtain green cards, rolled back protections for immigrant victims of domestic violence and human trafficking, and created an immigration system based on the lives of men by not giving points for caring for children and elderly or disabled family members.

President Barack Obama promised that he would enact sweeping immigration legislation when he ran for the presidency in 2008 but failed to undertake this task, to the chagrin of many Latino/as and immigration advocates, partly because he was preoccupied with policies to address the Great Recession of 2007 to 2009 as well as the Affordable Care Act and banking regulations. He renewed this pledge in his inaugural address and his State of the Union address in early 2013—but it soon became obvious that Republicans would not cooperate with him and Democratic leaders.

Why shouldn't social workers be leaders in seeking comprehensive immigration reforms during the coming years?

Discussion Questions

1. What kind of sweeping immigration legislation should social workers support in light of their Code of Ethics, with special reference to vulnerable populations and social justice?

2. What provisions should protect immigrants' civil rights so that immigrants do not continue to be subject to poor working conditions and low wages?

3. Can the social work profession be a leader in developing support for comprehensive immigration reform?

4. Drawing on materials in this chapter, list groups likely to oppose major immigration reforms, like granting amnesty to roughly 10 million persons and establishing a visa status for many working immigrants that would allow them to remain in the United States for extended periods.

5. Identify power resources that Obama and his allies—or the successor to Obama in the presidential elections of 2016—would need to use to obtain immigration reforms, including the growing electoral power of Latino/a voters.

LEARNING OUTCOMES

You are now equipped to:

1. Discuss how specific social problems are shaped by migration

2. Critically analyze key developments in the evolution of American immigration policies

3. Analyze the causes of migration across national boundaries

4. Discuss how immigrants' poverty and other social problems are linked to economic inequality in the United States

5. Discuss how immigration reform is often stymied by conflict between competing interest groups, political parties, and ideologies

6. Analyze seven core problems in the immigration and global sector, as well as selected Red Flag Alerts

REFERENCES

20 U.S. cities with the most immigrants. (n.d.). *The Daily Beast.* Retrieved from http://www
.thedailybeast.com/articles/2010/07/29/us-cities-with-the-most-immigrants.html

ACLU. (n.d.). *Human trafficking: Modern enslavement of immigrant women in the United States.*
Retrieved October 12, 2011, from http://www.aclu.org/immigrants-rights

ACLU. (2006). *Undocumented workers bring plea for non-discrimination to human rights body.*
Retrieved October 12, 2011, from http://www.aclu.org/immigrants-rights/undocumented
-workers-bring-plea-non-discrimination-human-rights-body

ACLU. (2008). *Immigration myths and facts.* Retrieved October 12, 2011, from http://www.aclu
.org/immigrants-rights/immigration-myths-and-facts

ACLU. (2009). *U.S.–Mexico border crossing deaths are a humanitarian crisis, according to
report from the ACLU and CNDH.* Retrieved October 12, 2011, from http://www.aclu.org/
immigrants-rights/us-mexico-border-crossing-deaths-are-humanitarian-crisis-according
-report-aclu-and

ACLU. (2010). *Immigration reform must respect civil liberties, says ACLU.* Retrieved October 12,
2010, from http://www.aclu.org/immigrants-rights/immiogration-reform-must-respect-civil
-liberties-says-aclu

ACLU. (2011a, October 12). *ACLU and Civil Rights Coalition file lawsuit against South
Carolina's anti-immigrant law.* Retrieved from https://www.aclu.org/immigrants-rights/aclu
-and-civil-rights-coalition-file-lawsuit-against-south-carolinas-anti

ACLU. (2011b). *DHS announces indefinite suspension of controversial and ineffective immigrant registration and tracking system.* Retrieved October 12, 2011, from http://www.aclu.org/immigrants
-rights/dhs-announces-indefinite-suspension-controversial-and-ineffective-immigrant-regist

Capps, R., Casteneda, R. M., Chaudry, A., & Santos, R. (2007). *Paying the price: The impact of
immigration raids on America's children.* Washington, DC: Urban Institute.

Chaudry, A., Capps, R., Pedroza, J. M., Castaneda, R. M., Santos, R., & Scott, M. (2009). *Facing our
future: Children in the aftermath of immigration enforcement.* Washington, DC: Urban Institute.

Congressional Budget Office. (2010). *Cost Estimate S. 3992 Development, Relief, and Education
for Alien Minors Act of 2010.* Retrieved October 12, 2011, from http://www.cbo.gov/
ftdocs/119xx?doc11991/s3992.pdf

Delgado, M., Jones, K., & Rohani, M. (2005). *Social work practice with refugee and immigrant
youth.* Boston, MA: Pearson.

Demleitner, N. V. (2003). How much do Western democracies value family and marriage:
Immigration law's conflicted answers. *Hofstra Law Review, 31,* 270–280.

Finno, M. (2010). *Immigration enforcement in the U.S. and its impact on family separation and
child trauma: The Spanish Model as a solution.* Paper written for doctoral policy class,
University of Southern California, School of Social Work.

Fores, G. (2005). She walked from El Salvador. *Health Affairs, 24,* pp. 5-6-510.

International Organization for Migration. (2011). *Facts & figures.* Retrieved from http://www
.iom,int/jahia/jahia/about-migration/facts-and-figures/lang/en

Kao, D. & Jansson, B. S. (2011). Advocacy to promote culturally competent health services.
In B. Jansson, *Improving healthcare through advocacy* (pp. 179–210). Hoboken, NJ: John
Wiley & Sons.

Leicher, H. (2004). Ethnic politics, policy fragmentation, and dependent health care access in
California, *Journal of Health Politics, Policy, and Law, 29,* 177–201.

Los Angeles Almanac. (2011). *Languages spoken at home by individual Los Angeles communities.* Retrieved from http://www.laalmanac.com/LA/la10b.htm

Los Angeles Coalition to End Hunger and Homelessness. (2010). *The people's guide to welfare, health, and other services,* (33rd ed.). Retrieved from http://www.lacehh.org/tpg/documents/english10PeoplesGuide.pdf

McGreevy, P., & York, A. (October, 2011). Brown signs California Dream Act. *Los Angeles Times,* p. 1.

Morawetz, N. (2000). Understanding the impact of the 1996 deportation laws and the limited scope of proposed reforms. *Harvard Law Review, 113,* 1950–1954.

Marshall, G. (2005). Mental health of Cambodian refugees two decades after resettlement in the United States. *Journal of the American Medical Society, 294,* 571–579.

Migration Policy Institute. (2011). *Frequently requested statistics on immigrants and immigration in the United States.* Migration Information Source. Retrieved from http://www.migration information.org/feature/display.cfm?ID=818

National Immigration Law Center. (2005). *Overview of immigrant eligibility for federal programs.* Resource Manual: Low-Income Immigrant Rights Conference.

National Immigration Law Center. (2011, October). *Supplemental Security Income (SSI) for refugees, asylees, and other humanitarian immigrants.* Retrieved October 25, 2011, from http://www.nilc.org

Pew Hispanic Center. (2011). *The toll of the Great Recession.* Retrieved from http:/www.pewhispanic.ort/2011/07/26/the-toll-of-the-great-recession/

Pew Hispanic Center. (2012, April 23). *Net migration from Mexico falls to Zero—and perhaps less.* Retrieved May 24, 2012, from homepage of Pew Hispanic Center website: http://pew hispanic.org/2012/04/23/net-migration-from-mexico-falls-to-zero-and-perhaps-less/

Stanford Law School. (n.d.). *Immigrants' rights clinic.* Retrieved from www.law.stanford.edu/program/clinics/immigrantsrights/

United Nations High Commissioner for Refugees. (n.d.) *UNHCR global trends 2010.* Retrieved from http://unhcr.org/4dfa11499.html

U.S. Department of Homeland Security, Office of the Inspector General. (2009). *Removals involving illegal alien parents of United States citizen children.* Washington, DC: U.S. Department of Homeland Security.

U.S. Department of State, Bureau of Consular Affairs, U.S. Visas. (n.d.). *Employment-based immigrant visa.* Retrieved from http://travel.state.gov/visa/immigrants/types/types_1323.html

Vega, W., Kolody, B., Aguilar-Gaxiola, S., & Catalona, R. (1999). Gaps in service utilization by Mexican Americans with mental health problems. *Psychiatry Online, 156*(6), 928–934.

VisaPro Immigration Attorneys. (n.d.). *Immigration law FAQ.* Retrieved from http://FAQ.VisaPro.com/

Weiland, J., & Sylvester, A. (2008, May 6). Unlawful immigration raids should trouble all Americans. *San Francisco Daily Journal,* p. 6.

Yoshikawa, H. (2011). *Immigrants raising citizens: Undocumented parents and their young children.* New York, NY: Russell Sage.

Chapter 14

BECOMING POLICY ADVOCATES IN THE CRIMINAL JUSTICE SECTOR

Bruce S. Jansson,
Gretchen Heidemann, and Elaine Sanchez Wilson

LEARNING OBJECTIVES

In this chapter, you will learn how to:

1. Understand the evolution of the criminal justice system in the United States

2. Understand how mass incarceration is powerfully linked to economic inequality in the United States

3. Describe the political economy of the corrections sector, including powerful players and interests, as well as underrepresented ones

4. Identify seven problems encountered in the criminal justice sector, as well as the policies, regulations, and organizational factors pertinent to them

5. Develop Red Flag Alerts for each of the seven problems at the micro advocacy level

6. Identify policy resources available to policy advocates with respect to each of the seven core problems

7. Identify strategies for moving from micro policy advocacy to mezzo and macro policy advocacy in the criminal justice sector

8. Engage the eight challenges in the multilevel policy empowerment framework in the criminal justice sector

Although instrumental in developing the policy of probation and the establishment of juvenile justice, social work has recently reduced its presence in corrections, as the sector has become more punitive and less rehabilitative. As Gumz (2004) noted, "The tenets of social work practice—the innate dignity of the individual, self-determination of the client, confidentiality, moral neutrality, and social justice—were, and are, challenged by a criminal justice system that values order, control, and punishment" (p. 451). As you read this chapter, reflect on ways that social workers can engage in the eight challenges of the multilevel policy advocacy framework in the criminal justice sector.

ANALYZING THE EVOLUTION OF THE AMERICAN CRIMINAL JUSTICE SECTOR

▶ VIDEO LINK 14.1
Youth in Gangs
and Reentry

Figure 14.1 depicts the evolution of the correctional systems in America, beginning with the antiquated notion of "an eye for an eye" as the appropriate

Figure 14.1 Evolution of the criminal justice sector

1750 BC
King Hammurabi of Babylon's Code imposes "an eye for an eye, and a tooth for a tooth" as punishment for crime.

1890s
During the reformatory era, criminals are largely seen as disadvantaged persons who require better education and training, especially in vocational and occupational skills.

1933
Alcatraz becomes the nation's first "supermax" prison, housing the country's most notorious convicted felons.

Early 1800s
Elam Lynds, warden of Auburn State Prison in Pennsylvania, subjects prisoners to harsh and humiliating punishments in the name of discipline, including floggings, prison stripes, and lockstep formation.

1920–1930s
The medical model becomes popular; offenders are viewed as being reformable with proper diagnosis and treatment. Treatment ideology encourages offenders to realize the benefits and rewards of positive behavior.

1935–1960
Public sentiment shifts against prisoners, due in part to the excessive debauchery of the Prohibition Era and reduced opportunities for inmate labor. Rioting takes place in many prisons due to overcrowding, neglect, harsh conditions, and lack of opportunities for rehabilitation.

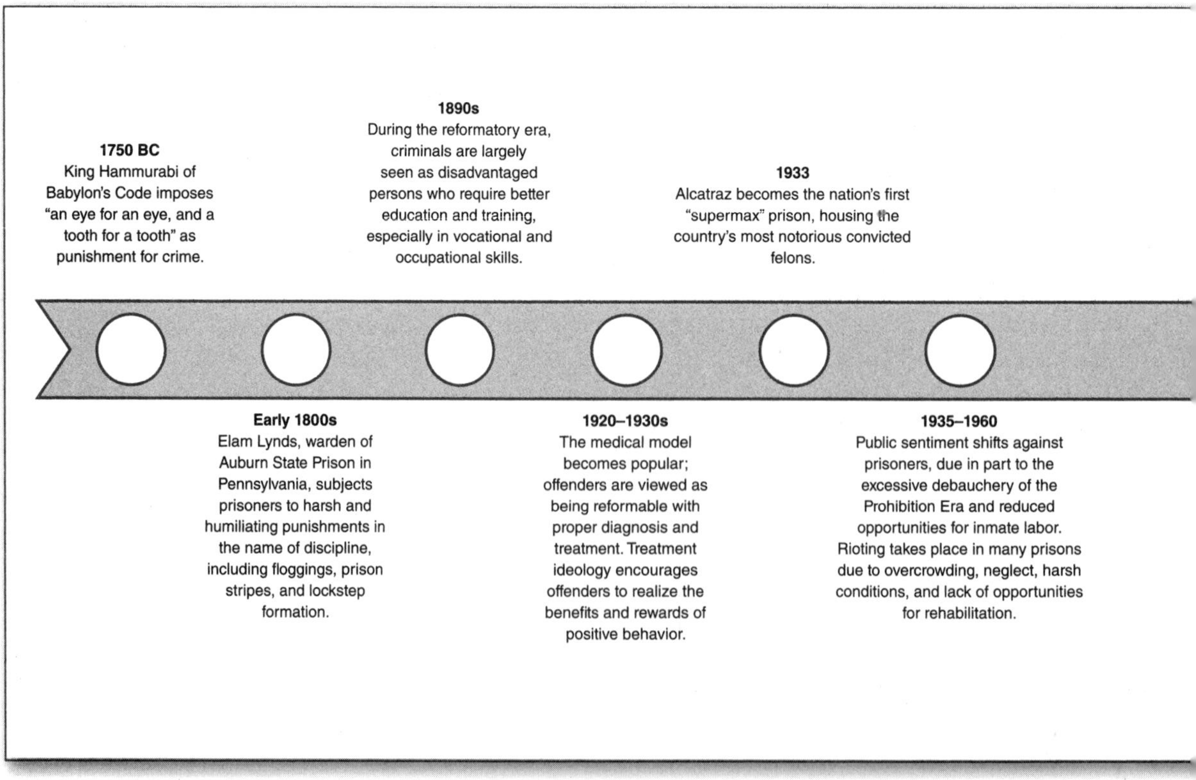

punishment for crime up through the present era of "mass incarceration" in the United States.

Of note in the history of corrections in America are prevailing notions of the reformability of those who violate the law, what behaviors constitute criminal behavior, and the appropriate amount of public spending on enforcement, punishment, and surveillance versus services to address social ills and public health problems that contribute to crime.

IDENTIFYING CONNECTIONS BETWEEN MASS INCARCERATION AND ECONOMIC INEQUALITY

An understanding of the criminal justice sector would be incomplete absent a discussion of mass incarceration and its connection to two phenomena: the deindustrialization that occurred in the 1970s and 1980s and the so-called "War on Drugs."

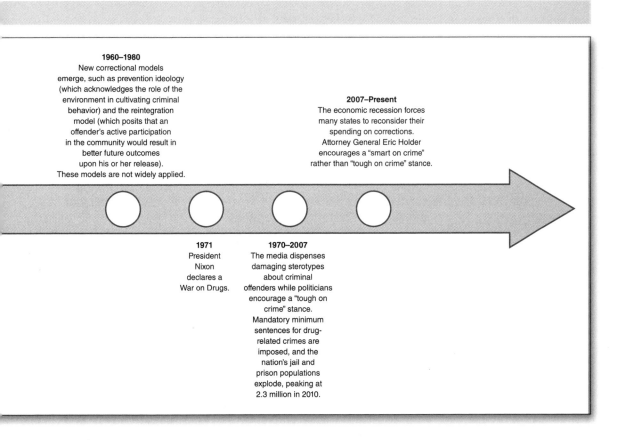

1960–1980
New correctional models emerge, such as prevention ideology (which acknowledges the role of the environment in cultivating criminal behavior) and the reintegration model (which posits that an offender's active participation in the community would result in better future outcomes upon his or her release). These models are not widely applied.

2007–Present
The economic recession forces many states to reconsider their spending on corrections. Attorney General Eric Holder encourages a "smart on crime" rather than "tough on crime" stance.

1971
President Nixon declares a War on Drugs.

1970–2007
The media dispenses damaging sterotypes about criminal offenders while politicians encourage a "tough on crime" stance. Mandatory minimum sentences for drug-related crimes are imposed, and the nation's jail and prison populations explode, peaking at 2.3 million in 2010.

Unemployment rates skyrocketed in the mid-1970s to early 1980s, when many manufacturing facilities pulled out of urban centers and moved their operations overseas, where labor was cheaper (Western & Wildeman, 2009). Unemployment benefits and the shrinking welfare state were insufficient to handle the social problems that arose from mass unemployment among men, who, at that time, were often the family "breadwinners." The drug trade became a source of economic opportunity where a vacuum of legitimate employment existed.

When President Richard Nixon characterized the abuse of illicit substances as "America's public enemy number one" in 1971, a wave of antidrug legislation ensued (Nixon, 1971). The Comprehensive Crime Control Act of 1984 and the Anti-Drug Abuse Act of 1986 reclassified drug users as "criminals" rather than persons in need of treatment, imposed tougher and longer mandatory sentences for drug-related crime (even for first-time offenders), provided the opportunity for higher-level traffickers and dealers to receive lesser sentences by turning in their accomplices, and targeted low-income communities through the crack/powder cocaine disparity (Sudbury, 2002). Individual states also enacted mandatory sentencing laws (i.e., "mandatory minimums") that removed judicial discretion and required automatic prison terms for drug offenses.

This "tough on crime" mentality thus criminalized certain segments of the U.S. population—namely, poor persons and persons of color who used and sold illicit substances—and contributed to skyrocketing levels of incarceration. According to the Bureau of Justice Statistics (BJS), in 1980, U.S. prisons held roughly 330,000 inmates. By 1990 that number had doubled to 774,000, and by 2010 the number of people incarcerated in the U.S. topped 1.5 million (Beck & Gilliard, 1995; Carson & Golinelli, 2013). Today, the United States incarcerates more of its citizens than any other country in the world, and its prison population makes up nearly one quarter of the world's 8.5 million total prisoners (Nation Master, n.d.). These dramatic statistics have led some to call this the "era of mass incarceration" (Alexander, 2010; Western & Wildeman, 2009; Wacquant, 2002).

Racial and ethnic minorities were disproportionately swept up in the broad net cast by the "War on Drugs." While Caucasian Americans represent about 73% of the total U.S. population, they represent only 32% of the prison population. African Americans, on the other hand, comprise only about 13% of the total U.S. population but 38% of all prisoners, and while Latino/as/Hispanics comprise 16% of the total U.S. population, they make up 22% of the prison population (Guerino, Harrison, & Sabol, 2011; Humes, Jones, & Ramirez, 2011). Indeed, one in three African American males will go to prison at some point in his lifetime. Some have argued that the disproportional representation of racial and ethnic minorities in our nation's criminal justice system is akin to, and even an outgrowth of, the slavery and Jim Crow eras (Alexander, 2010; Blackmon, 2009; Davis, 2003; Oshinsky, 1996).

Many advocacy groups are working to reform the criminal justice system, advocate more just correctional policies, and address the effects of mass incarceration on individuals, families, and communities. We provide just a snapshot of them here:

Some Criminal Justice Advocacy Groups.

All of Us or None: This is a national organizing initiative of prisoners, former prisoners, and felons to combat many forms of discrimination that people confront as the result of felony convictions.

America Civil Liberties Union (ACLU): The ACLU aims to ensure that American prisons, jails, and juvenile facilities comply with the Constitution, federal law, and international human rights principles.

American Friends Service Committee (AFSC): The AFSC runs numerous projects that advocate prisoners' rights. Its STOPMAX program works to eliminate the use of isolation and segregation in U.S. prisons through grassroots organizing, public education, and policy advocacy.

Amnesty International: This organization seeks to protect human rights, stop torture, defend women's rights, and abolish the death penalty.

NAACP Legal Defense Fund: This organization seeks to advance social justice and fairness in the criminal justice system, with a focus on African Americans.

National Coalition to Abolish the Death Penalty: This organization serves as a clearinghouse for advocacy groups seeking to end the death penalty and has a network of 100 state and national affiliates.

National Legal Aid and Defender Association: This organization provides resources for advocates seeking equity in the criminal justice system and as a resource to persons seeking more information about equal justice in the U.S.

The Sentencing Project: This project seeks a fair and effective criminal justice system by seeking alternatives to incarceration.

ANALYZING THE POLITICAL ECONOMY OF THE CRIMINAL JUSTICE SECTOR

The criminal justice system is a complex web of entities, including law enforcement agencies, courts, attorneys, local jails, state and federal prisons, and probation and parole entities. We briefly describe here main players, and how an individual typically is processed through the criminal justice system.

Law enforcement agencies include local police and sheriffs, highway patrol, and federal agencies that are tasked with enforcing laws at local, state, and federal levels. Law enforcement is typically the first point of contact for individuals involved in the criminal justice system, and usually this contact comes in the form of an arrest. According to the Federal Bureau of Investigations (2010), law enforcement officials made an estimated 13,687,241 arrests nationwide (not including traffic violations) in 2009. The offense categories representing the largest proportion of cases were larceny–theft at 10% (more than 1.3 million arrests), driving under the influence at 11% (more than 1.4 million arrests), drug abuse violations at 12% (more than 1.6 million arrests), and property crimes at 13% (more than 1.7 million arrests; U.S. Department of Justice, 2010).

Individuals are processed through the criminal justice system via courts. All persons suspected of committing a crime are officially charged with that crime (typically by a prosecutor) and offered an opportunity to either admit guilt, accept a plea deal, or take their case to trial in order to let a jury decide. While the vast majority (94%) of persons charged with a felony plead guilty (Durose, Farole, & Rosenmerkel, 2009), those who deny guilt must retain either a defense attorney or a public defender to represent them. Many advocates argue that the quality of defense is greatly limited for individuals of limited means, thus increasing the likelihood that poor persons will be convicted compared to persons who can afford private representation.

A felony or misdemeanor conviction is typically accompanied by a sentence, which is issued by a judge. Sentences typically match the severity of the crime, and can range from restitution and fines to community service or probation to serving time in local jail or state or federal prison. Many advocates argue that the imposition of mandatory minimum sentences for drug-related crime (discussed above), "three-strikes-you're-out" laws, and other similar sentences that remove judicial discretion are unfitting for the crime.

Jails and prisons are major figures in the political economy of the criminal justice system. More than 2 million people are currently confined in U.S. jails and prisons combined. Future sections of this chapter will discuss a vast array of issues confronting these entities—which are designed to house and punish convicted persons—including overcrowding, lack of proper healthcare and mental health care, sexual assault of inmates, and solitary confinement. Jails and prisons stand in stark contrast to the social welfare entities found in other sectors (discussed in Chapters 7 through 13 of this text) that are designed to serve, treat, and assist individuals.

Finally, the political economy of the criminal justice sector includes the entities of probation and parole. Probation offices (operated by counties) and parole offices (operated by states) supervise persons who are sentenced to serve a portion of time in the community, either instead of or in addition to jail or prison time. The Bureau of Justice Statistics reports that nearly 5 million adults were under the supervision of probation or parole at year-end 2010—the equivalent of about one in every 48 adults in the U.S. (Glaze & Bonczar, 2011).

ANALYZING SEVEN CORE PROBLEMS IN THE CRIMINAL JUSTICE SECTOR

Core Problem 1: Engaging in Advocacy to Improve Prisoners' and Former Prisoners' Ethical Rights—With Some Red Flag Alerts

The concepts of "ethical rights" (Core Problem 1), "quality care" (Core Problem 2), and "culturally appropriate services" (Core Problem 3) are difficult to apply to the criminal justice sector, given that persons involved in corrections are viewed not as consumers but rather as "deviants" or persons who have violated the social contract, and are thus subject to prevailing notions of punishment and retribution. This is not to say that the criminal justice system itself is not bound by important "quality assurance" mechanisms. Indeed, the Bill of Rights, comprising the first 10 amendments of the United States Constitution, serves to protect the natural rights of its citizens. It guarantees, among other things, protection against cruel and unusual punishment (Eighth Amendment); the due process of law, including the right to a speedy trial and the right to legal counsel (Fifth and Sixth Amendments); protection from unreasonable searches and seizures; the right of people "to be secure in their persons, houses, papers, and effects" (Fourth Amendment); and a public trial by an impartial jury, both in criminal cases (Sixth Amendment) and in common law civil suits (Seventh Amendment).

Yet the rights enshrined in the Constitution initially only applied to land-owning white men. Women and racial minorities were excluded. It took additional Constitutional amendments and numerous Supreme Court cases to extend the same rights to all U.S. citizens. Even since the passage of the Thirteenth, Fourteenth and Fifteenth Amendments, which abolished slavery and granted rights and citizenship to former slaves, and the Nineteenth Amendment, which extended rights to women, countless advocates have challenged the criminal justice system on grounds that the rights ensured in the U.S. Constitution and the Bill of Rights have been violated. One historical example is Dorothea Dix, who advocated better conditions for indigent, mentally ill detainees in the mid-1800s (see Core Problem 6). This section will discuss current efforts to ensure the rights of those involved in the criminal justice system.

- **Red Flag Alert 14.1.** A prisoner is labeled as a gang member and is threatened with solitary confinement unless he informs officials about gang leadership and planned activities.
- **Red Flag Alert 14.2.** A prisoner held in solitary confinement for five years becomes increasingly disoriented and lethargic, yet she has not been seen by a certified mental health professional.

- **Red Flag Alert 14.3.** An illiterate prisoner with limited English speaking ability is given a form that authorizes his inclusion in a pharmaceutical study.
- **Red Flag Alert 14.4.** Food is routinely withheld from a prisoner who refuses to work.
- **Red Flag Alert 14.5.** A female prisoner is "groped" by a male guard during a routine strip-search.
- **Red Flag Alert 14.6.** Prison guards look the other way while a male inmate is sexually assaulted by other inmates.

Background

Like many of the populations discussed in this text, prisoners housed in this country's correctional facilities are vulnerable to experiencing violations of their ethical rights. Yet, unlike students, seniors, and foster youth, prisoners carry with them a unique stigma; it is not politically incorrect for society to ignore or even discriminate against incarcerated individuals. There are numerous areas within the criminal justice sector—from the point of arrest through incarceration to reentry—where ethical violations are rife. We touch on just a few of them here.

One of those areas includes the use of controversial "stop-and-frisk" policies as a law enforcement mechanism for maintaining social order. At the present time in New York City, lawsuits have been filed against the NYPD for their use of the practice, which primarily targets young men of color. These tactics have been ruled by district courts to violate residents' constitutional rights.

A second area of great concern to many advocates is the sexual assault that takes place within the walls of many prisons, and is perpetrated by both guards and by fellow inmates (often while guards "look the other way"). The advocacy group Just Detention reports that 200,000 adults and children are sexually abused behind bars every year (Just Detention, n.d.).

Long-term segregation (i.e., solitary confinement) is another area that is considered a violation of prisoners' rights by some. Depending on the institution, the experience of solitary confinement can range from limited contact with other persons, including the general population of prisoners and family visitors, to complete sensory deprivation for 23 hours each day. Prisoners can be held in solitary confinement for months and years. Although its devastating psychological impacts have been widely documented (Arrigo & Bullock, 2008), few policies exist to regulate the practice. Human Rights Watch (2012) is currently working to end the practice of solitary confinement for incarcerated juveniles under the age of 18, while the American Civil Liberties Union seeks reforms to solitary confinement practices generally across the U.S. (American Civil Liberties Union, n.d.b).

Other violations of ethical rights include (but are not limited to) the disproportionate imposition of capital punishment sentences on members of ethnic minority groups; prison overcrowding that leads to inadequate health and mental health services; the elimination of educational and vocational training programs for inmates; the denial of employment, housing, and educational opportunities to persons with drug convictions; and lifetime disenfranchisement of formerly incarcerated people in many states (i.e., eliminating their right to vote because of a prior conviction).

Resources for Advocates

Court Rulings. Court decisions have played key roles in the formulation of correctional policies regarding prisoners' ethical rights. In its 1964 *Cooper v. Pate* decision, the Court held that prisoners are persons whose rights are protected by the Constitution, and they can challenge the conditions of their confinement. Under *Hudson v. Palmer* (1984), prison officials are permitted to search cells and confiscate items without violating the Fourth Amendment's prohibition of unreasonable search and seizures. Also, in the 1974 *Wolff v. McDonnell* case, the Court ruled that inmates have due process rights under the Fourteenth Amendment when being disciplined.

The constitutionality of the death penalty has also been discussed and debated in the courts. In *Furman v. Georgia* (1972), the Supreme Court found that capital punishment was imposed unpredictably and infrequently. As such, the Court ruled that the death penalty amounted to cruel and unusual punishment and should be ceased. However, four years later, in *Gregg v. Georgia*, the Court allowed executions to continue after a few states revised their death penalty statutes. Specifically, the Court upheld death penalty laws that require the sentencing judge or jury to take into account specific aggravating and mitigating factors in deciding which convicted murderers should be sentenced to death. In recent cases, the Court has ruled that the execution of mentally disabled individuals (*Atkins v. Virginia*, 2002) and the execution of offenders for crimes committed under the age of 18 (*Roper v. Simmons*, 2005) are unconstitutional.

Legislation. In 1996, Congress enacted the Prison Litigation Reform Act in an effort to curb the increase in prisoner litigation that was finding its way into the federal courts, including claims of physical and sexual abuse, mistreatment of confined individuals, and prison officials' indifference to inmate-to-inmate assault. Under the law, prisoners must exhaust all available administrative avenues before challenging a condition of their confinement. Prisoners must also pay court filing fees in full, either up front or through monthly installments, and this process requires the coordination and cooperation of the prison in handling the transaction (American Civil Liberties Union, n.d.a). Lawsuits or appeals that a judge rules are frivolous or without merit count as strikes; after three strikes, prisoners are unable to file additional lawsuits without up-front payment of filing fees. Also, prisoners seeking monetary damages for mental or emotional injury must provide proof of physical injury.

POLICY ADVOCACY LEARNING CHALLENGE 14.1

Connecting Micro, Mezzo, and Macro Policy Interventions

By Marilyn Montenegro, PhD, MSW

2002 NASW Social Worker of the Year recipient

Stella is a 62-year-old woman with a long history of addiction and convictions for drug-related violations. When she was released from prison in 2010, she was able to enter a drug treatment program. She said that she had been trying to get into treatment for some time and that this was her first opportunity to change her life. While she was in the treatment program, a social worker assisted her in applying for Supplemental Security Income (SSI) based on her mental illness, diabetes, and hepatitis C. Stella graduated from the treatment program in 2011 and decided to move into the agency's sober living facility. A few months later she was approved for SSI and now receives $854 a month.

As a result of her sobriety, she reestablished relationships with her family. Stella and her sister decided that since they were both eligible for low-income housing, they would get an apartment together in a building for low-income seniors. The women applied at a number of senior buildings; often they were placed on a waiting list, but two of the buildings had immediate openings, and the sisters filled out rental applications and agreed to a background check. In addition to a credit history, a criminal history was obtained for both women. Stella was denied housing based on her criminal history (Code of Federal Regulations 24 C.F.R 982.553). Her sister, who has no criminal history, was approved and has since moved into the senior building.

Stella says she is tired of sharing a room with strangers and has been looking for an unsubsidized single apartment, hoping that they will not check her criminal history. So far she has been summarily rejected.

LEARNING EXERCISE

1. What are some of the ethical violations that Stella experienced?
2. If you were the social worker assigned to Stella's case, what could you have done at the micro policy level to avoid, or remedy, this situation?
3. Imagine that the California Department of Fair Employment and Housing has commissioned you to write a policy brief on housing practices affecting formerly incarcerated persons. Using Stella's case, outline some of the mezzo- or macro-level recommendations you would propose to reform current policy.

Core Problem 2: Engaging in Advocacy to Promote Quality Programs for Prisoners and Ex-Prisoners—With Some Red Flag Alerts

Although certain rights are granted to citizens who come into contact with the criminal justice system via the U.S. Constitution, "quality care" is a notion largely foreign to corrections. A meta-analysis of the effects of custodial versus noncustodial sentences found that the rate of reoffending after a noncustodial sanction is actually lower than after a custodial sanction (Villettaz, Killias, & Zoder, 2006). In other words, prison does not decrease future criminal activity. Rather, it may actually perpetuate it through the psychological damage it exacts, and by denying former prisoners opportunities for legitimate employment and self-sufficiency. Researchers and advocates from a broad spectrum of ideologies have concluded that the system, as currently constituted, does not serve the best interests of the public, but rather extracts from it valuable resources that could better be spent on social programs to address problems of drug abuse, social disorder, and poverty.

This state of affairs—a criminal justice system that routinely violates civil and human rights, does not effectively respond to social problems but may actually exacerbate them, and that costs taxpayers enormous valuable resources—has moved some advocates to want to fundamentally reform the criminal justice system.

- **Red Flag Alert 14.7.** A poor person suffering from drug addiction is sentenced to life in prison for petty theft—a nonviolent, nonserious third felony offense.
- **Red Flag Alert 14.8.** A crime victim wants to confront the perpetrator and the offender wants to make amends, but avenues through which to do so are not available in their jurisdiction.
- **Red Flag Alert 14.9.** A city council member wishes to implement criminal justice reforms in her jurisdictions based on evidence and best practices, but is lambasted by her opponents for being "soft on crime."
- **Red Flag Alert 14.10.** Resources in one's jurisdiction are spent on corrections at a rate many times the amount spent on social programs, such as housing, WIC, and drug treatment.

Background

Those who seek to transform the basic structure of the criminal justice system are met with formidable foes. These include powerful special interests as well as conservative scare tactics and the previously mentioned "law-and-order" mentality that hinders elected officials from accomplishing significant reforms for fear of being labeled "soft on crime."

Special Interests. Prisons are expensive to operate, yet they are quite profitable to many parties. First, rising incarceration rates require greater numbers of correctional staff. According to the Bureau of Justice Statistics, a total of 2.5 million persons were employed in the nation's justice system in 2007, and nearly half a million of those jobs were in state corrections (Kyckelhahn, 2011). Additionally, vendors who supply food, uniforms, commissary items, and collect phone calls from inmates to their families benefit from lucrative contracts with prison authorities (Dannenberg, 2011). Moreover, major manufacturers and retailers benefit from the free or cheap labor of the nation's 1.6 million inmates (Winter, 2008).

Examination of lobbying efforts on behalf of these special interests suggests that their level of investment is high. The California Correctional and Peace Officers Association (CCPOA), a 31,000-member-strong prison guards union, spends approximately $8 million of the annual $23 million it raises through membership dues on lobbying (Kowal, 2011). In a December 2009 report, the Pennsylvania State Corrections Officers Association touted the union's efforts to support a $500 million Pennsylvania prison expansion effort to build five new prisons with 12,000 total beds (Winter Group, 2009). Advocates seeking to reform the criminal justice system in their jurisdictions can expect to be met by these and other powerful special interests.

"Tough on Crime" Ideologies. At the time of the initiation of the War on Drugs and massive prison buildup, considerable media attention was focused on the so-called "dangerous class" (Golden, 2005). Nightly news programs portrayed images of inner-city residents, usually black men, as violent outlaws, drug dealers, rapists, and murderers. Black women, on the other hand, were portrayed as "welfare queens" and crack addicts who exposed their fetuses (so-called "crack babies") to drugs. These spectacles of the gangster and the unfit mother were given tremendous national media attention while similar attention was not given to white-collar crime (Golden, 2005). This prompted a dramatic rise in the fear of crime, and more and more politicians sought to align their platforms with popular views. "Tough on crime" rhetoric was subsequently translated into policies such as mandatory minimum sentencing for drug-related crime and "three strikes you're out" legislation, which mandated a life sentence for any person convicted of a third felony (Sudbury, 2002).

Resources for Advocates

There has been a shift in recent years away from the "tough on crime" stance and toward a "smart on crime" approach. In a 2009 address, Attorney General Eric Holder argued,

Getting smart on crime requires talking honestly about which policies have worked and which have not, without fear of being labeled as too hard or, more likely, as too soft on crime. Getting smart on crime means moving beyond useless labels and instead embracing science and data, and relying on them to shape policy. And it means thinking about crime in context—not just reacting to the criminal act, but developing the government's ability to enhance public safety before the crime is committed and after the former offender is returned to society. (Vera Institute of Justice, 2009)

Efforts have been initiated at local, state and federal levels to reverse some of the trends of the harsh sentencing era, and to challenge prevailing systems of punishment.

Restorative Justice. A growing movement favors the restorative justice approach as an alternative to incarceration. Restorative justice emphasizes repairing the harm caused by crime. Howard Zehr, a pioneer of the American restorative justice movement, defines restorative justice as processes "to involve, to the extent possible, those who have a stake in a specific offense to collectively identify and address harms, needs, and obligations, in order to heal and put things as right as possible" (Zehr, 2002). In the U.S., numerous restorative justice programs exist (see, e.g., Bishop, 2012, and Mills, Maley, & Shy, 2009). Advocates tout the benefits of the approach as humanizing in comparison to the harsh and stifling conditions of prison. A meta-analysis of restorative justice programs found that they were more effective than traditional sanctions in reducing recidivism and ensuring restitution compliance (Latimer, Dowden, & Muise, 2005).

Prison Abolition. Some advocates argue that prisons should be done away with entirely. The preeminent organization working to abolish the prison system and replace it with a system of community accountability is Critical Resistance (Critical Resistance, n.d.). Formed in 1997 by activists challenging the idea that imprisonment and policing are the best solution for social, political, and economic problems, Critical Resistance seeks to build a movement to abolish the prison industrial complex (for more information, go to www.criticalresistance.org). Through local chapters, Critical Resistance advocates systems of harm prevention that build community and provide for basic needs, and systems of accountability that address the root causes of harm.

POLICY ADVOCACY LEARNING CHALLENGE 14.2

Connecting Micro, Mezzo, and Macro Policy Interventions

Discussing the Ethics of "Three Strikes"

Visit the website of Families to Amend California's Three Strikes (www.facts1.org) and read one of the "3 Strikes Stories." In small groups, discuss the following:

1. Do you think this person deserves to be sentenced to life in prison? If so, why?
2. If not, what would be a fair or more appropriate sentence?
3. In what ways could social workers intervene at the micro and mezzo levels to help individuals keep from repeating crimes?
4. In what ways could social workers intervene at the macro level to change three-strikes laws in their state?

Core Problem 3: Engaging in Advocacy to Promote Culturally Competent Services and Policies for Prisoners and Ex-Prisoners—With Some Red Flag Alerts

The U.S. criminal justice system is not set up to "serve" those who come into contact with it, but rather to punish them, *but* there is growing recognition that certain vulnerable groups, such as women, the elderly, the indigent, and mentally ill persons, have unique needs and circumstances and require specialized attention at various stages of the criminal justice process. This section will address advocates' attempts to reform the criminal justice system by changing specific laws and policies pertaining to marginalized or vulnerable groups. Specific focus will be paid to women, the elderly, and the ill, as issues concerning mentally ill prisoners will be discussed later.

- **Red Flag Alert 14.11.** A woman is given a mandatory minimum sentence for her role as an accomplice to her abusive boyfriend who sells drugs out of the couple's home. She was aware of the drug activity, but not directly involved. He was given a reduced sentence of probation for turning in his accomplices (including her).
- **Red Flag Alert 14.12.** A woman inmate is handcuffed and shackled to her bed while giving birth, and the child is immediately removed and placed in foster care.
- **Red Flag Alert 14.13.** A woman inmate serving a two-year sentence for a first-time drug offense is not informed that the state has moved to permanently terminate her parental rights.

- **Red Flag Alert 14.14.** An elderly man serving a life sentence for murder is diagnosed with brain cancer and will probably die within six months. His in-prison medical care costs $100,000 per year.
- **Red Flag Alert 14.15.** Persons of color comprise the vast bulk of prison populations in the United States, including African Americans, Latino/as, and Native Americans. They receive disproportionate convictions and sentences as compared to the white population.

Background

Three kinds of prisoners and ex-prisoners have drawn considerable attention in policy debates about the criminal justice sector: women, the elderly and individuals with medical problems, and people of color.

▶

VIDEO LINK 14.2
Women's
Rehabilitation
Program

Women. Women are the fastest-growing prisoner population in the United States, and their rate of incarceration has increased by 840% since 1980 (Gilliard & Beck, 1994; West & Sabol, 2010). Women are more likely to be sentenced for drug-related crime and less likely to be sentenced for violent crime than men (Guerino et al., 2011). Women prisoners report significantly higher rates of prior physical and sexual abuse as well as higher rates of mental illness and substance abuse than their male counterparts (Harlow, 1999; James & Glaze, 2006; Mumola & Karberg, 2006). In addition, women prisoners are more likely than their male counterparts to have lived at or below the poverty level, less likely to have been employed prior to their incarceration, more likely to have been receiving welfare assistance prior to incarceration, and more likely than men to engage in criminal behavior for economic reasons (Lewis, 2006; O'Brien & Harm, 2002; Covington & Bloom, 2006). Yet current sentencing laws and standard management strategies, which include surveillance, searches, restraints, infractions, and isolation, are based on male characteristics and crime and fail to take into account women's characteristics, responsibilities, and roles in crimes (Covington & Bloom, 2003).

Female prisoners are also more likely to be parents of dependent children than are male prisoners (Glaze & Maruschak, 2008). Correctional practices and policies governing contact between prisoners and their children often impede, rather than support, the maintenance of family ties (Hairston, 2004). Most children are unable to visit their mothers due to the remote locations of prisons. Those who are able to visit often experience long waits, rude treatment by staff, and physical environments that restrain mother–child interaction (Arditti & Few, 2006). Phone calls placed to correctional facilities or received as collect calls from prisons are up to six times more expensive than the typical long-distance call, making this form of communication difficult for poor families (Dannenberg, 2011). Moreover, pregnant inmates in many states face the dehumanizing prospect of being shackled to their beds during childbirth and of having their infant taken from them within hours of delivery (Women's Prison Association, n.d.).

The Elderly and the Ill. Prisoners sentenced to death, to life without the possibility of parole, or to consecutive or lengthy sentences (such as those mandated by three-strikes laws) often grow old and/or ill in prison. In recent years, the number and proportion of older inmates has grown. There were more than 25,000 inmates aged 65 and older in state and federal prisons at year-end 2010 (Guerino, Harrison, & Sabol, 2010), and 89% of all inmate deaths are attributable to medical conditions (Mumola, 2007). For inmates who serve at least 10 years in state prison, the mortality rate due to illness is triple that of inmates who serve less than five years (Mumola, 2007).

The ever-expanding prison population places a strain on prison healthcare systems to provide basic medical services, as well as specialty services for the above populations. This strain is felt not only by prison physicians and nurses; elected officials struggle to justify rising correctional budgets to weary taxpayers. The ultimate impact, however, is experienced by a population that is too often invisible to society—the inmates themselves. Among them, terminally ill prisoners are perhaps the most vulnerable of all. Typically, terminally ill prisoners are isolated, without access to visitors, and often fear dying alone (Snyder, van Wormer, Chadha, & Jaggers, 2009). Social workers who are able to visit terminally ill patients report that these prisoners are subjected to body cavity searches after visits (Snyder et al., 2009). Many terminally ill prisoners report feeling shame that they will die as a prisoner (Wahidin, 2004). The National Institute of Justice in 2004 reported that only half of the 50 U.S. states operate hospice programs in their prisons (Anno, Graham, Lawrence, & Shansky, 2004).

People of Color. We have discussed how male persons of color constitute the overwhelming majority of inmates in the United States at greatly disproportionate levels as compared to the white population. Considerable evidence suggests that they are subject to the death penalty, as well as long sentences, far more than whites who commit similar crimes.

Resources for Advocates

Policy Reforms Targeting Females. In 1997, the U.S. Federal Bureau of Prisons (BOP) issued a formal policy on the management of female offenders that mandated all Board of Prison programs and services to "consider and address" the unique treatment needs of female offenders (General Accounting Office, 1999). It also requires each applicable BOP facility to develop and document programs and services that meet women's needs, prepare them to function in an institutional environment, and return them to the community. The BOP's "gender-responsive" mandate, although difficult to enforce, nonetheless recognizes that a "one-size-fits-all" correctional system is insensitive to the differential needs and characteristics of women, who often leave behind children for whom they were the primary caregiver, and who often become involved in crime for reasons related to economic marginality and drug addiction. The gender-responsive philosophy promotes "creating an environment through site selection, staff selection, program development, content, and material that reflects an understanding of the realities of the lives of women in criminal justice settings and addresses their specific challenges and strengths" (Covington & Bloom, 2006, p. 19).

Unfortunately, this ideal model is far from the norm. In 2010, of the 93,000 total women incarcerated in state prisons, nearly one in 12 was confined in California's "supermax" women's prisons. The largest women's prison in the world—Central California Women's Facility (CCWF)—had a design capacity of 2,004 and a population of 3,736 on September 30, 2011. Its neighbor across the street—Valley State Prison for Women (VSPW)—is the second-largest women's prison in the world. It had a design capacity of 1,980 and a population of 3,496 on September 30, 2011 (California Department of Corrections and Rehabilitation, 2011). Far from being nurturing environments designed to address women's trauma and promote healthy relationships, these facilities have instead been described as "suicide cities" (Olson, 2007). In writing about her experience as an inmate at CCWF, Olson recounts how the overcrowded conditions inside the facility led to frequent lockdowns and inadequate mental health care, all of which precipitated a number of attempted and successful suicides (Olson, 2007). Clearly, there is much work to be done to properly address women prisoners' unique needs. Advocates, including the Women's Prison Association, are working to ensure that the needs of women prisoners and their families are addressed (see Table 14.1).

Table 14.1 Advocacy Groups Focusing on Women and Children

Women's Prison Association (www.wpaonline.org)

The Family and Corrections Network (https://www.prisonactivist.org/resources/family-and -corrections-network)

Legal Services for Prisoners with Children (www.prisonerswithchildren.org)

The Center for Community Alternatives (www.communityalternatives.org)

The Justice Policy Institute (www.justicepolicy.org/index.html)

The Sentencing Project (www.sentencingproject.org)

The Vera Institute of Justice (www.vera.org)

Policy Reforms Targeting the Elderly and Ill. Advocates concerned with issues confronting elderly and terminally ill prisoners often argue for compassionate release of these vulnerable populations. Compassionate release—a program that allows some eligible, seriously ill prisoners to die outside of prison before sentence completion—is permitted under the Sentencing Reform Act of 1984 (Williams, Sudore, Greifinger, & Morrison, 2011), and all but five states have some mechanism through which dying prisoners can seek release (Anno et al., 2004). Advocates of compassionate release argue that releasing prisoners with life-limiting illnesses who no longer pose a threat to society is both the ethical and moral thing to do, and that the financial costs to society of continuing to incarcerate such persons outweigh the benefits. Medical eligibility guidelines vary by jurisdiction, but most states require that the prisoner have a diagnosed terminal or severely debilitating medical condition that cannot be appropriately cared for within the prison, and that the prisoner pose no further threat to society (Williams et al., 2011).

However, a recent study of compassionate release in practice found that only 36 requests for compassionate release in the Federal Bureau of Prisons in 2008 made it to the final review stage, and 27 were approved. The Vera Institute of Justice cites narrow eligibility criteria, complicated and lengthy referral and review processes, political considerations, and public opinion as barriers to compassionate release (Chiu, 2010). Those in the medical field concur that eligibility guidelines are too stringent, requiring a short prognosis (e.g., six months) that excludes prisoners with severe dementia, those in a persistent vegetative state, or those with end-stage organ disease who may actually live longer, although they pose no threat to society (Williams et al., 2011). However, the power of the "court of public opinion" and political motivations for the denial of compassionate releases should not be discounted. Advocates, including family members of dying prisoners, as well as those in the medical profession, continue to fight for the rights of terminally ill and severely incapacitated prisoners by challenging the necessary qualifications for compassionate release.

Prison Reforms Targeting Persons of Color. Considerable attention has been given to greatly decreasing the incarceration rates of African American, Latino, and Native American males by decreasing them for nonviolent crimes—and by greatly shortening sentences for nonviolent offenders. Some states have abolished the death penalty in the wake of evidence that many innocent males of color receive this sentence.

POLICY ADVOCACY LEARNING CHALLENGE 14.3

Connecting Micro, Mezzo, and Macro Policy Advocacy

Should They Be Released?

Material drawn from The Real Cost of Prisons Project website: realcostofprisons .org/writing/Muise_Compassionate_Release.pdf

Picture 92-year-old Nick leaning on his cane, out of breath, in the quad at the largest men's prison in Massachusetts. Nick is making one of his three trips a day across the prison complex to get his life-sustaining medications, and is forced to ask another prisoner to dig nitroglycerin out of his pocket so he can address the heart episode he is experiencing. Nick was sentenced to life in prison more than 40 years ago for murdering his wife when he caught her with another man. He was drunk at the time. He had no prior criminal history, and has expressed remorse for his crime.

Also picture Frank, a 70-year-old diabetic and Vietnam War veteran, in his wheelchair. Frank has had both legs amputated and is unable to see well enough to write his son to tell him about a guard in the assisted care facility at the prison who would not allow him to be wheeled over to a church service. Frank was sentenced to life in prison 27 years ago on a third strike for armed robbery. His previous convictions include unarmed robbery and petty theft. As a young father, Frank had been laid off and resorted to stealing to support his wife and three kids. His wife is now deceased. Like Nick, Frank has also expressed remorse for his crimes.

Both men are model prisoners, with no infractions in the past 25 years. The family members of both men are fighting for their release, but Massachusetts is one of only a few states that does not have some type of compassionate/medical release law that allows seriously ill prisoners to be released to more appropriate care. The cost to care for aging MA prisoners ranges from $75,000 to $115,000 per prisoner per year, as opposed to about $44,000 for a healthy man or woman. The managed care these men would receive outside of prison walls is a fraction of the cost of in-prison care.

LEARNING EXERCISE

Consider the following questions from the points of view of (1) a terminally ill prisoner's doctor, (2) a terminally ill prisoner's son or daughter, (3) a member of the victim's family, and (4) a concerned taxpayer:

1. Should prisoners like Frank and Nick be granted compassionate release?
2. What guidelines do you think should be used to determine the release of elderly or severely/terminally ill prisoners?
3. Who should ultimately get to decide the fate of terminally ill prisoners?
4. Do the risks of releasing prisoners like Nick and Frank outweigh the benefits in terms of the healthcare savings?
5. How might you engage in micro, mezzo, and/or macro level policy advocacy to improve the situation of terminally ill prisoners?

Core Problem 4: Engaging in Advocacy to Promote Prevention for Prisoners and Ex-Prisoners—With Some Red Flag Alerts

Prison affects an individual not only during the time he or she spends there; it also carries lasting financial, emotional, and social effects. For example, black men without high school diplomas have a 60% chance of being sent to jail, which is associated with a reduction in their annual employment by nine weeks and a 40% drop in their yearly income (Romano, 2011). The stigma of a criminal record can haunt an individual for life, despite his or her best efforts to change. Therefore, it is crucial that efforts be made to strengthen preventive services targeted at those at risk of entering the system. Additionally, preventive services can do much to reduce recidivism and promote successful reentry into society.

- **Red Flag Alert 14.16.** A prisoner who has been in jail for years is up for parole and will return to his impoverished neighborhood with few skills or resources.
- **Red Flag Alert 14.17.** A soon-to-be released prisoner has never had any visits from family or made calls to home. His only known support system was the gang of which he was previously a member.
- **Red Flag Alert 14.18.** A prisoner is unable to attain his certification while incarcerated because the vocational training program was cut due to budgetary constraints.

Background

The implementation of evidence-based practices has been shown to reduce recidivism rates by 50% (Andrews et al., 1990). Early intervention programs have also kept vulnerable youth from entering into gangs and their spiraling life of crime. Replacing a once-size-fits-all approach with a flexible model for responding to ex-offenders' individual situations can yield more positive outcomes. For example, the National Institute of Corrections and Crime and Justice Institute presented eight evidence-based practices that aim to improve reentry outcomes (Bogue et al., 2004), including assessing risks and needs, enhancing intrinsic motivation, targeting interventions, using cognitive behavioral treatment methods for skill-building purposes, increasing positive reinforcement, engaging with natural communities, measuring practices, and providing feedback.

Gang Involvement. According to figures from the Office of Juvenile Justice and Delinquency Prevention, there were 800,000 gang members active in more than 3,000 gangs in the year 2000. A number of risk factors are correlated with gang involvement, including but not limited to low household incomes, single-parent households, low academic achievement, identification as learning disabled, and accessibility to marijuana (Hill, Howell, Hawkins, & Battin-Pearson, 1999). Early childhood, school-based, and after-school programs have been used to prevent adolescents from entering into gangs as well as to disrupt and dismantle existing gangs. However, the most effective programs involve the community at large and require multiagency coordination and integration among a variety of stakeholders, such as youth services, police, parole, and grassroots organizations.

Recidivism. Upon their release from prison, ex-offenders face the challenge of figuring out where to live, where to work, and where to seek or continue their medical care. The lack of resources and employment opportunities, limited supervision, and inadequate collaboration between parole agencies and community partners lead many to commit crimes and find themselves back in jail. The Bureau of Justice Statistics published a 2002 report on recidivism rates of prisoners who had been released in 1994. The study showed that in the first six months, 30% had been rearrested; within the first year, 44%; and within three years, 67.5% (Langan & Levin, 2002).

Resources for Advocates

The Racketeer Influenced and Corrupt Organizations (RICO) Act has been used against youth and adult gang members by 17% of local prosecutors in large counties and less than 10% of prosecutors in small counties (Howell, 2006). A number of states, including California, Florida, and Illinois, have enacted policies that impose stiffer penalties for crimes affiliated with identified gangs. For example, under California's Street Terrorism, Enforcement, and Prevention (STEP) Act of 1988, gang members receive written documentation that they have been identified as part of a particular gang and can face harsher penalties for any crimes committed. In Hawaii's Youth Gang Response System, prosecutors focus on high-level gang leadership, while youth members have access to prevention and education services. Furthermore, many cities have turned to curfew laws to curb gang activity. Yet, this policy does little to address the fundamental problem of gang recruitment and membership.

A number of states have passed measures seeking to reduce ineffective and inappropriate policies that favor incarceration rather than treatment, in the case of those convicted of simple drug possession. For example, Arizona passed the Drug Medicalization, Prevention, and Control Act in 1996, allowing nonviolent drug offenders to undergo drug treatment and education services rather than incarceration. In November 2000, California passed the Substance Abuse and Crime Prevention Act, also known as Proposition 36. Citing that substance abuse treatment "is a proven public safety and health measure," the act enabled first- and second-time nonviolent, drug possession offenders to undergo a treatment program instead of jail time. It continued to state that "non-violent, drug dependent criminal offenders who receive drug treatment are much less likely to abuse drugs and commit future crimes, and are likelier to live healthier, more stable and more productive lives" (National Families in Action, 2000). Furthermore, the Act pointed out that replacing incarceration with appropriate community-based treatment not only improves community safety and health but also saves taxpayer dollars.

POLICY ADVOCACY LEARNING CHALLENGE 14.4

Connecting Micro, Mezzo, and Macro Policy Advocacy

Improving the Rights of Prisoners

By Marilyn Montenegro, PhD, MSW
2002 NASW Social Worker of the Year recipient

Manuel was raised in an urban community, and most of the young people identified to some extent with the neighborhood gang. After a series of encounters with law enforcement, he was sent to prison for a four-year term, not an unusual progression for young Latinos from his neighborhood. Once in prison, he found old friends, gang members from his community. He was quickly identified as a gang member and confined in the Security Housing Unit (SHU). He was placed in a windowless, soundproof 8-by-10-foot concrete cell (about the size of a small bathroom). On a good day he remained in the cell for only 22 hours; often it was longer. He was told that the only way he could return to the "general population" was to "debrief" or identify fellow prisoners as gang members. He knew that Hugo Pinell had been held in the SHU for over 40 years and was overwhelmed with fear that he would live the rest of his life in the SHU.

Manuel joined approximately 6,000 other prisoners in the SHU hunger strike in 2011, supporting the five key demands to (1) end group punishment, (2) abolish the debriefing policy, (3) end long-term solitary confinement, (4) provide adequate food, and (5) provide constructive programming.

After three weeks, prison officials agreed to consider the demands but asked for time. The strike stopped, and many, including Manuel, were filled with hope. But even after a legislative hearing and a second hunger strike, nothing changed. Two attorneys, members of the mediation team, were barred from the prison pending investigation. Investigative journalists became interested in the story of torture and attempted to visit the SHU and interview prisoners involved in the hunger strike. The prison refused to allow media to conduct face-to-face interviews with specific prisoners or even individuals involved in the strike (Title 15, Section 3261 (a)(2) and 3261.5(a)(1)). A prison spokesperson later said, "The department is not going to be coerced or manipulated."

Manuel remains in solitary confinement, exhibiting symptoms of severe depression interrupted by bouts of rage.

LEARNING EXERCISE

1. Imagine that you are a social worker who has decided to become Manuel's advocate. What are some avenues you would explore at the micro level to help his current situation?
2. What might be done additionally at the mezzo level to improve conditions and change regulations within individual prisons related to solitary confinement and hunger strikes?
3. A local senator has agreed to meet with you regarding Manuel and the ethical concerns you've raised about his solitary confinement. Develop a 15-minute PowerPoint presentation about macro-level correctional polices for youth gang members, including preventative services.

Core Problem 5: Engaging in Advocacy to Promote Decreased Spending on Prisons and Increased Spending on Affordable and Accessible Services for Prisoners and Ex-Prisoners—With Some Red Flag Alerts

As we have seen, the seven problems identified in other social welfare sectors are difficult to apply to corrections, since its purpose—punishment of offenders—is antithetical to service provision. This section will instead discuss the exorbitant cost of the U.S. correctional system to taxpayers, and what advocacy groups are doing to shift resources away from corrections and into prevention and community-based services that address the root causes of crime.

- **Red Flag Alert 14.19.** A 14-year-old male from the inner city is exposed daily to violence and gangs. The city in which he lives has done little to invest in gang prevention or reduction programs, parks, recreational facilities, or other opportunities for youth. Instead, the city has invested in maintaining a strong police presence in inner city neighborhoods.
- **Red Flag Alert 14.20.** A formerly incarcerated woman who was recently released from state prison returns to the community to find there are no services to assist her with housing, job training, or child reunification. Her parole officer seems to be more interested in the results of her mandatory drug test than in assisting her to get back on her feet. This dearth of programs to help prisoners and ex-prisoners extends as well to males, persons of color, youthful persons, and other kinds of prisoners and ex-prisoners.

Background

Figure 14.2 displays total national spending (by local, state, and federal governments combined) in billions on prisons during the 20-year period between 1992 and 2012 (Government Spending, n.d.). It shows a sharp and steady increase from $30 billion in 1992, a slight dip from 2010 to 2011, and another increase in 2012 when total spending reached $84 billion.

With approximately 313,190,500 total U.S. residents in 2014, the $84 billion prison price tag represents $268 per person. Many prison reform advocates feel this figure is too high, given the lack of evidence that prisons deter crime, nor that they rehabilitate offenders. Yet advocates for reform face some of the same powerful interests and ideologies described under Core Problem 2 (advocacy to reform the criminal justice system), including those who believe prisons are necessary for public safety and those who profit from the ever-expanding prison population.

Resources for Advocates

Local, state, and federal budgets are considered by many to be social contracts. Influencing how governments invest public dollars is no simple task. Yet many advocates and groups are attempting to do just that, in hopes that resources will be channeled away from prisons and into social programs and education.

Figure 14.2   Spending on prisons in the U.S. from 1992 to 2012

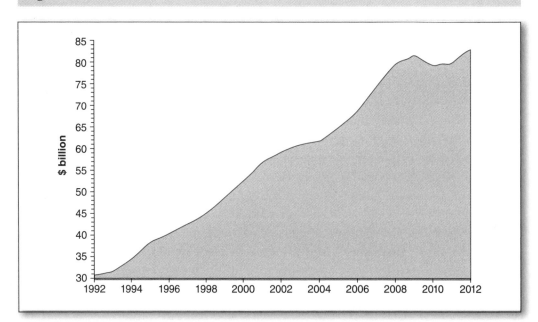

One of the most active of such spending reform advocacy groups is Californians United for a Responsible Budget (CURB). CURB is a coalition of more than 40 organizations that work to reduce spending on prisons. The organization seeks a "budget for humanity" that stops all prison and jail construction, reduces prison overcrowding through sentencing reform and reentry support, and instead invests in education, affordable housing, jobs, and mental and medical healthcare. According to its website, CURB has helped defeat over 140,000 new prison and jail beds proposed since 2004 (Californians United for a Responsible Budget, n.d.).

POLICY ADVOCACY LEARNING CHALLENGE 14.5

Connecting Micro, Mezzo, and Macro Policy Advocacy

The Impact of Prisons on the Communities That Surround Them

View the four-minute trailer for the film Prison Town, USA (it can be accessed at http://www.pbs.org/pov/prisontown/). Download the discussion guide to learn more about the town portrayed in the film and the impacts of the Susanville prison on residents of the town. Pay particular attention to the economic impact that building the prison had on the community (p. 9 of the discussion guide). Think about what the possible micro, mezzo, and macro implications of building a prison would be in your town.

Core Problem 6: Engaging in Advocacy to Promote Care for the Mental Distress of Prisoners and Ex-Prisoners—With Some Red Flag Alerts

Dorothea Dix was a famous advocate for mentally ill persons in the United States in the middle portion of the 19th century. She launched a legendary battle to rescue them from poorhouses, where they were often shackled to their beds and forced to deal with vermin and feces. Fast forward 150 years from the mid-1800s to the early 21st century, where contemporary prisons have become "the new poorhouses."

What would Dix find if she were to reappear and visit the jails of today? According to the Department of Justice, the number of U.S. residents being held in federal and state correctional facilities and municipal jails soared to 2.2 million by the end of 2005 (Bureau of Justice Statistics, 2006). Although this statistic in itself is alarming, of greater concern is the issue highlighted by Human Rights Watch, the largest human rights organization in the United States, that of those incarcerated in prisons today, about half the jail and prison population in the United States, 1,254,800 men and women, have a mental health problem (Fellner, 2007).

- **Red Flag Alert 14.21.** A new inmate with a history of substance abuse and depression was not told about the institution's mental health services.
- **Red Flag Alert 14.22.** A prisoner is shown to be developmentally disabled.
- **Red Flag Alert 14.23.** An inmate has been experiencing panic attacks for the past week. She requested an evaluation by a qualified mental health professional four days ago.
- **Red Flag Alert 14.24.** A mental health professional asks a prisoner about his past suicide attempts in front of other prisoners.
- **Red Flag Alert 14.25.** A prison guard routinely places inmates in solitary confinement as a means of punishment.
- **Red Flag Alert 14.26.** A prisoner receives no continuing or follow-up treatment services upon parole.

Background

As a result of inadequate and inaccessible mental health treatment in the community, people with mental illness often engage in behavior deemed illegal, thus thrusting them into the criminal justice system—a system not designed to deal with mental health issues. The availability of adequate mental health services in the community prior to the criminal offense could have acted as a deterrent to behavior that resulted in incarceration. Further, even though prisons are housing men and women suffering from serious mental health disorders, including schizophrenia, bipolar disorder, and major depression, Bureau of Justice records indicate that federal prisons have provided treatment to only about 24% of the inmates identified as having mental health problems (Fellner, 2007).

Prisons have become the last stop for many Americans with severe mental illness (Gilligan, 2001). In fact, the country's largest psychiatric inpatient facility is the Los Angeles County Jail, which has 3,400 inmates with mental illness (Torrey, 1999). It comes as no surprise that the correctional system is not conducive to treating persons with psychiatric symptoms. Not only are correctional employees oftentimes ill equipped to recognize or help prisoners with mental illness, but the prison environment itself can intensify emotional and physical distress. For example, the American Correctional Association has recognized that holding mentally challenged individuals in isolation can exacerbate their problems and bring about additional mental problems.

Within the population of incarcerated persons with mental illness, a vast majority also battle substance use disorders; one study found that 90% of mentally ill inmates had struggled with substance abuse at some point in their lifetimes. Only 11% of inmates with substance use disorders receive any type of treatment during incarceration; few of those receive evidence-based care (Columbia University,

2010). Not to be forgotten is the increased number of offenders in community settings, such as those in parole, probation, or other forms of supervised release.

Moreover, other major players in the criminal justice system—such as police officers who are dispatched to respond to mentally ill persons, as well as judges and attorneys who prosecute and sentence mentally ill defendants—are oftentimes not sufficiently trained to deal with those with psychiatric issues. The recent beating of mentally ill homeless person Kelly Thomas by two Fullerton, California, law enforcement officers is an egregious example of these inadequacies in training. Persons who exhibit signs of a mental disorder are associated with a 67% increased likelihood of being arrested, compared to persons without an apparent disorder (Teplin, 2000). Explicitly stated guidelines, outlining protocols for situation assessment and safety management, should be developed in order to educate law enforcement on how to respond appropriately.

Last, another important issue involves releasing mentally ill individuals back into society without a mandate to participate in continuing treatment. Although some persons are offered discharge planning services, many reenter communities without having their post-release mental health needs addressed.

Resources for Advocates

In taking inmates into custody, the United States government has a special legal obligation to protect them from harm (Cohen & Gerbasi, 2005). According to the American Psychiatric Association (2000),

> the fundamental policy goal for correctional mental health is to provide the same level of mental health services to each patient in the criminal justice process that should be available in the community. This policy goal is deliberately higher than the "community standard" that is called for in various contexts.

In other words, incarcerated persons should experience no discrimination in their mental health services.

No court-mandated guidelines exist in terms of a single mental health service delivery model. Instead, national organizations have created their own sets of policy recommendations. The American Psychiatric Association and the National Commission on Correctional Health Care, for example, published a comprehensive set of guidelines to expand and improve mental health services for prisoners (Hills, Siegfried, & Ickowitz, 2004).

Court Rulings. While numerous court rulings have held that inmates should receive mental healthcare equivalent to that available in the community, the vast majority of prisons are unable to offer a comprehensive array of services. Because of constrained resources and time, corrections personnel must prioritize individuals with the most serious, dangerous, or disruptive conditions. Persons with milder problems or adjustment disorders are likely to receive delayed treatment or no treatment at all.

After the passage of the Ku Klux Klan Act in 1871, inmates were able to sue correctional officials for neglecting to provide constitutionally adequate care. In particular, the federal statute enabled incarcerated persons to sue providers for violating their Eighth Amendment rights if their care or lack of care amounted to cruel and unusual punishment. Under the 1976 *Estelle v. Gamble* case, the U.S. Supreme Court ruled that corrections personnel must exhibit "deliberate indifference" to an incarcerated person's "serious illness or injury." Deliberate indifference can be shown by prison doctors' response to an individual's needs, correctional personnel who intentionally deny or delay access to care, or corrections officers who intentionally interfere with a prisoner's treatment.

Mental health needs fall under *medical* needs, according to lower courts. Incarcerated persons are entitled to psychological or psychiatric treatment if a physician observes that the prisoner's symptoms are indicative of a serious disease or injury that could be significantly remedied and that the denial of care could substantially cause harm to the individual.

The Federal Bureau of Prisons. In a 2010 national study commissioned by the Justice Department's National Institute of Corrections, research showed that the suicide rate in county jails has had a dramatic decrease during the past 20 years. According to the Bureau, its staff members receive annual training—some semiannual training—on suicide prevention. Inmates are provided with information on mental health services upon admission. Since 1982, the Bureau has used the following five-step suicide prevention program (Hills et al., 2004).

1. The initial screening of all inmates for suicidal potential

2. Criteria for the treatment and housing of suicidal inmates

3. Standardized record-keeping, follow-up procedures, and collection of data relevant to suicides

4. Staff training

5. Periodic reviews and audits

In the first decade after the five-step program's launch, inmate suicides within the Bureau of Prisons decreased by 43% (White & Schimmel, 1995). Still, suicide remains the third leading cause of death for prison inmates. No mandated standards exist for suicide prevention policies, but organizations like the American

Correctional Association and National Commission on Correctional Health Care have issued their own suicide prevention plans. Included in these plans are more frequent observation and monitoring of inmates with violent tendencies or mental illness, intake screening assessments for at-risk inmates, ensuring that suicidal inmates are not placed in isolation, staff training, and procedures for notifying family, prison administrators, and other authorities.

POLICY ADVOCACY LEARNING CHALLENGE 14.5

Connecting Micro, Mezzo, and Macro Policy Advocacy

Go to the PBS archives of *Frontline* and access its documentary "The New Asylums" (2005). After watching the one-hour documentary, discuss these questions:

1. Why do such a large proportion of inmates suffer from substance abuse and mental health problems?
2. Why is it difficult to engage many inmates in mental health interventions in prison settings?
3. Why don't prisons provide better mental health and substance abuse services?
4. Do you think released prisoners receive follow-up mental health and substance abuse treatment in the community?
5. Does evidence exist regarding whether mental health and substance abuse services decrease the likelihood that prisoners will be repeat offenders?
6. What micro, mezzo, and/or macro level advocacy interventions might help to reduce the number of people suffering from substance abuse and mental health issues who become involved in the criminal justice system?

Core Problem 7: Engaging in Advocacy to Promote Linkages With Communities of Prisoners and Ex-prisoners—With Some Red Flag Alerts

All prisoners except those sentenced to death or life without the possibility of parole are eventually released (Hughes & Wilson, 2002). Only in the past two to three decades has attention been focused on the topic of prisoner reentry. Few formalized interventions or evidence-based practices exist to address the needs of this growing population. Instead, formerly incarcerated people return to their communities to face a host of barriers to successful reentry (discussed below). These barriers wreak devastating consequences for individuals, families, communities, and society as a whole, and contribute to soaring rates of recidivism.

- **Red Flag Alert 14.27.** A formerly incarcerated woman wishes to begin the process of reunification with her children, and she files papers with the court to obtain visitation rights.
- **Red Flag Alert 14.28.** A formerly incarcerated person is frustrated because he is unable to find work and believes he is being discriminated against by potential employers.
- **Red Flag Alert 14.29.** A formerly incarcerated person is homeless on the streets and does not qualify for public housing because of a drug conviction.
- **Red Flag Alert 14.30.** A formerly incarcerated woman is unable to obtain food stamps or welfare to support herself and her two children because of a drug conviction.
- **Red Flag Alert 14.31.** A formerly incarcerated person is unsure about his right to vote in his state.

Background

No federal guidelines exist with regard to the release of prisoners. Many released inmates are sent back to their communities without any form of identification, which would have been confiscated by authorities upon arrest. Without ID, former prisoners must first locate a birth certificate and social security card, which can take weeks if they do not have copies stored in safe locations. Those with diagnosed mental health conditions are typically released with only two weeks' worth of medication (O'Shea, 2012), and obtaining an appointment to see a psychiatrist or mental health professional can take a month or more.

The majority of released prisoners are released on parole, and are typically required to report to their parole officer within 24 hours. Requirements of parole vary from state to state, but in virtually all cases, persons on parole do not enjoy the rights of free citizens. Parolees are entitled to only limited Fifth Amendment due process rights before having their parole revoked; and in most jurisdictions, parolees are subject to search and seizure at any time, without a warrant and without cause. Such searches, however, must be made on "reasonable" suspicion of criminal activity (Koshy, 1987). In addition, parolees typically cannot leave their county of residence or go beyond a prescribed area (such as a 50-mile radius) without the prior approval of their parole officer. They must inform the parole officer of any change of address or of new employment, and they are restricted from owning or carrying weapons. They must also comply with individualized requirements, such as to complete substance abuse treatment programs.

Parole can be revoked for any violation of parole conditions, and parole officers enjoy wide discretion in determining parole revocations (California Department of Corrections and Rehabilitation, 2012). Nationwide, approximately 23% of all adults on parole return to incarceration due to parole revocation (Glaze & Bonczar, 2011).

Social workers are likely to encounter formerly incarcerated people in various settings, including in child welfare, healthcare settings, WIC programs, public assistance offices, drug rehabilitation and treatment programs, homeless shelters, and mental health facilities. Social workers should be aware of the formidable reentry barriers that formerly incarcerated people face. Supplemental material for this chapter documents the many policy barriers to successful reunification, including barriers to housing, public assistance, employment, education, civic participation, and reunification.

Resources for Advocates

In recognition of the "reentry crisis" posed by half a million inmates returning to communities unprepared and without support every year, Congress enacted the Second Chance Act in April 2008. It authorized $25 million in grants to state, local, and tribal agencies and community organizations in FY 2009 to provide vital services for recently released prisoners, and an average of $82 million in each subsequent year (Reentry Policy Council, 2012). Since 2009, over 300 government agencies and nonprofit organizations from 48 states have received grant awards for reentry programs serving adults and juveniles.

Formerly incarcerated people and their allies feel, however, that these efforts do not go far enough. Instead, they are working to change policies that hinder successful reentry, as well as public perceptions of formerly incarcerated people, in the hope of diminishing barriers and reclaiming their civil rights. One of those groups is All of Us or None (AOUON), a national organizing initiative of former prisoners that works "to combat the many forms of discrimination that we face as the result of felony convictions" (All of Us or None, n.d.). Through local chapters, AOUON is working to implement strategies that ensure that former prisoners are able to participate in the democratic process through public education and voter registration drives. They are also working to eliminate barriers to employment through their "Ban the Box" campaign, which seeks to remove the question about prior conviction from application for employment. Moreover, AOUON's clean slate work provides training on the legal remedies available to people with convictions, such as expungements and certificates of rehabilitation.

POLICY ADVOCACY LEARNING CHALLENGE 14.6

Connecting Micro, Mezzo, and Macro Policy Interventions

View the video *Enough is Enough* (available at http://www.facebook.com/video/video.php?v=1371013354970) about formerly incarcerated people. In small groups, discuss the following:

1. At what point do you think a person has paid his or her debt to society?
2. Should restrictions be placed on convicted felons, even after they have completed their sentence (including parole/probation)? If so, what types, and why?
3. Should people with previous convictions be allowed to re-acquire rights they possessed prior to their conviction?
4. What types of micro, mezzo, and/or macro level advocacy might you engage in to help formerly incarcerated people become successful after release?

"THINKING BIG" AS POLICY ADVOCATES IN THE CRIMINAL JUSTICE SECTOR

Several major proposals for reforming the criminal justice system currently exist. These include legalization of marijuana, ending capital punishment, and helping persons who have been imprisoned find jobs.

These individual reforms can be viewed as a larger movement to decrease the number of imprisoned persons drastically due to the cost of the prison system, its negative effects on the economy by taking thousands of persons out of the labor force, its discriminatory patterns of sentencing, and its executions of innocent persons. *Does the United States want the dubious distinction of incarcerating more persons as a percentage of its population than any other industrialized nation?*

Develop a broad program to decrease the size of prisons. It can be multifaceted. For example, look at the website ProCon (http://medicalmarijuana.procon.org/), which offers a detailed summary of passed and pending legislation to further decriminalize marijuana use for medical purposes. Look at efforts to terminate capital punishment on the website ProCon (http://deathpenalty.procon.org/) Google California's drastic cuts in the state's prison populations with changes in sentencing laws. Consider working to convert some penalties that incarcerate persons to home arrest options.

Identify specific programs that might be developed for ex-prisoners, such as visiting the National Employment Law Project at http://www.nelp.org/index.php/content/content_issues/category/criminal_records_and_employment/.

LEARNING OUTCOMES

You are now equipped to:

- Describe how members of specific populations receive harsh and often inequitable treatment from the criminal justice sector
- Identify key eras in the evolution of the criminal justice sector
- Identify and analyze the seven problems in the criminal justice sector
- Apply the eight challenges of the multilevel policy empowerment framework to the criminal justice sector with respect to the "thinking big" exercise

REFERENCES

Alexander, M. (2010). *The new Jim Crow: Mass incarceration in the age of colorblindness.* New York, NY: New Press.

All of Us or None (n.d.). *All of Us or None.* Retrieved from www.allofusornone.org

American Civil Liberties Union. (n.d.a). *Know your rights: The Prison Litigation Reform Act.* Retrieved from http://www.aclu.org/images/asset_upload_file79_25805.pdf

American Civil Liberties Union. (n.d.b). *We can stop solitary.* Retrieved from https://www.aclu .org/we-can-stop-solitary

American Psychiatric Association. (2000). *Psychiatric services in jails and prisons: A task force report of the American Psychiatric Association* (2nd ed.). Washington, DC: American Psychiatric Association.

Andrews, D. A., Zinger, I., Hoge, R. D., Bonta, J., Gendreau, P., & Cullen, F. T. (1990). Does correctional treatment work: A clinically relevant and psychologically informed meta-analysis. *Criminology, 28,* 369–404.

Anno, J., Graham, C., Lawrence, J., & Shansky, R. (2004). *Correctional health care: Addressing the needs of elderly, chronically ill and terminally ill inmates.* Washington, DC: National Institute of Corrections.

Arditti, J., & Few, A. (2006). Mothers' reentry into family life following incarceration. *Criminal Justice Policy Review, 17*(1), 103–123.

Arrigo, B. A., & Bullock, J. L. (2008). The psychological effects of solitary confinement on prisoners in supermax units: Reviewing what we know and recommending what should change. *International Journal of Offender Therapy and Comparative Criminology, 52*(6), 622–640.

Beck, A., & Gilliard, D. (1995). *Prisoners in 1994.* Washington, DC: Bureau of Justice Statistics.

Bishop, J. (2012, February 2). Restorative justice provides new path for prisoners. *Vox Magazine.* Retrieved from http://www.voxmagazine.com/stories/2012/02/02/restorative-justice-provides -new-path-prisoners/

Blackmon, D. A. (2009). *Slavery by another name: The re-enslavement of black Americans from the Civil War to World War II.* Harpswell, ME: Anchor.

Bogue, B., Campbell, N., Carey, M., Clawson, E., Faust, D., Florio, K., . . . Woodward, W. (2004). *Implementing evidence-based practice in community corrections: The principles of effective intervention*. Washington, DC: National Institute of Corrections. Retrieved from http://www.nicic.org/pubs/2004/019342.pdf

Bureau of Justice Statistics. (2006). *Bureau of Justice Statistics press release*. Retrieved from http://www.ojp.usdoj.gov/bjs/pub/press/pripropr.htm

California Department of Corrections and Rehabilitation. (2011). *Prison census data as of June 30, 2011*. Sacramento, CA: Department of Corrections and Rehabilitation, Offender Information Services Branch.

California Department of Corrections and Rehabilitation. (2012). *Division of adult parole operations: Parole requirements*. Retrieved from http://www.cdcr.ca.gov/parole /Parole_Requirements/index.html

Californians United for a Responsible Budget. (n.d.). *Californians United for a Responsible Budget*. Retrieved from www.curbprisonspending.org

Carson, A., & Golinelli, D. (2013). *Prisoners in 2012: Trends in admissions and releases, 1991–2012*. Washington, DC: Bureau of Justice Statistics.

Chiu, T. (2010). *It's about time: Aging prisoners, increasing costs, and geriatric release*. New York, NY: Vera Institute of Justice.

Cohen, F., & Gerbasi, J. (2005). Legal issues. In C. L. Scott & J. B. Gerbasi (Eds.), *Handbook of correctional mental health* (pp. 259–283). Washington, DC: American Psychiatric Publishing.

Columbia University, National Center on Addiction and Substance Abuse. (2010). *Behind bars II: Substance abuse and America's prison population*. New York, NY. Retrieved from http://www.casacolumbia.org/articlefiles/575-report2010behindbars2.pdf

Covington, S., & Bloom, B. (2003). Gendered justice: Women in the criminal justice system. In B. Bloom (Ed.), *Gendered justice: Addressing female offenders*. Durham, NC: Carolina Academic Press.

Covington, S., & Bloom, B. (2006). Gender-responsive treatment and services in correctional settings. *Women and Therapy, 29*(3–4), 9–33.

Critical Resistance. (n.d.). Retrieved from www.criticalresistance.org

Dannenberg, J. (2011, April). Nationwide PLN survey examines prison phone contracts, kickbacks. *Prison Legal News, 22*(4). Retrieved from https://www.prisonlegalnews .org/23083_displayArticle.aspx

Davis, A. (2003). *Are prisons obsolete?* New York, NY: Seven Stories Press.

Durose, M., Farole, D, & Rosenmerkel, S. (2009). *Felony sentences in state courts, 2006–statistical tables*. Rockville, MD: Bureau of Justice Statistics.

Federal Bureau of Investigations. (2010, September). Arrests by Race, 2009. Retrieved from http://www2.fbi.gov/ucr/cius2009/data/table_43.html

Fellner, J. (2007). *Prevalence and policy: New data on the prevalence of mental illness in US prisons*. Retrieved from http://hrw.org/English/docs/200701/10/usdom15040.htm

General Accounting Office. (1999). *Women in prison: Issues and challenges confronting U.S. correctional systems*. Washington, DC: Author.

Gilliard, D., & Beck, A. (1994). *Prisoners in 1993*. Washington, DC: Bureau of Justice Statistics.

Gilligan, J. (2001). The last mental hospital. *Psychiatric Quarterly, 72*(1), 45–61.

Glaze, L., & Bonczar, T. (2011). *Probation and parole in the United States, 2010*. Washington, DC: Bureau of Justice Statistics.

Glaze, L., & Maruschak, L. (2008). *Parents in prison and their minor children.* Washington, DC: Bureau of Justice Statistics.

Golden, R. (2005). *War on the family: Mothers in prison and the families they leave behind.* New York, NY: Routledge.

Government Spending. (n.d.). *Government spending details.* Retrieved from www.usgovernment spending.com

Guerino, P., Harrison, P., & Sabol, W. (2011). *Prisoners in 2010.* Washington, DC: Bureau of Justice Statistics.

Gumz, E. J. (2004). American social work, corrections and restorative justice: An appraisal. *International Journal of Offender Therapy and Comparative Criminology, 48*(4), 449–460.

Hairston, C. (2004). Prisoners and their families: Parenting issues during incarceration. In J. Travis & M. Waul (Eds.), *Prisoners once removed: The impact of incarceration and reentry on children, families, and communities.* Washington, DC: Urban Institute Press.

Harlow, C. (1999). *Prior abuse reported by inmates and probationers.* Washington, DC: Bureau of Justice Statistics.

Hill, K. G., Howell, J. C., Hawkins, J. D., & Battin-Pearson, S. R. (1999). Childhood risk factors for adolescent gang membership: Results from the Seattle Social Development Project. *Journal of Research in Crime and Delinquency, 36*(3), 300–322.

Hills, H., Siegfried, C., & Ickowitz, A. (2004). *Effective prison mental health services: Guidelines to expand and improve treatment* (NIC Accession Number 018604). Washington, DC: U.S. Department of Corrections, National Institute of Corrections.

Howell, J. C. (2006). *Youth gang programs and strategies.* Washington, DC: U.S. Department of Justice, Office of Juvenile Justice and Delinquency Prevention. Retrieved from https://www .ncjrs.gov/pdffiles1/ojjdp/171154.pdf

Hughes, H., & Wilson, D.J. (2002). *Reentry trends in the United States.* Washington, DC: Bureau of Justice Statistics.

Human Rights Watch. (2012). *Teens in solitary confinement.* Retrieved from http://www.hrw.org /news/2012/10/10/us-teens-solitary-confinement

Humes, K., Jones, N., & Ramirez, R. (2011). *Overview of race and Hispanic origin: 2010.* Washington, DC: U.S. Census Bureau.

James, D., & Glaze, L. (2006). *Mental health problems of jail and prison inmates.* Washington, DC: Bureau of Justice Statistics.

Just Detention. (n.d.). *Learn the basics.* Retrieved from http://www.justdetention.org/en/learn _the_basics.aspx

Koshy, S. (1987). The right of (all) the people to be secure: Extending fundamental Fourth Amendment rights to probationers and parolees. *Hastings Law Journal, 39,* 449.

Kowal, T. (2011, June 5). *The role of the Prison Guards Union in California's troubled prison system. The League of Ordinary Gentlemen.* Retrieved from http://ordinary-gentlemen.com /blog/2011/06/the-role-of-the-prison-guards-union-in-californias-troubled-prison-system/

Kyckelhahn, T. (2011). *Justice expenditures and employment, FY 1982–2007: Statistical tables.* Washington, DC: Bureau of Justice Statistics.

Langan, P. A., & Levin, D. J. (2002). Recidivism of prisoners released in 1994. *Federal Sentencing Reporter, 15*(1), 58–65.

Latimer, J., Dowden, C., & Muise, D. (2005). The effectiveness of restorative justice practices: A meta-analysis. *The Prison Journal, 85*(2), 127–144.

Lewis, C. (2006). Treating incarcerated women: Gender matters. *Psychiatric Clinics of North America, 29*(3), 773–789.

Mills, L., Maley, M. H., & Shy, Y. (2009). Circulos de Paz and the promise of peace: Restorative justice meets intimate violence. *NYU Review of Law and Social Change, 33,* 127–152.

Mumola, C. (2007). *Medical causes of death in state prisons, 2001–2004.* Washington, DC: Bureau of Justice Statistics.

Mumola, C., & Karberg, J. (2006). *Drug use and dependence, state and federal prisoners, 2004.* Washington, DC: Bureau of Justice Statistics.

Nation Master. (n.d.). *Crime statistics: Prisoners by country.* Retrieved from http://www.nation master.com/graph/cri_pri-crime-prisoners

National Families in Action. (2000). *A guide to drug-related state ballot initiatives.* Retrieved from http://www.nationalfamilies.org/guide/california36-full.html

Nixon, R. (1971, June 17). *Remarks about an intensified program for drug abuse prevention and control.* The American Presidency Project. Retrieved from http://www.presidency.ucsb.edu /ws/?pid=3047

O'Brien, P., & Harm, N. (2002). Women's recidivism and reintegration: Two sides of the same coin. In J. Figueira-McDonough & R. Sarri (Eds.), *Women at the margins: Neglect, punishment, and resistance.* New York, NY: Haworth.

Olson, S. (2007, November 17). Suicide city. *Indy Bay.* Retrieved from http://www.indybay.org/ newsitems/2007/11/17/18461835.php

O'Shea, B. (2012, February 18). Psychiatric patients with no place to go but jail. *The New York Times,* p. A25A.

Oshinsky, D. (1996). *Worse than slavery.* New York, NY: Free Press.

Reentry Policy Council. (2012). *The Second Chance Act.* Retrieved from http://www.reentry policy.org/government_affairs/second_chance_act

Romano, A. (2011, September 19). Jim Webb's last crusade. Newsweek, 158(12).

Snyder, C., van Wormer, K., Chadha, J., & Jaggers, J. (2009). Older adult inmates: The challenge for social work. *Social Work, 54*(2), 117–124.

Sudbury, J. (2002). Celling black bodies: Black women in the global prison industrial complex. *Feminist Review, 70,* 57–74.

Teplin, L. A. (2000). Keeping the peace: Police discretion and mentally ill persons. *National Institute of Justice Journal.* Retrieved from http://www.ncjrs.org/pdffiles1/jr000244c.pdf

Torrey, E. F. (1999, Autumn). Reinventing mental health care. *City Journal.* Retrieved from http://www.city-journal.org/html/9_4_a5.html

U.S. Department of Justice. (2010). *Uniform crime report: Arrests, by race, 2009.* Washington, DC: Author.

Vera Institute of Justice. (2009, July 9). *Remarks as prepared for delivery by Attorney General Eric Holder at the Vera Institute of Justice's third annual justice address.* Retrieved from http://www.vera.org/?q=events/justice-address-2009

Villettaz, P., Killias, M., & Zoder, I. (2006). The effects of custodial vs. non-custodial sentences on re-offending: A systematic review of the state of knowledge. *Campbell Systematic Reviews, 13.*

Wacquant, L. (2002). From slavery to mass incarceration: Rethinking the "race question" in the US. *New Left Review, 13,* 41–60.

Wahidin, A. (2004). *Older women in the criminal justice system: Running out of time.* London, UK: Jessica Kingsley.

West, H., & Sabol, W. (2010). *Prisoners in 2009.* Washington, DC: Bureau of Justice Statistics.

Western, B., & Wildeman, C. (2009). Punishment, inequality, and the future of mass incarceration. *Kansas Law Review, 57,* 851–877.

White, T., & Schimmel, D. (1995). Suicide prevention in federal prisons: A successful five step program. In L. M. Hayes, (Project Director), *Prison suicide: An overview and guide to prevention.* Mansfield, MA: National Center for Institution and Alternatives.

Williams, B., Sudore, R., Greifinger, R., & Morrison, R. S. (2011). Balancing punishment and compassion for seriously ill prisoners. *Annals of Internal Medicine, 155,* 122–126.

Winter, C. (2008, July/August). What do prisoners make for Victoria's Secret? *Mother Jones.* Retrieved from http://www.motherjones.com/politics/2008/07/what-do-prisoners-make -victorias-secret

Winter Group. (2009). *PSCOA: Past accomplishments & current projects.* Retrieved from www .pscoa.org/wp-content/uploads/WG_Dec_2009.pdf

Women's Prison Association. (n.d.). *Laws banning shackling during childbirth gaining momentum nationwide.* Retrieved from http://66.29.139.159/pdf/Shackling Brief_final.pdf

Zehr, H. (2002). *The little book of restorative justice.* Intercourse, PA: Good Books.

Index

ABOUT THE AUTHOR

Bruce S. Jansson (MA, University of Chicago and Harvard University; PhD, University of Chicago) is the Driscoll/Clevenger professor of social policy in the School of Social Work at the University of Southern California (USC). He joined the USC faculty in 1973 after working in Michigan as a community organizer and planner for tenant rights. He also has served as the Moses distinguished research professor at the City University of New York (CUNY) Graduate Center. His scholarly interests focus on advancing case advocacy and policy advocacy in social work, as well as examining the history and practice of social welfare policy. He invented the term "policy practice" in the 1984 release of *The Theory and Practice of Social Policy*, which was succeeded by other titles, including *Becoming an Effective Policy Advocate* (1999, 2003, 2008, 2011, and 2014). Policy practice has since emerged as a recognized intervention, with the Council on Social Work Education now requiring social work schools to teach policy practice.